Functional Histology

Functional Histology

A TEXT AND COLOUR ATLAS

Paul R. Wheater
BA Hons (York), B Med Sci Hons (Nott), BM BS (Nott)
The Queen's Medical Centre, University of Nottingham

H. George Burkitt
BDSc Hons (Queensland), M Med Sci (Nott) FRACDS
The Queen's Medical Centre, University of Nottingham

Victor G. Daniels
BSc Hons (Lon), MB BChir (Cam), PhD (Sheff)
Lecturer in medical education, University of Dundee

Illustrated by

Philip J. Deakin
BSc Hons (Sheff), MB ChB (Sheff)
The Medical School, University of Sheffield

Prepared in the Department of Pathology, University of Nottingham

Foreword by

Roger Warwick, BSc, PhD, MD
Professor of Anatomy
Guy's Hospital Medical School
University of London

CHURCHILL LIVINGSTONE
EDINBURGH LONDON AND NEW YORK 1979

CHURCHILL LIVINGSTONE
Medical Division of Longman Group Limited

Distributed in the United States of America by Churchill
Livingstone Inc., 19 West 44th Street, New York, N.Y. 10036,
and by associated companies, branches and representatives
throughout the world

First published 1979
  Reprinted 1980
  Reprinted 1981

ISBN 0 443 01658 5 (cased)
ISBN 0 443 01657 7 (limp)

British Library Cataloguing in Publication Data
Wheater, Paul R
  Functional histology.
  1. Histology
  I. Title II. Burkitt, H George
  III. Daniels, Victor G
  599'.08'24   QM551   79–40314

Printed in Great Britain by Jarrold & Sons Ltd, Norwich

Foreword

A new book, added to the current spate of publications, must offer some special qualities to commend it amongst its rivals—perhaps a newness of approach to its subject, perhaps an unusual excellence in content. This volume satisfies both criteria.

Firstly, it is deliberately planned to assist the reader not only as an armchair textbook but equally as a book for work in the laboratory. The main text, succinct and not over-burdened with details, deals primarily with principles, generalisations, and functional considerations, but is nevertheless closely linked to appropriate illustrations. The captions to these, being chiefly concerned with structural details, directly adjoin the corresponding illustrations.

Secondly, the illustrations are indeed of unusual excellence. The diagrams are clear, concise and well conceived and are a credit to the illustrator and, of course, to the advice of the three other members of the authorship. These three authors are almost entirely responsible for all the photographs (except for those taken by electron microscope) and also for the preparation of materials for them. As a result of these efforts they have assembled, specifically for this book, a magnificent display of mammalian cells and tissues (largely from human sources), which in clarity and accuracy, in scope and quality, surpasses any similar series of illustrations in books of such moderate size.

The volume is most interesting and attractive in conception and format. It has freshness and yet authority, which doubtless are derived from the comparative youthfulness of its originators and from their collectively wide and varied experience of teaching and research in biology and medicine. Evidently also, they have not forgotten the problems of student days, and have therefore produced a book which, without obscurity or condescension, both instructs and stimulates. Its appeal should be wide in biological, medical and ancillary fields, and I wish its authors much success.

London, 1979   Roger Warwick

Preface

Histology has bored generations of students. This is almost certainly because it has been regarded as the study of structure in isolation from function; yet few would dispute that structure and function are intimately related. Thus, the aim of this book is to present histology in relation to the principles of physiology, biochemistry and molecular biology.

Within the limits imposed by any book format, we have attempted to create the environment of the lecture room and microscope laboratory by basing the discussion of histology upon appropriate micrographs and diagrams. Consequently, colour photography has been used since it reproduces the actual images seen in light microscopy and allows a variety of common staining methods to be employed in highlighting different aspects of tissue structure. In addition, some less common techniques such as immunohistochemistry have been introduced where such methods best illustrate a particular point.

Since electron microscopy is a relatively new technique, a myth has arisen amongst many students that light and electron microscopy are poles apart. We have tried to show that electron microscopy is merely an extension of light microscopy. In order to demonstrate this continuity, we have included resin-embedded thin sections photographed around the limit of resolution of the light microscope; this technique is being applied increasingly in routine histological and histopathological practice. Where such less conventional techniques have been adopted, their rationale has been outlined at the appropriate place rather than in a formal chapter devoted to techniques.

The content and pictorial design of the book have been chosen to make it easy to use both as a textbook and as a laboratory guide. Wherever possible, the subject matter has been condensed into units of illustration plus relevant text; each unit is designed to have a degree of autonomy whilst at the same time remaining integrated into the subject as a whole. Short sections of non-illustrated text have been used by way of introduction, to outline general principles and to consider the subject matter in broader perspective.

Human tissues were mainly selected in order to maintain consistency, but when suitable human specimens were not available, primate tissues were generally substituted. Since this book stresses the understanding of principles rather than extensive detail, some tissues have been omitted deliberately, for example the regional variations of the central nervous system and the vestibulo-auditory apparatus.

This book should adequately encompass the requirements of undergraduate courses in medicine, dentistry, veterinary science, pharmacy, mammalian biology and allied fields. Further, it offers a pictorial reference for use in histology and histopathology laboratories. Finally, we envisage that the book will also find application as a teaching manual in schools and colleges of further education.

Nottingham, 1979

Paul R. Wheater
H. George Burkitt
Victor G. Daniels

Acknowledgements

With few exceptions, each of the illustrations was specially prepared for the book. Whilst accepting full responsibility for the entire contents, the authors are indebted to many individuals who have made invaluable contributions in their specialised fields.

Most of the tissue preparation and photomicrography was performed within the Departments of Pathology and Human Morphology of the Queen's Medical Centre, University of Nottingham. The authors are thus extremely grateful for the generous co-operation of Professors I. M. P. Dawson and R. E. Coupland. Special thanks are due to Mrs Janet Palmer of the Department of Pathology, who gave tireless assistance in the preparation of many of the tissues for light microscopy which were used in this book and many more preparations, for which space was not available. Similarly, our thanks are conveyed to Mr Paul Beck of the Department of Human Morphology for producing a large number of valuable specimens. Many of the electron micrographs were made available by Mr John Kugler and Mrs Annette Tomlinson, also of the Department of Human Morphology; to both we are deeply indebted.

Other people freely made available their resources: Mr Peter Crosby of the Department of Biology, University of York provided all the scanning electron micrographs, and his colleague Mr Brian Norman provided several light microscopic sections; Dr Robert Lang, also of York University, provided the freeze-etched preparation used in Figure 1.8; Mr Donald Canwell of the Physiological Laboratory, University of Cambridge contributed several sections from his personal collection; Mr Nigel Cooper of the Department of Zoology, University of Cambridge, provided the electron micrographs for Figure 13.18; Dr Graham Robinson and Mr Stan Terras of the Department of Pathology, University of Nottingham each provided several electron micrographs, and they and their colleague, Miss Linda Burns, provided all the thin resin sections used for light microscopy; Dr David Tomlinson and Dr Terry Bennett of the Department of Physiology, University of Nottingham contributed Figures 7.14 and 7.17 respectively; Dr Pat Cooke of the Department of Genetics, City Hospital, Nottingham lent the chromosome preparation used in Figure 1.19; Dr David Ansell of the Department of Pathology, City Hospital, Nottingham, Dr Hugh Rice and Dr Peter James of the Department of Pathology, Nottingham General Hospital, and Dr Pauline Cooper of the Department of Pathology, Addenbrooke's Hospital, Cambridge made available various tissue specimens and slides. Mr Peter Squires and Mr Hugh Pulsford of Huntingdon Research Centre, Cambridgeshire were a great source of help in providing the primate tissues used when suitable human tissues were unavailable. To all of these kind and co-operative people we express our sincere thanks.

Mr Bill Brackenbury of the Department of Pathology, University of Nottingham very skilfully performed all the macrophotography. All the remaining colour photomicrography was performed by one of the authors (P.R.W.). The onerous task of typing the manuscript was carried out with skill and great patience by Mrs Christine Stevens.

The authors express their warmest thanks to Dr Alan Stevens of the Department of Pathology, University of Nottingham who performed the role of scientific editor with seemingly limitless dedication, insight and enthusiasm.

Finally, we would like to express our thanks to the staffs of Churchill Livingstone and Jarrold & Sons Ltd for their unstinting assistance.

P.R.W.
H.G.B.
V.G.D.

Contents

1. The cell

Introduction

The cell, the functional unit of all tissues, has the capacity to perform individually all the essential life functions. Within the various tissues of the body, the constituent cells exhibit a wide range of specialisations which are, nevertheless, merely amplifications of one or more of the fundamental cellular processes. Reflecting their particular functional specialisations, mammalian cells have an extraordinary range of morphological forms yet all cells conform to a basic model of cell structure.

Even with primitive light microscopy, it was evident that cells were divided into at least two components, the *nucleus* and the *cytoplasm*, and as microscopical techniques advanced it became increasingly obvious that both the cytoplasm and the nucleus contained a number of subcellular elements which were called *organelles*. The advent of electron microscopy (EM) permitted description of the ultrastructure of these and many more organelles beyond the limit of resolution of the light microscope; the light microscope cannot resolve structures smaller than $0.5\,\mu m$ (500nm). Much of present knowledge about cell structure is based upon electron microscopy, but most cellular functions take place at the biochemical level which is even beyond the resolving capacity of the electron microscope; currently, structures smaller than about 1.0nm (10Å) are not generally resolvable. Microscopy is only one of many techniques which have been used to further the understanding of cell function and structure.

Fig. 1.1 The cell *(illustration opposite)*
(EM × 15000)

The basic organisational features common to all cells are illustrated in this electron micrograph of a hormone-secreting cell from the pituitary gland. All cells are bounded by an external limiting membrane called the *plasma membrane* or *plasmalemma* **PM** which serves as a dynamic interface between the internal environment of the cell and its various external environments. In this particular example, the cell interacts with two types of external environment: adjacent cells **C** and intercellular spaces **IS**.

The nucleus **N** is the largest organelle and its substance, often referred to as the *nucleoplasm*, is bounded by a membrane system called the *nuclear envelope* **NE**. The cytoplasm contains a variety of organelles most of which are also bounded by membranes. A diffuse system of membrane-bound tubules, saccules and flattened cisterns, collectively known as the *endoplasmic reticulum* **ER**, pervades the cytoplasm. A more distended system of membrane-bound saccules, the *Golgi apparatus* **G**, is usually found close to the nucleus. Scattered free in the cytoplasm are a number of relatively large, elongated organelles called *mitochondria* **M** which have a smooth outer membrane and a convoluted inner membrane system. In addition to these major organelles, the cell contains a variety of other membrane-bound structures, an example of which are the numerous, electron-dense *secretory vacuoles* **V** seen in this micrograph. Thus the cell is divided into a number of membrane-bound compartments each of which has its own particular biochemical environment. The organelles are suspended in a fluid medium called the *cytosol* which itself constitutes a discrete biochemical environment.

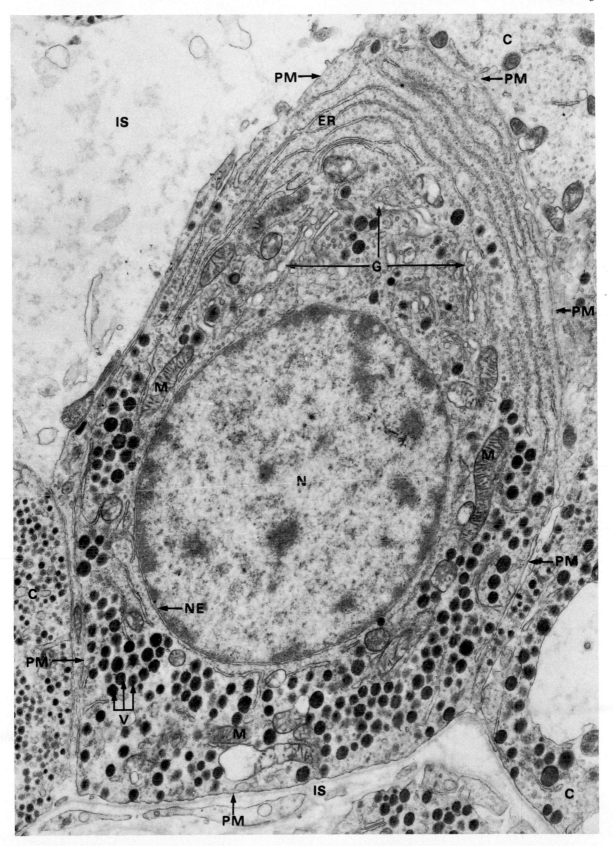

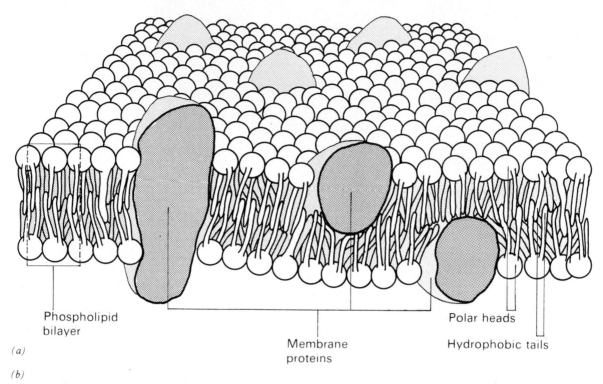

(a)

Phospholipid
bilayer

Membrane
proteins

Polar heads

Hydrophobic tails

(b)

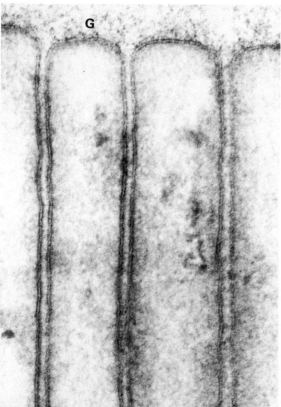

Fig. 1.2 **Membrane structure**

(a) Schematic diagram (b) EM × 167 400

Despite intensive investigation, the structure of cell
membranes is still not known with certainty; however, a
theoretical model has been progressively developed which
satisfactorily incorporates much of the currently available
biochemical and histological evidence.

Towards the end of the last century, it was observed that
lipids rapidly gain entry into cells, and it was postulated
that the 'cell boundary' was composed of lipid. In the 1920s
it was found that, by measuring the minimum area that
could be occupied by a monolayer of lipids extracted from a
defined number of red blood cells, there was enough lipid
present in the monolayer to cover each cell twice. From
this it was concluded that the cells were bounded by a
double layer of lipid. Later, it was proposed that cell
membranes are symmetrical structures consisting of a
bilayer of phospholipid molecules sandwiched between two
layers of protein. This model, however, failed to explain the
selective permeability of most cell membranes to molecules
which are not lipid soluble such as glucose, sodium ions and
potassium ions. These difficulties were theoretically
overcome by postulating the existence of 'pores' composed
of protein, through which hydrophilic molecules could
readily be transported by passive or active mechanisms. As
a result of electron microscopic studies in the late 1950s, the
concept of the 'unit membrane' was devised, in which it was
envisaged that all cell membranes have the same structure,
since they all appeared to have the same trilaminate
ultrastructure.

The current concepts of membrane structure are shown
diagrammatically above. In this model, cell membranes are
considered to consist of a bilayer of phospholipid
molecules; the hydrophilic (lipid-insoluble) portions of the

phospholipid molecules of each layer are aggregated at the surface with their hydrophobic 'tails' projecting into the centre of the membrane where they interact with the hydrophobic 'tails' of the opposed phospholipid layer. The weak intermolecular forces which hold the bilayer together allow individual molecules of phospholipid to move relatively freely within each layer. Cell membranes are therefore highly fluid in nature, yet have the ordered structure of a crystal. Cholesterol molecules are incorporated in the hydrophobic regions of the membrane and modify the fluidity of the membrane. In this model, proteins are scattered in the phospholipid bilayer, some of them extending through the entire thickness of the membrane to be exposed to each surface; it is proposed that these molecules function as 'pores' through which hydrophilic molecules are transported either passively or actively. These proteins, and others which do not span the whole width of the membrane, are also freely mobile within the plane of the phospholipid bilayer. This model is known as the *'fluid mosaic model'* of membrane structure.

On the external surface of the plasma membranes of animal cells, many of the membrane proteins and some of the membrane lipids are conjugated with short chains of polysaccharide; these glycoproteins and glycolipids project from the surface of the bilayer forming an outer coating (glycocalyx)

which may be analogous to the cell walls of plants, bacteria and fungi. This polysaccharide layer has been termed the *glycocalyx* and appears to vary in thickness in different cell types; whether an analogous layer exists on all membranes or only at the external surface is unknown. The function of the glycocalyx is obscure, but there is evidence that it may be involved in cell recognition phenomena, in the formation of intercellular adhesions, and in the adsorption of molecules to the cell surface. Alternatively, the glycocalyx may simply provide mechanical and chemical protection for the plasma membrane.

The electron micrograph in (b) provides a high magnification view of a plasma membrane; this example illustrates the minute surface projections of a lining cell from the small intestine. All membranes have a characteristic trilaminate appearance comprising two electron-dense layers separated by an electron-lucent layer. The outer dense layers are thought to correspond to the hydrophilic 'heads' of phospholipid molecules whilst the electron-lucent layer is thought to represent the intermediate hydrophobic layer mainly consisting of fatty acid side chains. On the external surface of the plasma membrane an outer fibrillar coat, called the *'fuzzy coat'*, represents the glycocalyx **G**. This is an unusually prominent feature of small intestinal lining cells.

Transport across plasma membranes

Plasma membranes mediate the continuous exchange of metabolites between the internal and external environments of the cell in four principal ways. These mechanisms enable the cell to control the quality of its internal environment with a high degree of specificity.

(i) Passive diffusion: this type of transport is entirely dependent on the presence of a concentration gradient across the plasma membrane. Lipids and lipid-soluble metabolites such as ethanol pass freely through plasma membranes; plasma membranes also offer little barrier to the diffusion of gases such as oxygen and carbon dioxide. The plasma membrane is, in general, impermeable to hydrophilic molecules; nevertheless some small molecules including water and urea, and inorganic ions such as bicarbonate, are able to pass down osmotic or electrochemical gradients through the membrane via hydrophilic regions, the nature of which remains obscure.

(ii) Facilitated diffusion: this type of transport is also concentration-dependent and involves the transport of larger hydrophilic metabolites such as glucose and amino-acids. The process is strictly passive but requires the presence of so-called 'carriers' to which the metabolites bind specifically but reversibly in a manner analogous to the binding of substrate with enzyme.

(iii) Active transport: this mode of transport is not only independent of concentration gradients but also often operates against extreme concentration gradients. The classical example of this form of transport is the continuous transport of sodium out of the cell by the so-called 'sodium pump'; this process requires the expenditure of energy provided in the form of ATP. It is postulated that this form of transport occurs through 'dynamic pores' consisting of proteins or protein systems which span the plasma membrane. Both active and passive transport processes are enhanced by increasing the area of the plasma membrane by folds or projections of the cell surface as exemplified by the absorptive cells lining the small intestine (see Fig. 1.2).

(iv) Bulk transport: bulk transport involves engulfment of large molecules or small particles by cytoplasmic extensions, thus forming membrane-bound vacuoles within the cytoplasm. When this process involves the creation of small vacuoles it is known as *pinocytosis*, and when large vacuoles are formed it is called *phagocytosis*. The term *endocytosis*, encompassing both processes, is probably a more appropriate term for bulk transport into the cell. Endocytotic vesicles either discharge their contents directly into the cytoplasm or fuse with membrane-bound organelles called *lysosomes*; lysosomes contain more than twelve different enzymes which are capable of degrading carbohydrates, lipids, proteins, nucleic acids and other organic molecules. Lysosomal enzymes digest engulfed material which is then made available for metabolic processes. In many secretory processes, bulk transport also occurs in the opposite direction when it is termed *exocytosis*.

Histologically, the passive and active processes of transport can only be observed indirectly; for example, cells suspended in hypotonic solutions swell due to passive uptake of water whereas cells placed in hypertonic solutions tend to shrink due to outflow of water. Radio-isotope labelling techniques can be used to follow active transport processes. Bulk transport, however, is readily observable by microscopy.

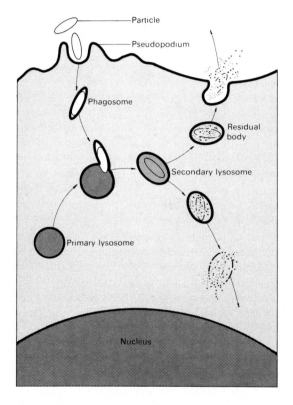

Fig. 1.3 Endocytosis

This diagram summarises the main steps in endocytosis of particulate matter. The first stage of phagocytosis involves recognition of a particle; this then becomes surrounded by cytoplasmic extensions called *pseudopodia*. When the particle is completely surrounded, the plasma membrane fuses and the membrane surrounding the engulfed particle forms a vesicle, known as a *phagosome* or *endocytotic vesicle*, which detaches from the plasma membrane to float freely within the cytoplasm. The phagosome is then in some way recognised by one or more *primary lysosomes* which fuse with the phagosome to form a *secondary lysosome*. This exposes the engulfed material to a battery of lysosomal enzymes. When digestion is complete, the lysosomal membrane may rupture, discharging its contents into the cytoplasm. Undigested material may remain within membrane-bound vesicles called *residual bodies*, the contents of which may be discharged at the cell surface by exocytosis; alternatively residual bodies may accumulate in the cytoplasm.

Lysosomes are also involved in the degradation of cellular organelles, many of which have only a finite lifespan and are therefore replaced continuously; this lysosomal function is termed *autophagy*. Most autophagocytic degradation products are reutilised by the cell, but some indigestible products accumulate and become indistinguishable from the residual bodies of endocytosis. With advancing age, residual bodies accumulate in the cells of some tissues and appear as brown so-called *lipofuscin granules*.

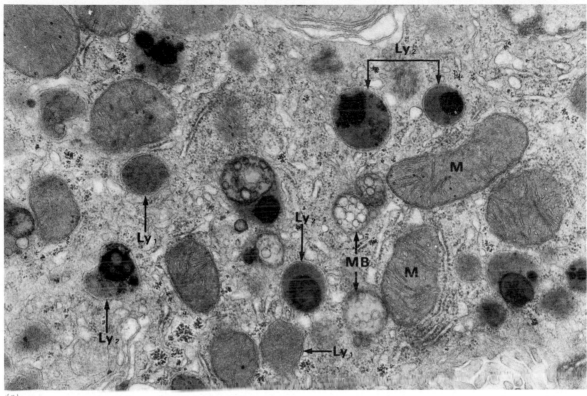

(a)

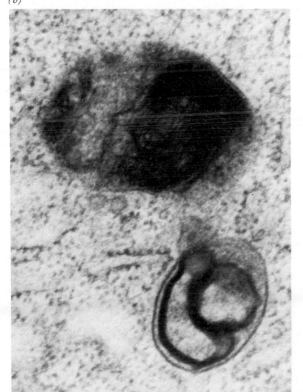

(b)

Fig. 1.4 Lysosomes

(EM (a) ×27000 (b) ×95000)

These micrographs show the typical appearance of lysosomes and residual bodies. Micrograph (a) shows part of the cytoplasm of a liver cell. Primary lysosomes **Ly₁** vary greatly in size and appearance but they are recognised as membrane-bound organelles containing a granular, amorphous material. Secondary lysosomes **Ly₂** are even more variable in appearance but are recognisable by their diverse particulate content some of which is extremely electron-dense. The distinction between residual bodies and secondary lysosomes is often difficult, but one distinctive type of residual body, the so-called *multivesicular body* **MB**, is seen in this micrograph. Multivesicular bodies are membrane-bound vesicles containing a number of smaller vesicles which are thought to represent the debris of cell membrane degradation. Note the size of lysosomes relative to mitochondria **M**.

In micrograph (b), two residual bodies, also from a liver cell, are shown at high magnification.

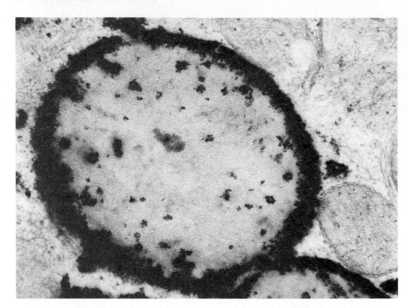

Fig. 1.5 Lysosomes

(EM histochemical method for acid phosphatase × 45000)

Histochemical methods can be used to demonstrate sites of enzyme activity within cells. Such a method has been used in this preparation to demonstrate the presence of *acid phosphatase* within lysosomes; the enzyme activity is represented by a very dense deposit within lysosomes. Acid phosphatase is one of several hydrolytic enzymes characteristic of lysosomes which can be used as histochemical markers for these organelles.

Protein synthesis

Proteins are not only a major structural component of cells but, in the form of enzymes, mediate every metabolic process within the cell. Thus the nature and quantity of proteins present within any individual cell determines the activity of that cell. Both the structural proteins and enzymes of the cell are subject to wear and tear and are replaced continuously. Many cells also synthesise proteins for export; such proteins include glandular secretions and extracellular structural components of tissues. Protein synthesis is, therefore, an essential and continuous activity of all cells and the major function of some cells.

The principal organelles involved in protein synthesis are the *nucleus* and *ribosomes*. The nucleus of every cell contains within its complement of DNA a template for each protein that can be made by that individual as a whole. However, most cells only synthesise a certain defined range of proteins which are characteristic of the particular cell type and therefore only part of the DNA template is utilised. The process of protein synthesis involves *transcription* of the DNA code for a particular protein by synthesis of the specific, complementary messenger RNA (mRNA) molecule. The mRNA molecule then enters the cytoplasm to associate with ribosomes upon which protein synthesis occurs; the amino-acid sequence of the resulting protein is determined by *translation* of the mRNA code.

Ribosomes are minute cytoplasmic organelles, each composed of two subunits of unequal size. Each subunit consists of a strand of RNA (ribosomal RNA) with associated ribosomal proteins; the ribosomal RNA strand and associated proteins are folded to form a condensed, globular structure. Ribosomes are highly active structures with specific receptor proteins which align mRNA strands so that transfer RNA (tRNA) molecules carrying the appropriate amino-acids may be brought into position prior to the addition of their amino-acids to the growing polypeptide chain. Other ribosomal proteins are involved in catalysing peptide bond formation between amino-acids. Individual ribosomes are too small to be clearly resolved by electron microscopy although they are visible as small electron-dense masses at high magnification; nevertheless, the detail of ribosome structure and function are well established at the molecular level. Ribosomes are found free in the cytoplasm either singly or as small aggregations called *polyribosomes* or *polysomes*; ribosomes are also attached to the surface of the extensive intra-cytoplasmic membrane system known as the endoplasmic reticulum (see Fig. 1.9).

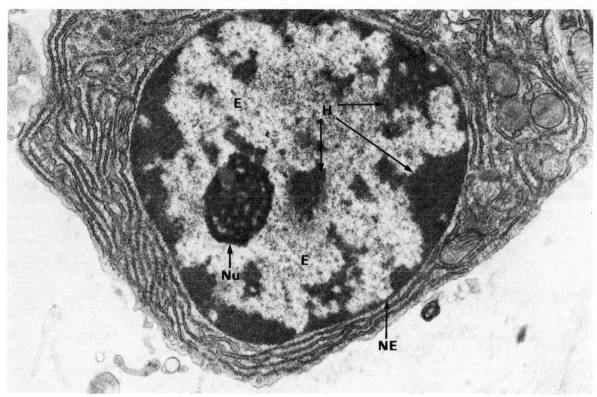

Fig. 1.6 Nucleus

(EM × 15400)

This micrograph illustrates the typical nucleus of a highly active, protein-secreting cell. The nuclear envelope **NE**, separating the nuclear contents from the cytoplasm, is barely visible at this magnification. The nucleus not only contains DNA, which comprises less than twenty per cent of its mass, but also contains a large quantity of protein called *nucleoprotein*, and some RNA. Most of the nucleoprotein is intimately associated with DNA; the remainder consists of enzymes responsible for RNA and DNA synthesis. The nuclear RNA represents newly synthesised messenger, transfer and ribosomal RNA which has not yet passed into the cytoplasm.

Except during cell division, the chromosomes, each comprising a discrete length of the DNA complement, exist as tangled strands which extend throughout the nucleus and cannot be visualised individually by direct electron microscopy. Nuclei appear as heterogeneous structures with electron-dense and electron-lucent areas. The dense areas, called *heterochromatin*, represent that portion of the DNA complement and its associated nucleoprotein which is not active in protein synthesis. Heterochromatin **H** tends to be clumped around the periphery of the nucleus but also forms

irregular clumps throughout the nucleus. In females, the quiescent X-chromosome (equivalent to the Y-chromosome of the male) forms a small discrete mass known as a *Barr body*; Barr bodies are seen at the edge of the nucleus in a small proportion of female cells when cut in a favourable plane of section. The electron-lucent nuclear material, called *euchromatin* **E**, represents that part of the DNA which is active in protein synthesis. Collectively, heterochromatin and euchromatin are known as *chromatin*, a name derived from the strongly coloured appearance of nuclei when stained for light microscopy.

Many nuclei, especially those of cells highly active in protein synthesis, contain one or more extremely dense structures called *nucleoli* **Nu** which are the sites of ribosomal RNA synthesis. Each cell type has a characteristic nucleolar morphology. In general, the degree of activity of any cell may be judged by the ultrastructural appearance of its nucleus. Relatively inactive cells have small nuclei in which the chromatin is predominantly in the condensed form (heterochromatin) and in which the nucleolus is small or absent.

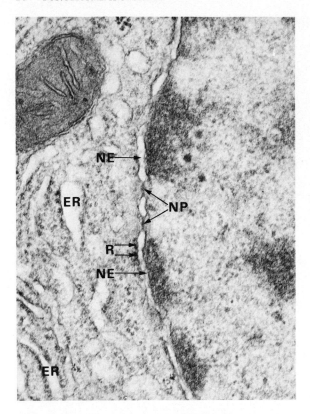

Fig. 1.7 Nuclear envelope

(EM ×67500)

The nuclear envelope **NE** consists of two layers of membrane. The space between these layers is known to be continuous, in places, with cisternae of the endoplasmic reticulum; thus the nuclear envelope may be considered as a specialised region of the endoplasmic reticulum. Like the endoplasmic reticulum **ER**, the outer surface of the outer nuclear membrane is often studded with ribosomes **R**. A considerable proportion of the nuclear envelope contains apparent perforations called *nuclear pores* **NP**, at the margins of which the inner and outer membranes become continuous. The membrane at the periphery of each pore is thickened and each pore appears to be closed by a diaphragm of unknown structure. Nuclear pores may permit the exchange of metabolites between the nucleus and cytoplasm; it is suggested that the pores are the sites through which RNA molecules enter the cytoplasm.

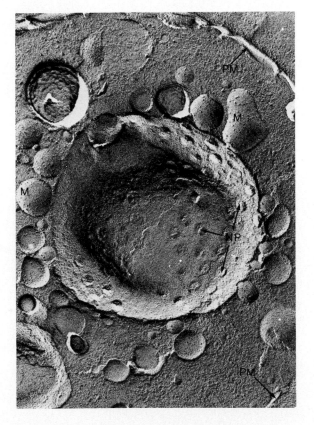

Fig. 1.8 Nuclear pores

(Freeze-etched preparation ×34000)

This micrograph shows an example of a technique called *freeze-etching*. Briefly, this method involves the rapid cooling of cells to subzero temperatures; the frozen cells are then fractured. This exposes internal surfaces of the cell in a somewhat random manner although the fracture lines tend to follow natural planes of weakness. Further surface detail is obtained by 'etching' or subliming excess water molecules from the specimen at low temperature. A thin carbon impression is then made of the surface and this mirror image is viewed by conventional electron microscopy. Freeze-etching provides a valuable tool for studying internal cell surfaces at high resolution.

In this preparation, the plane of cleavage has included part of the nuclear envelope and nuclear pores **NP** are clearly demonstrated. Note also the outline of the plasma membrane **PM** and mitochondria **M**.

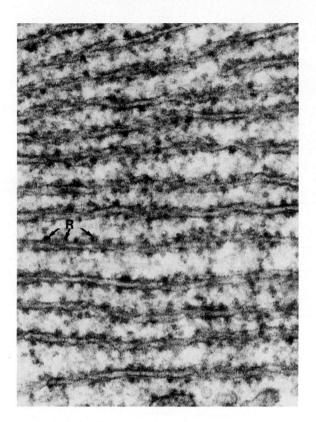

Fig. 1.9 Rough endoplasmic reticulum
(EM × 103400)

As previously described, the endoplasmic reticulum consists of an anastomosing network of tubules, vesicles and flattened cisternae which ramifies throughout the cytoplasm. Much of the surface of the endoplasmic reticulum is studded with ribosomes **R** giving the reticulum a rough or granular appearance; such endoplasmic reticulum is therefore called *rough* or *granular endoplasmic reticulum* (rER or gER). This micrograph illustrates rough ER in a cell which is specialised for the synthesis and secretion of protein; in such cells, rough ER tends to be profuse and to form closely packed, parallel laminae of flattened cisternae. It has been proposed that protein is synthesised on the ribosomes of the external surface of rough ER and then passed into the cisternal cavity; the interconnected cisternal cavities may act as intracellular pathways for the transport of newly synthesised protein.

Lipid biosynthesis

Lipids are synthesised by all cells in order to repair and replace damaged or worn membranes. Many cells also synthesise lipid as a means of storing excess energy; in such cells lipid is stored as cytoplasmic droplets. The synthesis of all classes of lipid is based on the precursor molecules fatty acids, triglycerides and cholesterol. These precursors are available to the cell from dietary sources or as a result of mobilisation of lipid stores in other cells. Fatty acids, triglycerides and cholesterol, however, can be synthesised by most cells using simple sources of carbon such as acetyl-CoA and other intermediates of glucose catabolism. Fatty acids and triglycerides are mostly synthesised within the cytosol, whereas cholesterol and phospholipids are synthesised in areas of endoplasmic reticulum devoid of ribosomes called *smooth endoplasmic reticulum* (sER). Cells which are highly active in lipid biosynthesis, such as liver cells, tend to have well developed networks of smooth ER.

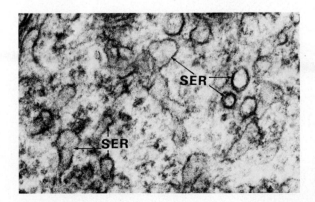

Fig. 1.10 Smooth endoplasmic reticulum
(EM × 92400)

This micrograph shows part of the prolific smooth ER **SER** of a steroid hormone secreting cell; steroid hormones are lipids derived from the precursor cholesterol. Smooth ER usually consists of an irregular network of tubules and vesicles rather than flattened cisternae as in rough ER. In addition to its role in lipid biosynthesis, smooth ER is also thought to be part of the intracellular transport system since it is continuous with rough ER and with the Golgi apparatus (see Fig. 1.11). A modified form of smooth ER is present in nerve and muscle cells (see Chapters 5 and 7) where it is believed to have specialised storage and transport functions.

Secretion

The export from cells of materials, which may be excretory waste products or secretory products, involves the four principal mechanisms outlined earlier for the transport of materials into cells. Excretion or secretion of small molecular weight compounds or lipid-soluble materials rarely involves bulk transport, whereas secretion of proteins and protein complexes almost exclusively involves bulk transport. Prior to release from the cell, proteins and other secretory products are packaged within membrane-bound vesicles which then fuse with the surface plasma membrane thus releasing their contents by the process of exocytosis. The Golgi apparatus (also called *Golgi body* or *Golgi complex*) is the organelle primarily responsible for the packaging process. During the secretory process in highly secretory cells, large amounts of intracellular membrane become incorporated into the plasma membrane; there must be, therefore, a complementary mechanism for reabsorbing excess plasma membrane and returning it to the internal pool of membrane.

An unexplained finding is that certain cell types have a well developed Golgi apparatus but are manifestly not involved in secretory activities. A possible explanation for this finding may be that the primary function of the Golgi apparatus in all cells is the production of new membrane necessary for cell growth and to replace membrane lost or damaged during normal metabolic activities; the well established packaging role of the Golgi apparatus may represent a specialisation of the suggested primary function.

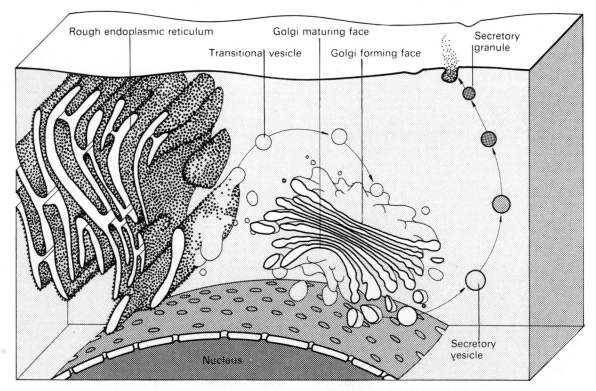

Fig. 1.11 Golgi apparatus

This schematic diagram illustrates the main structural features of the Golgi apparatus and summarises the probable mechanism by which secretory products are packaged within membrane-bound vesicles. The Golgi apparatus consists of a stacked system of saucer-shaped cisternae, with the concave surface facing the nucleus.

Proteins, synthesised on ribosomes of the rough ER, are transported within the endoplasmic reticulum to the region of the Golgi apparatus. Membrane-bound vesicles containing protein, known as *transitional vesicles*, bud off from the endoplasmic reticulum and then coalesce with the convex surface of the Golgi apparatus, an area of the Golgi apparatus known as the *forming face*. By a mechanism still unresolved, secretory product is passed towards the concave surface, the *maturing face*, where new vesicles containing secretory product are formed. Some proteinaceous secretion products consist of protein-carbohydrate complexes; it is known that the carbohydrate component is added during passage through the Golgi apparatus. After release from the maturing face the contents of *secretory vesicles* become condensed to form mature secretory vesicles, often termed *secretory granules*, which are then liberated at the cell surface by exocytosis.

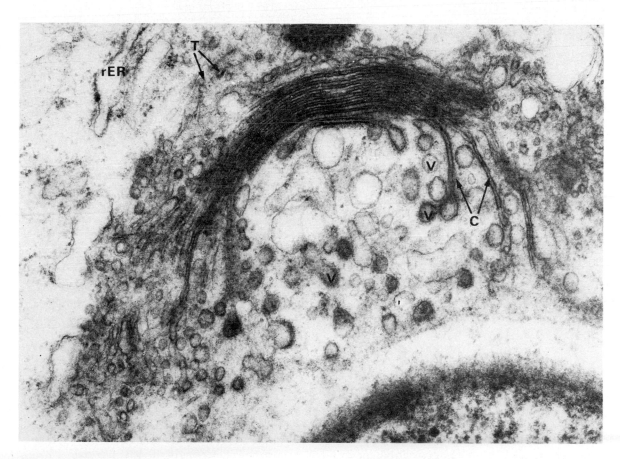

Fig. 1.12 Golgi apparatus

(EM ×49950)

The Golgi apparatus is a dynamically changing structure, the appearance of which varies enormously according to the functional state of the cell; for this reason the 'classical' appearance of the Golgi apparatus is, in practice, rarely seen. This micrograph illustrates a particularly well developed Golgi apparatus; transitional vesicles **T** and elements of the rough endoplasmic reticulum **rER** are seen adjacent to the forming face. A variety of larger vesicles **V** can be seen in the concavity of the maturing face, some of which appear to be budding from the Golgi cisternae **C**. A large number of intermediate vesicles can be seen close to the periphery of the cisternal stack.

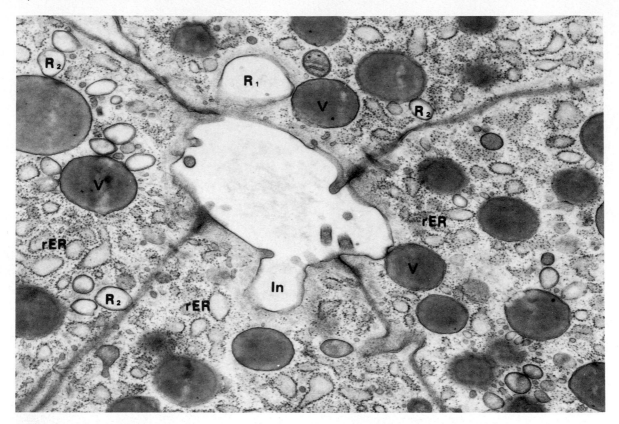

Fig. 1.13 Exocytosis

(EM × 28 900)

This micrograph shows the apical regions of four secretory cells converging on a central channel. Large, membrane-bound secretory vesicles **V** are seen approaching the lumen, one of which appears to be fusing with the surface plasma membrane. A deep invagination **In** in one of the plasma membranes probably represents a secretory vesicle which has just discharged its contents. Although the fate of membrane from discharged vesicles is not clear, a large vesicle R_1, and numerous smaller, apparently empty vesicles R_2 may represent vesicle membrane in the process of being recycled. Note also in this micrograph a well developed system of rough endoplasmic reticulum **rER** with dilated cisternae; numerous free ribosomes are present in the cytoplasm.

Energy production and storage

All cellular functions are dependent on a continuous supply of energy. Energy is derived from the sequential breakdown of organic molecules during the process of *cellular respiration*; the energy released from the breakage of chemical bonds during this process is ultimately stored in the form of ATP molecules. In actively respiring cells, ATP forms a pool of readily available energy for all the metabolic functions of the cell. The main substrates for cellular respiration are simple sugars and lipids, particularly glucose and fatty acids. Cellular respiration of glucose begins in the cytosol where it is partially degraded to form pyruvic acid by the process known as glycolysis, which yields a small amount of ATP. Pyruvic acid then diffuses into specialised organelles called *mitochondria* where, in the presence of oxygen, it is degraded to carbon dioxide and water in a process which yields a large quantity of ATP. In contrast, fatty acids pass directly into mitochondria where they are also degraded to carbon dioxide and water; this process also yields a large amount of ATP. Glycolysis may occur in the absence of oxygen and is therefore termed anaerobic respiration, whereas mitochondrial respiration is dependent on a continuous supply of oxygen and is therefore termed aerobic respiration. Mitochondria are the principal organelles involved in cellular respiration in mammals, and are found in large numbers in metabolically active cells as in the liver.

Under favourable nutritional conditions, most cells generate and store excess glucose and fatty acids in the relatively insoluble and non-toxic forms glycogen and triglyceride respectively. Cells vary greatly in their content of stored carbohydrate and lipid; extreme examples are nerve cells which contain almost no intracellular glycogen or triglyceride, and fat cells, the cytoplasm of which is almost entirely filled with stored lipid.

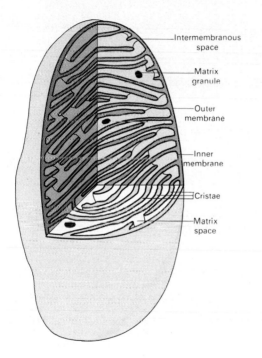

Intermembranous space

Matrix granule

Outer membrane

Inner membrane

Cristae

Matrix space

Fig. 1.14 Mitochondrion

Mitochondria vary enormously in size and shape but are most often elongated, cigar-shaped organelles. Each mitochondrion consists of two layers of membrane; the inner membrane is thrown into folds, called *cristae*, projecting into the inner cavity which is filled with an amorphous substance called *matrix*. The matrix contains a number of dense *matrix granules* the nature and function of which are unclear. The inner mitochondrial membrane is closely applied to the outer membrane leaving a narrow intermembranous space which extends into each crista.

Aerobic respiration takes place within the matrix and inner mitochondrial membranes. The matrix contains most of the enzymes involved in oxidation of fatty acids and the enzymes of the tricarboxylic acid cycle (Krebs cycle). The inner membrane contains the cytochromes, the carrier molecules of the electron transport chain, and the enzymes involved in ATP production. There is evidence that these molecules are arranged in an ordered manner as discrete functional units called *respiratory assemblies* within the mitochondrial inner membrane, but whether these units have a structure which is discernible with the electron microscope is in dispute.

Mitochondria, as organelles, have several most unusual features. The mitochondrial matrix contains a strand of DNA arranged as a circle in a manner analogous to the chromosomes of bacteria. The matrix also contains ribosomes which have a similar structure to bacterial ribosomes. There is evidence that mitochondria synthesise at least some of their own constituent proteins, others being synthesised by the cell in which they reside. In addition, mitochondria undergo self-replication by a process which is similar to bacterial cell division. On the basis of these features, it has been proposed that mitochondria are semi-autonomous organelles which arose during evolution as bacterial intracellular parasites of larger, more advanced cells.

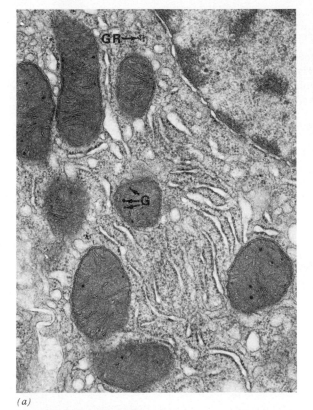

(a)

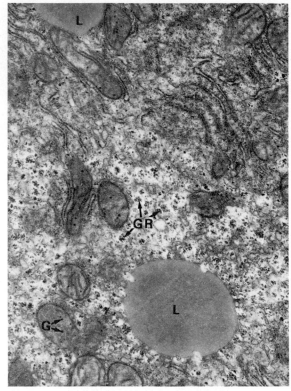

(b)

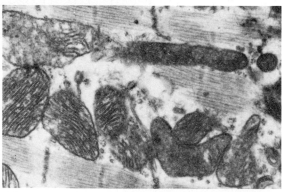

(c)

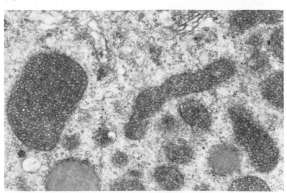

(d)

Fig. 1.15 Mitochondria, lipid droplets and glycogen

(EM (a) × 21 200 (b) × 18 200 (c) × 21 300 (d) × 16 200)

All mitochondria conform to the same general structure but vary greatly in size, shape and arrangement of cristae; these variations often reflect the metabolic status of the cell type in which mitochondria are found. Mitochondria move freely within the cytosol and tend to aggregate in intracellular sites with high energy demands where their shape often conforms to the available space. Micrographs (a) and (b), both of liver cell cytoplasm, show the typical appearance of mitochondria when cut in different planes of section; note the relatively dense matrix containing a few matrix granules **G**. Glycogen and lipid droplets are also seen in (a) and (b); glycogen appears either as single, minute dense granules (called α *particles*) or as aggregations termed *glycogen rosettes* **GR**, also called *β particles*. Lipid droplets **L** are of variable size and electron density and are not bounded by a membrane. Mitochondria from heart muscle and steroid-secreting cells can be seen in (c) and (d) respectively; in each, the cristae are densely packed, reflecting the metabolic activity of the cell, and have a characteristic shape. The cristae of heart muscle mitochondria are laminar whereas those of steroid-secreting cells are tubular.

The cytoskeleton and cell movement

The concept of a *cytoskeleton* has been evolved to explain how cell shape is maintained and altered during such processes as endocytosis, amoeboid movement and cell division. The cytoskeleton is thought to consist of an internal framework of minute filaments and tubules which may not only provide structural support but also may direct intracellular movement of organelles and metabolites. Cell movement would thus depend on rearrangement of the supporting elements, a process termed *contractility*. In muscle cells, which are highly specialised contractile cells, the contractile mechanism is thought to involve the movement of minute filaments relative to one another, according to the *sliding filament theory* (see Chapter 5), but this mechanism may not be wholly applicable to all cell types.

The minute filaments of the cytoskeleton, called *microfilaments*, are probably a mixed population of filamentous proteins of which the protein *actin* is the major constituent. Since actin is known to be one of the major filament types involved in muscle contraction, it may have a similar role in the cytoskeleton of other cell types. In some cells, microfilaments are arranged as bundles called *tonofibrils*; tonofibrils appear to converge upon the plasma membrane in the region of certain types of intercellular junctions (see Chapter 4) thus integrating the plasma membrane into the cytoskeleton.

The tubular structures of the cytoskeleton, *microtubules*, are demonstrable in the cytoplasm of many cell types where they may provide the major elements of a supporting framework. Microtubules are composed of subunits of a globular protein called *tubulin* arranged in a closely packed, helical manner. Tubulin subunits appear to disaggregate and reaggregate readily, thereby providing a dynamic, rather than static, framework.

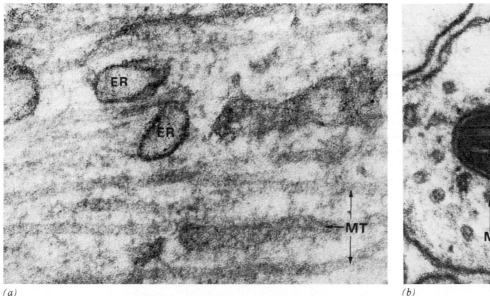
(a)

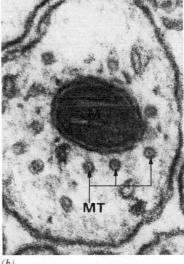
(b)

Fig. 1.16 Microtubules
(EM (a) LS × 171 500 (b) TS × 171 500)

These micrographs illustrate microtubules within nerve cells; each nerve cell has an extremely elongated cytoplasmic extension called an axon (see Chapter 7) in which microtubules are unusually prominent. The axonal microtubules probably provide structural support and direct intra-axonal transport. In longitudinal section, microtubules **MT** appear as straight, unbranched structures and in transverse section appear hollow. The small diameter of microtubules is evident when compared with an adjacent small mitochondrion **M** and elements of smooth endoplasmic reticulum **ER**. Microtubules may direct intracellular transport by acting as 'guide rails' for the movement of organelles such as mitochondria or secretory vesicles; alternatively microtubules may merely act as a system of internal tubes for conveying molecules within the cytoplasm.

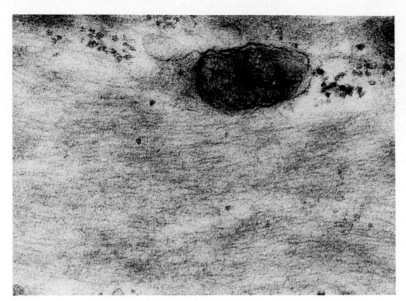

Fig. 1.17 Microfilaments
(EM × 76 500)

In general, individual microfilaments are difficult to demonstrate because of their small diameter and diffuse arrangement amongst other cytoplasmic components. In this example from a smooth muscle cell, a cell type in which cytoplasmic filaments are a predominant feature, parallel arrays of microfilaments are readily seen. The diameter of microfilaments may be compared with the diameter of a mitochondrion **M**.

The cell cycle and cell replication

The development of a single, fertilised egg cell to form a complex, multicellular organism involves cellular replication, growth and progressive specialisation for a variety of functions. The mechanism of cellular replication in all but the male and female germ cells (see Chapter 15) is known as *mitosis*. Mitosis or *mitotic division* of a single cell results in the production of two daughter cells, each genetically identical to the parent cell. After the period in which mitosis takes place, the daughter cells enter a period of growth and metabolic activity prior to further mitotic division. The time interval between mitotic divisions, that is the life cycle of an individual cell, is called the *cell cycle*. As development of the fertilised ovum progresses to produce a multicellular embryo, groups of cells and their progeny become increasingly specialised to form tissues each with different specific functions. The process whereby cells become specialised is called *differentiation*. In the fully developed organism, the differentiated cells of some tissues, such as the neurones of the nervous system, lose the ability to undergo mitosis, whereas certain cells of other tissues, such as the epithelial cells lining the gastro-intestinal tract, undergo continuous cycles of mitotic division throughout the lifespan of the organism. Between these extremes, other cells, such as liver cells, do not normally undergo mitosis in the fully developed organism but retain the capacity to undergo mitosis should the need arise.

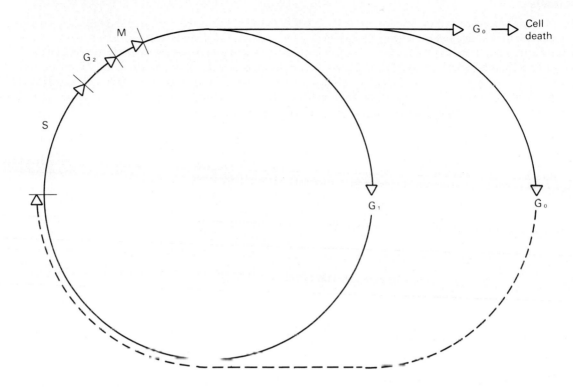

Fig. 1.18 The cell cycle

Historically, only two phases of the cell cycle were recognised, the phase during which mitosis takes place, which in general occurs in a relatively short time, and the phase in which cell division does not take place. This second phase, called *interphase*, usually occupies most of the life cycle of an individual cell. With the development of radio-isotopes it was found that, in cells which undergo mitosis, there is a discrete period during interphase when nuclear DNA is replicated; this phase, described as the *synthesis* or *S phase* of the cell cycle, is completed some time before the onset of mitosis (also called the *M phase*). Thus interphase may be divided into three separate phases. Between the end of the M phase and the beginning of the S phase, the *first gap* or G_1 *phase* occurs; this is usually much longer than the other phases of the cell cycle. During the G_1 phase, cells grow and perform their specialised functions with respect to the tissue as a whole. The interval between the end of the S phase and the beginning of the M phase, the *second gap* or G_2 *phase*, is of relatively short duration and is the period in which cells prepare for mitotic division.

Some cell types progress continuously through the cell cycle in situations where tissue growth or cell turnover is occurring. Cell types which lose the capacity for mitotic division, for example nerve cells, leave the cell cycle after the M phase and enter a protracted functional state designated as the G_0 *phase*. Some other cell types enter the G_0 phase but retain the capacity to re-enter the cell cycle when suitably stimulated. Some liver cells appear to enter a protracted G_2 phase in which they are fully functional cells despite the presence of more than the usual complement of DNA.

The M phase is usually relatively short and is the period in which DNA, duplicated during the S phase, is equally distributed between the two daughter cells as cell division occurs.

In general, the S, G_2 and M phases of the cell cycle are relatively constant in duration, each taking up to several hours to complete whereas the G_1 phase is highly variable, in some cases lasting for several days or even longer. The G_0 phase may last for the entire lifespan of an individual.

The cell cycle, and hence the rate of cell division, is controlled by both extrinsic and intrinsic factors. Hormones are extrinsic factors which regulate the cell cycles of many cells and thus co-ordinate tissue growth and function. At present, little is known about the intrinsic factors which control the cell cycle. An understanding of all the factors which control the cell cycle is likely to be a prerequisite for elucidation of the primary defect which occurs in conditions of uncontrolled cell division such as cancer.

Mitosis

The process of somatic cell division, or mitosis, occurs in the M phase of the cell cycle and takes approximately 30 to 60 minutes in mammals. Mitosis has two main functions. Firstly, it is the phase in which the chromosomes duplicated in the S phase are distributed equally and identically between the two potential daughter cells; this process is called *karyokinesis*. Secondly, mitosis is the phase in which the dividing cell is cleaved into genetically identical daughter cells by cytoplasmic division or *cytokinesis*. Although karyokinesis is always equal and symmetrical, cytokinesis may, in some situations, result in the formation of two daughter cells with grossly unequal amounts of cytoplasm or cytoplasmic organelles.

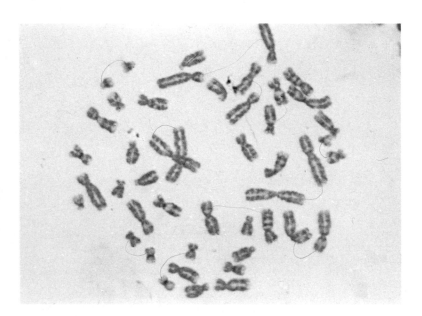

Fig. 1.19 Mitotic chromosomes

(Giemsa × 1200)

In general, the nuclei of all cells contain the same fixed complement of DNA, a quantity called the *genome*. The genome is identical in every cell (except the germ cells, see Chapter 15, and a few odd exceptions) of the same individual. The DNA of the genome is intimately associated with proteins, called nucleo-proteins, and is arranged as a number of discrete strands called *chromosomes*. The cells of each species have a characteristic, fixed number of chromosomes (46 in man) known as *the diploid number*. Chromosomes function in pairs, called *homologous pairs*, the members of each pair having a similar length of DNA and a similar structure.

During interphase, chromosomes exist as an unravelled mass within the nucleus; this arrangement may facilitate gene expression, a process which takes place mainly within the G_1 and G_0 phases of the cell cycle. Histologically, chromosomes are not usually visible within the nucleus of cells in interphase. During the S phase, each chromosome is duplicated and the two identical chromosomes remain attached to each other. At the onset of mitosis, the duplicated chromosomes become tightly coiled and

condensed such that they are readily visible with the light microscope. This arrangement of chromosomes during mitosis is merely a mechanism for packaging the duplicated genome which may then be distributed identically and equally between the two daughter cells during mitosis.

This micrograph illustrates the chromosomes of a human cell cultured *in vitro* and arrested at the onset of mitosis; the chromosomes have been treated with the enzyme trypsin, thus revealing a cross-banding pattern along the length of each chromosome. Chromosomes, as seen at mitosis, each consist of a duplicated chromosome, each member of the duplicate being referred to as a *chromatid*. The two so-called chromatids of each chromosome are joined at a point called *the kinetochore* (or *centromere*); this appears as a constriction in each mitotic chromosome.

Each member of a homologous pair of chromosomes is similar in length, kinetochore location and banding pattern. The significance of trypsin-induced chromosomal banding is not understood but the phenomenon provides a useful technique for the identification of chromosomes, especially in the investigation of chromosomal abnormalities.

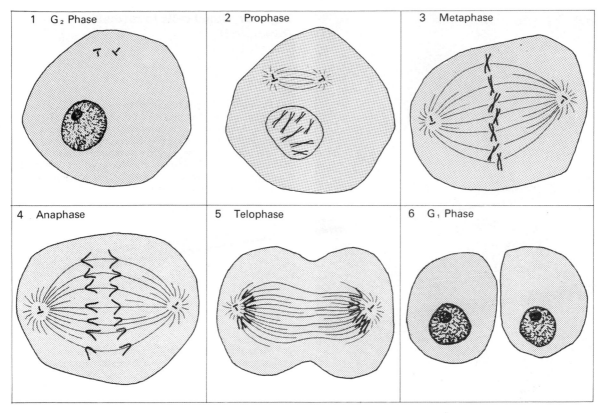

Fig. 1.20 Mitosis

Mitosis is a continuous process which is traditionally divided into four phases: *prophase*, *anaphase*, *metaphase* and *telophase*, each stage being readily recognisable with the light microscope. In mammalian cells, both karyokinesis and cytokinesis require the presence of a structure called the *mitotic apparatus*. This structure, which is more fully discussed with Fig. 1.22, consists of longitudinally arranged microtubules which extend between paired organising centres called *centrioles* at the two poles of the dividing cell. Centrioles are discussed further with Fig. 1.22. The mitotic apparatus is visible within the cytoplasm only during the M phase of the cell cycle since it disaggregates shortly after the completion of mitosis.

Prophase: the beginning of this stage of mitosis is defined as the moment when chromosomes first become visible within the nucleus. As prophase continues, the chromosomes become increasingly condensed and shortened and the nucleoli disappear. Dissolution of the nuclear envelope marks the end of prophase. During prophase, the two pairs of centrioles (duplicated earlier in interphase) migrate to opposite poles of the cell. The centrioles remain connected by numerous longitudinal microtubules, collectively forming the so-called *mitotic spindle*; the spindle tubules elongate as the centrioles move apart.

Metaphase: during the second stage of mitosis, the mitotic spindle is completed and the chromosomes become arranged at the equator of the spindle, a region known as the *equatorial* or *metaphase plate*. At this stage the two

chromatids of each chromosome are still joined at the kinetochore.

Anaphase: this stage of mitosis is marked by separation of the two chromatids of each chromosome, which then migrate along the spindle to opposite poles of the cell, thus achieving an exact division of the duplicated genetic material. By the end of anaphase, two groups of identical chromosomes (the former chromatids) are clustered at opposite poles of the cell.

Telophase: during the final phase of mitosis, the chromosomes begin to uncoil and to regain their interphase conformation. The nuclear envelope reforms and nucleoli again become apparent. The process of cytokinesis also takes place during telophase; the plane of cytoplasmic division is usually defined by the position of the spindle equator, thus producing two cells of equal size. The plasma membrane around the spindle equator becomes indented to form a circumferential furrow around the cell, the *cleavage furrow*, which progressively constricts the cell until it is cleaved into two daughter cells. In mammalian cells, a ring of microfilaments is present just beneath the surface of the cleavage furrow and it has been suggested that cytokinesis occurs as a result of contraction of this filamentous ring.

In the early G_1 phase, the mitotic spindle disaggregates and in many cell types the single pair of centrioles begins to duplicate in preparation for the next mitotic division. In Fig. 1.21 the four main stages of mitosis are illustrated in actively dividing, primitive blood cells from a smear preparation of bone marrow.

2. Blood

Introduction

Blood is a tissue which consists of a variety of cells suspended in a fluid medium called *plasma*. Blood functions principally as a vehicle for the transport of gases, nutrients, metabolic waste products, cells and hormones throughout the body. Thus any sample of blood is composed not only of cells and molecules involved in transport processes but also cells and molecules in the process of being transported.

Plasma is essentially an aqueous solution of inorganic salts which is constantly exchanged with the extracellular fluid medium of all body tissues. Plasma also contains proteins, the *plasma proteins*, of three main types: *albumins, globulins* and *fibrinogen*. Collectively, the plasma proteins exert a colloidal osmotic pressure within the circulatory system which helps to regulate the exchange of aqueous solution between plasma and extracellular fluid. The albumins, which constitute the bulk of plasma proteins, bind relatively insoluble metabolites such as fatty acids and thus serve as transport proteins. The globulins are a diverse group of proteins which include the antibodies of the immune system (see Chapter 10) and certain proteins responsible for the transport of lipids and some heavy metal ions. Fibrinogen is a soluble protein which polymerises to form the insoluble protein *fibrin* during blood clotting. In general, the molecular components of plasma cannot be demonstrated by light and electron microscopy.

The cells of blood are of three major functional classes: *red blood cells (erythrocytes), white blood cells (leucocytes)* and *platelets (thrombocytes)*. Erythrocytes are primarily involved in oxygen and carbon dioxide transport, the leucocytes constitute an important part of the defence and immune systems of the body, and platelets are a vital component of the blood clotting mechanism. All these cell types are formed in the bone marrow by a process called *haemopoiesis*. Erythrocytes and platelets function entirely within blood vessels whereas leucocytes act mainly outside blood vessels in the tissues. Thus the leucocytes found in circulating blood are merely in transit between their various sites of activity.

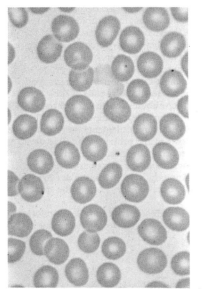

Fig. 2.1 Erythrocytes

(Giemsa × 800)

The erythrocyte is highly adapted for its principal function, that is, the transport of oxygen and carbon dioxide. The erythrocyte develops from precursors in the bone marrow. During differentiation, vast quantities of the iron-containing respiratory pigment *haemoglobin* are synthesised. Before release into the general circulation, the nucleus is extruded and, by maturity, all cytoplasmic organelles degenerate. The fully differentiated erythrocyte thus consists merely of an outer plasma membrane enclosing haemoglobin and the limited number of enzymes which are necessary for maintenance of the integrity of the plasma membrane and the gaseous transport function.

This micrograph demonstrates the characteristic appearance of erythrocytes in a stained smear of peripheral blood. The cells are stained pink due to their high content of haemoglobin. The pale staining of the central region of the erythrocyte is a result of its unusual biconcave disc shape.

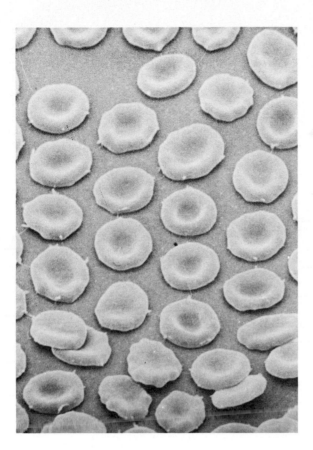

Fig. 2.2 Erythrocytes
(Scanning EM × 2400)

Scanning electron microscopy reveals the biconcave disc shape of erythrocytes. The unusual shape provides a large surface area relative to cell volume; this greatly enhances gaseous exchange. The fluidity of the plasma membrane, combined with its biconcave shape, allows the erythrocyte to deform readily; thus erythrocytes (average diameter 6 to 8 μm) are able to pass through the smallest capillaries (3 to 4 μm in diameter).

The means by which the erythrocyte maintains the biconcave shape is poorly understood. The shape is partly governed by the cell's water content and the volume of water in the cell is partially determined by the concentration of inorganic ions within the cell. As with all other mammalian cells, sodium ions must be pumped out of erythrocytes continuously. The energy required for this process is derived, in the form of ATP, from anaerobic metabolism of glucose. The absence of mitochondria precludes aerobic energy production; hence erythrocytes are totally dependent on glucose as an energy source.

The lifespan of an erythrocyte, 120 days on average, may be determined by its ability to maintain the biconcave shape. In the absence of appropriate organelles, erythrocytes are unable to synthesise new proteins to replace deteriorating enzymes and membrane proteins. This leads to diminished ability to pump sodium ions from the cell and results in uptake of water, thereby producing spheroidal erythrocytes. Such cells are removed from the circulation and destroyed by the spleen and liver

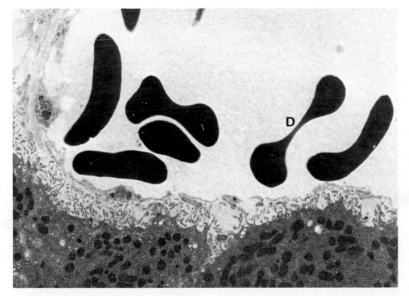

Fig. 2.3 Erythrocytes
(EM × 5700)

This micrograph illustrates the characteristic features of erythrocytes seen by transmission electron microscopy. With this technique, the observed shape of the erythrocyte depends on the plane of section through the cell. The classical dumb-bell shape **D** is only seen when the erythrocyte is cut through its thin central zone; more frequently irregularly shaped erythrocytes are seen due to the deformation which normally occurs in the bloodstream. The high electron density of erythrocytes is due to the iron atoms of haemoglobin. Note the total absence of cytoplasmic organelles.

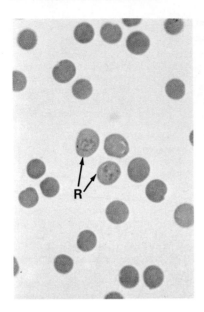

Fig. 2.4 Reticulocytes
(Cresyl blue/eosin × 800)

Reticulocytes are the immature form in which erythrocytes are released into the circulation from the bone marrow; they mature into erythrocytes within about one day of release. The rate of release of reticulocytes into the circulation generally equals the rate of removal of spent erythrocytes by the spleen and liver. Since the lifespan of circulating erythrocytes is about 120 days, reticulocytes constitute slightly less than one per cent of the circulating red blood cells.

Reticulocytes cannot be readily distinguished in routinely stained blood smears, but when fresh blood is incubated with the basic dye, brilliant cresyl blue, a blue-stained reticular precipitate is formed in the reticulocytes but not in mature erythrocytes. This is due to the interaction of the dye with ribosomal RNA still remaining in the immature cells. This technique, called *supravital staining*, is illustrated in this micrograph. Note that reticulocytes **R** are usually slightly larger than the surrounding mature erythrocytes.

When severe erythrocyte depletion occurs, such as after haemorrhage and in certain disease states, the rate of erythrocyte production in the bone marrow increases and the proportion of reticulocytes in circulating blood rises. Thus the reticulocyte count provides a convenient measure of the rate of red blood cell formation in the bone marrow.

phagocytic cells { *monocytes (macrophages)* / *neutrophils (microphages)* }

White cell series

There are five cell types in the white blood cell series and these are subdivided into two main classes, *granulocytes* and *agranulocytes*, according to the granularity of their cytoplasm and general nuclear characteristics:

(i) Granulocytes: the granulocytes are characterised by prominent cytoplasmic granules and a single, multilobed nucleus which may give the erroneous impression that granulocytes are multinucleate cells. The highly variable shape of granulocyte nuclei has given rise to the common name of *polymorphonuclear leucocytes* or *polymorphs*. Granulocytes contain granules of two types. Firstly, granulocytes are phagocytic and contain lysosomes which are known as *primary granules*. Secondly, each of the granulocytes has an additional class of granule which is specific to the cell; these are called *specific* or *secondary granules*. According to the staining characteristics of the specific granules, granulocytes are subdivided into three types: *neutrophils*, *eosinophils* and *basophils*. The specific granules of neutrophils have little affinity for either acidic or basic dyes whereas those of eosinophils are stained strongly by acidic dyes such as eosin, and those of basophils are stained intensely by basic dyes such as haematoxylin or methylene blue.

(ii) Agranulocytes: the agranulocytes, which comprise the *lymphocytes* and *monocytes*, were so named since they do not contain cytoplasmic granules readily visible with light microscopy. In contrast to the granulocytes, the nuclei of the agranulocytes are not lobed although they may be deeply indented; this nuclear feature led to the application of the misleading term *mononuclear leucocytes* in reference to the agranulocytes.

Leucocytes constitute an important part of the body's defences against foreign invaders. Granulocytes and monocytes are highly phagocytic and engulf micro-organisms, cell debris and particulate matter in a non-specific manner; this activity may be enhanced and directed by immune responses to specific foreign agents (see Chapter 10). Monocytes and neutrophils are the most active phagocytes and, on the basis of their relative sizes, are often referred to as *macrophages* and *microphages* respectively.

Lymphocytes play the key role in all immune responses and, in contrast to the other leucocytes, their activity is always directed against specific foreign agents.

In general, all the leucocytes perform their functions in the tissues and merely use the blood as a vehicle for passage between sites of formation, storage and activity. It follows, therefore, that increased demand for particular leucocytes in various sites is reflected in increased numbers in the circulation. All leucocytes exhibit amoeboid movement which provides the means for migration in and out of the circulatory system and through the tissues.

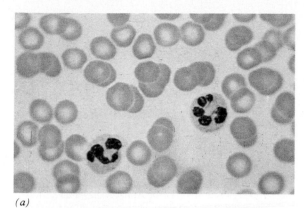

(a)

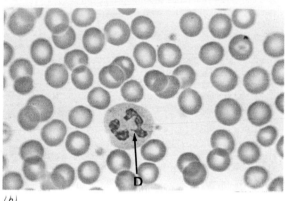

(b)

Fig. 2.5 Neutrophils

(Giemsa (a) and (b) × 800)

Neutrophils are the most common type of leucocyte in blood and constitute from forty to seventy-five per cent of circulating leucocytes. The most prominent feature of the neutrophil is the highly lobulated nucleus. In the mature neutrophil there are usually five lobes connected by fine strands of nuclear material, but in the less mature neutrophil the nucleus is generally not as lobulated. In micrograph (a) two neutrophils in different stages of maturity are illustrated.

In neutrophils of females, the condensed, quiescent X-chromosome or Barr body (see Fig. 1.6) exists in the form of a small drumstick-shaped appendage of one of the nuclear lobes. This appendage, known as the *drumstick chromosome* **D**, is visible in about three per cent of neutrophils in females as shown in micrograph (b).

The cytoplasm of neutrophils is lightly stippled with purplish granules called *azurophilic granules* which are merely large lysosomes (primary granules). The cytoplasm also contains numerous smaller granules, the specific granules, which are poorly stained and are thus not visible in this type of preparation.

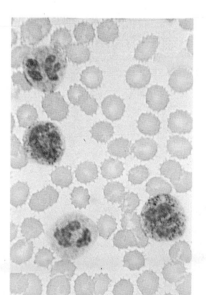

Fig. 2.6 Neutrophils

(Histochemical method for alkaline phosphatase × 800)

The specific granules of neutrophils contain a group of proteins with antibacterial action called *phagocytins* and the enzyme *alkaline phosphatase*, the function of which is not understood. Nevertheless, alkaline phosphatase activity is a useful marker for the specific granules of neutrophils and can be demonstrated by histochemical methods. In this preparation, enzyme activity is indicated by a brown, granular deposition in the neutrophil cytoplasm. Immature neutrophils, recognisable by their less lobulated nuclei, exhibit less enzyme activity since they contain fewer specific granules.

In contrast to the specific granules, the azurophilic primary granules, the lysosomes, contain a variety of hydrolytic enzymes plus potent antibacterial enzymes such as lysozyme, myeloperoxidase and D-amino-oxidase, enzymes which destroy bacterial cell walls. The principal function of neutrophils is to engulf invading micro-organisms, particularly bacteria; neutrophils are the main white cell type involved in acute inflammatory responses.

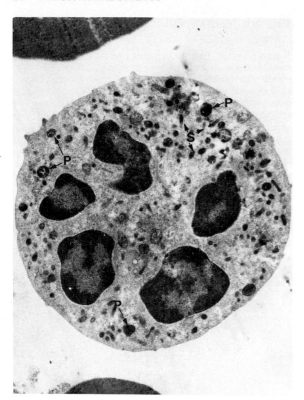

Fig. 2.7 Neutrophil

(EM × 11 300)

With electron microscopy, neutrophils have three distinguishing features. Firstly, the nucleus has up to five lobes which in section may appear as separate nuclei. Secondly, the cytoplasm contains numerous membrane-bound granules. The primary granules **P** are large, spheroidal and electron-dense, similar to the lysosomes of other cell types. The specific granules **S** are much more numerous, small and often rod-like, and of variable density and shape. Thirdly, all other cytoplasmic organelles are scarce although the cytoplasm is particularly rich in dispersed glycogen.

Neutrophils are the principal cells involved in the acute inflammatory response to tissue damage; they are highly mobile and migrate from small blood vessels to sites of tissue damage where they engulf and destroy cell debris and micro-organisms by phagocytosis. Since the mature neutrophil has few appropriate organelles for protein synthesis, it has very limited capacity to regenerate expended lysosomal and specific enzymes which are rapidly depleted by phagocytic activity; the neutrophil is thus incapable of continuous function and degenerates after a single burst of activity. Defunct neutrophils are the main cellular constituent of *pus* and are therefore sometimes referred to as *pus cells*. The paucity of mitochondria and the abundance of glycogen in neutrophils reflects the predominance of the anaerobic mode of metabolism; this permits neutrophils to function in the poorly oxygenated environment of damaged tissues.

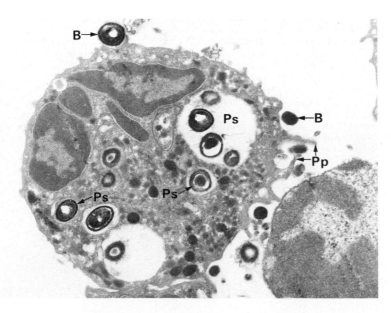

Fig. 2.8 Neutrophil: phagocytosis of bacteria

(EM × 11 750)

This micrograph illustrates a neutrophil in the process of engulfing and destroying several bacteria **B**. Note the manner in which pseudopodia **Pp** embrace bacteria before engulfment. Note also phagosomes **Ps** containing bacteria in various stages of degradation. Several prominent primary (lysosomal) granules and numerous smaller specific granules remain in the cytoplasm.

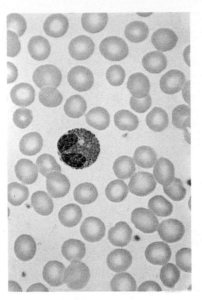

Fig. 2.9 Eosinophil

(Giemsa × 800)

Eosinophils are much less common than neutrophils and account for one to six per cent of leucocytes in circulating blood. Characteristically, eosinophils have a bilobed nucleus and the cytoplasm is packed with large, eosinophilic (dark-pink stained) specific granules of uniform size.

It has long been observed that the number of eosinophils in circulating blood increases in certain parasitic infestations such as hookworm, and in some hypersensitivity states such as hay fever, but the role of eosinophils in these processes is poorly understood.

During the last decade, the eosinophil has been found to have a variety of functions in inflammatory and immune responses, often in conjunction with other leucocytes. Eosinophils are highly phagocytic for antigen-antibody complexes (see Chapter 10) although they also exhibit some of the general phagocytic activity of neutrophils. Eosinophils are attracted to sites of inflammation by substances released from basophils and their connective tissue analogues, the mast cells (see Figs 2.11 and 2.12, and 3.17 and 3.18), and deactivate vasoactive substances such as histamine produced by these cells during the inflammatory response. More recent evidence suggests that eosinophils have a direct destructive effect on some parasites provided that specific antibodies are present (see also Chapter 10).

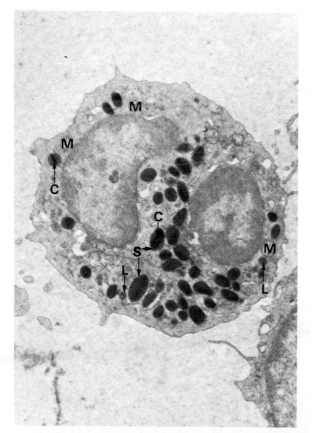

Fig. 2.10 Eosinophil

(EM × 10600)

The most characteristic ultrastructural feature of eosinophils are the large, ovoid, specific granules **S**, each containing a dense crystalloid **C** in the long axis of the granule; in man, as in this micrograph, the crystalloids are irregular in form but in many other mammals they have a regular, discoid shape. The specific granules are membrane-bound and the matrix contains a variety of hydrolytic enzymes including *histaminase*. The crystalloids are thought to be composed of basic proteins but these are of unknown function. Eosinophils also contain a small number of primary (lysosomal) granules **L** which are less electron-dense and lack crystalloids. Other cytoplasmic organelles such as mitochondria **M** are relatively sparse and rough endoplasmic reticulum is absent. Note the characteristic bilobed nucleus.

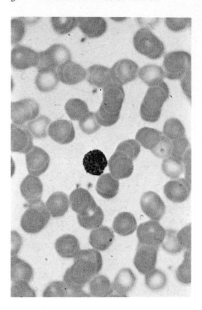

Fig. 2.11 Basophil

(Giemsa × 800)

Basophils are the least common leucocyte and constitute less than one per cent of leucocytes in circulating blood. Like eosinophils, basophils also have a bilobed nucleus but, in general, this is obscured by numerous, large, densely basophilic (deep blue) specific granules. These granules are highly soluble in water and tend to be dissolved away during common blood smear preparation, thus adding to the difficulty of finding these rare cells.

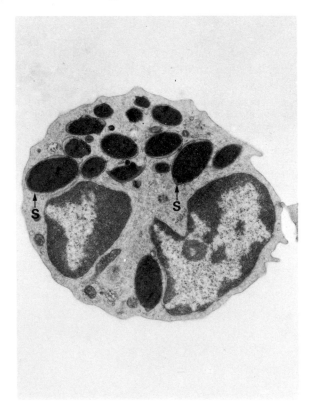

Fig. 2.12 Basophil

(EM × 10 500)

With electron microscopy, the characteristic bilobed nucleus of the basophil is easily recognisable. The large specific granules **S** are membrane-bound and are filled with a closely packed, electron-dense material which contains the vasoactive substances *histamine*, *heparin* and *slow reacting substance of anaphylaxis (SRS-A)*. Heparin is a potent anticoagulant, and histamine and SRS-A have a variety of effects on the muscle of blood vessel walls and on the permeability of capillaries. Certain inflammatory and immune responses stimulate discharge of the contents of specific granules into plasma by exocytosis.

Basophils bear a close resemblance to the fixed mast cells of connective tissue (see Figs. 3.17 and 3.18) in the structure and content of their specific granules, but there are important ultrastructural differences. Whilst basophils and mast cells are not thought to be two manifestations of the same cell type, they are considered to be functionally analogous since similar stimuli induce degranulation of both cell types producing similar physiological consequences.

Basophils are the least phagocytic of the granulocytes and thus contain few primary (lysosomal) granules.

Fig. 2.13 Lymphocytes

(Giemsa × 800)

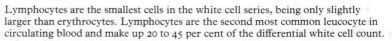

Lymphocytes are the smallest cells in the white cell series, being only slightly larger than erythrocytes. Lymphocytes are the second most common leucocyte in circulating blood and make up 20 to 45 per cent of the differential white cell count.

Lymphocytes are characterised by a round, densely stained nucleus and a relatively small amount of pale basophilic, non-granular cytoplasm. The amount of cytoplasm varies with the state of activity of the lymphocyte, and in circulating blood there is a predominance of 'small' lymphocytes; however, 'medium' and 'large' lymphocytes are also seen in peripheral blood. This micrograph illustrates small and medium lymphocytes. In the medium lymphocyte the cytoplasm is readily visible but in the small lymphocyte the cytoplasm is almost too sparse to be seen.

Lymphocytes play the central role in all immunological defence mechanisms; these are described in detail in Chapter 10. Blood provides the medium in which lymphocytes circulate between the various lymphoid tissues and all other tissues of the body.

Fig. 2.14 Lymphocyte

(EM × 15000)

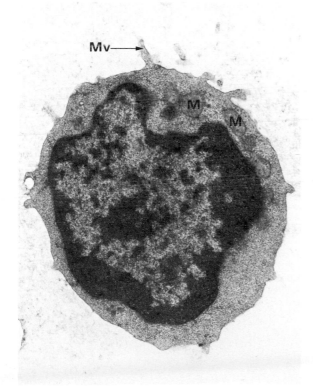

Most of the lymphocytes in the circulation are in a relatively inactive metabolic state; this is reflected in their ultrastructural appearance. The nucleus is small, rounded and often slightly indented and the chromatin is moderately condensed; nucleoli are not usually present. The sparse cytoplasm contains a few mitochondria **M**, a rudimentary Golgi apparatus, little or no endoplasmic reticulum and a comparatively large number of free ribosomes accounting for the basophilia of light microscopy. The plasma membrane has a few irregular microvilli **Mv**. When activated during the immune response, lymphocytes undergo remarkable morphological transformations into metabolically active cells with specific functions (see Chapter 10).

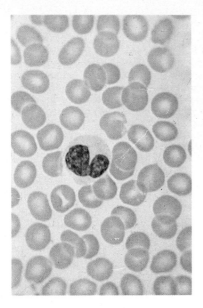

Fig. 2.15 Monocytes

(Giemsa × 800)

Monocytes are the largest members of the white cell series and constitute from two to ten per cent of leucocytes in peripheral blood. Monocytes are characterised by a large, eccentrically placed nucleus which is stained less intensely than that of other leucocytes. The nucleus is usually indented, a feature which becomes more pronounced as the cell matures, so as to give a horseshoe or even bilobed appearance. The extensive cytoplasm is filled with small lysosomes which, in light microscopy, confer a characteristic 'frosted-glass' appearance. Ultrastructural studies show that monocytes have two or more nucleoli, a well developed Golgi apparatus, relatively numerous mitochondria and a moderate amount of rough endoplasmic reticulum. Thus, in contrast to neutrophils, the monocyte is capable of continuous lysosomal activity and regeneration. Also in contrast to neutrophils, monocytes utilise both aerobic and anaerobic metabolic pathways depending on their location within the body. These features permit the monocyte to function over a long period which may be many months or years.

Monocytes appear to have little function in circulating blood. They are highly motile cells and migrate into connective tissues where they are termed *histiocytes* or *tissue fixed macrophages* (see Figs. 3.19 and 3.20).

A major function of macrophages is the destruction of cellular debris arising from normal turnover of cells within the tissues. Macrophages also play an important role in the immune defence system which is described in Chapter 10. The monocytes dispersed throughout the body collectively form the *macrophage-monocyte system*.

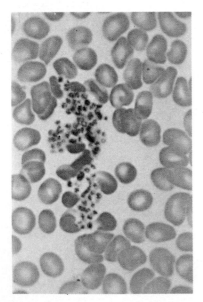

Fig. 2.16 Platelets

(Giemsa × 800)

Platelets or thrombocytes are small, non-nucleated cells formed in the bone marrow by budding from the cytoplasm of huge cells called megakaryocytes. Platelets are present in large numbers in circulating blood, from 150,000 to 400,000 per millilitre.

Platelets are round or oval, biconvex discs about 2 to 3 μm in diameter. In blood smears, their shape is not clearly seen and they are often partially clumped together, as in this micrograph. The shape of platelets is maintained by a bundle of microtubules arranged circumferentially around the equator. The cytoplasm has a purple-stained, granular appearance due to a high content of organelles which are concentrated towards the centre of the cell; the peripheral cytoplasm is very poorly stained and therefore barely visible.

Platelets are known to participate in haemostasis in two main ways. Firstly, in normal tissues, platelets clump together to plug small defects which appear continuously in the walls of small blood vessels. Secondly, when blood vessels are injured, platelets contribute to the processes of clot formation and retraction as well as releasing a substance called *serotonin* which reduces blood flow by constricting the damaged vessels.

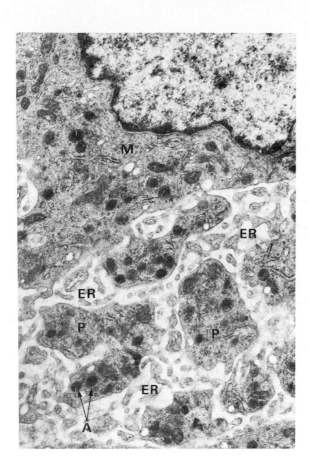

Fig. 2.17 Platelets

(EM ×15000)

This micrograph shows newly formed platelets just prior to being shed from a megakaryocyte **M** in the bone marrow. After release into the general circulation, platelets assume a regular, biconvex disc shape. By a most unusual process, the endoplasmic reticulum **ER** of the megakaryocyte proliferates to form a three-dimensional network which partitions the cytoplasm into areas corresponding to the future platelets **P**. Platelets contain a variety of cytoplasmic organelles derived from the megakaryocyte, including mitochondria, rough endoplasmic reticulum, ribosomes and membrane-bound granules. The main granules found in platelets are called *alpha granules* **A** but the nature and function of their contents is not known.

The mature, circulating platelets of man contain a few, small, very dense granules which are presumed to contain the blood vessel constrictor substances serotonin (5-hydroxytryptamine) and ATP. Biochemical analysis has shown that platelets also contain stores of ADP, fibrinogen, a phospholipid called *platelet factor III*, and a protein complex called *thrombosthenin* which is analogous to the actin and myosin contractile complex of skeletal muscle (see Chapter 5).

ADP is thought to promote platelet aggregation during the formation of a platelet plug. Platelet fibrinogen probably supplements plasma fibrinogen during the early stages of haemostasis. Platelet factor III is involved in activating the clotting mechanism. Thrombosthenin may mediate the process of clot retraction thus producing a more stable clot.

Haemopoiesis

Haemopoiesis is the process by which mature blood cells develop from precursor cells. In the human adult, haemopoiesis takes place in the marrow of certain bones, mainly the flat bones of the skull, the ribs and sternum, the vertebral column, the pelvis and the proximal ends of some long bones. Before maturity, however, haemopoiesis occurs in other sites at different stages in development. In the early embryo, primitive blood cells arise in the yolk sac; a little later, the liver becomes the major site of haemopoiesis, and during further development, the spleen and lymph nodes supplement this activity. As the bones develop during the fourth and fifth months of intra-uterine life, haemopoiesis begins in the marrow cavities and by birth, haemopoiesis is almost exclusively restricted to the bone marrow. From birth to maturity, the number of active sites of haemopoiesis in bone marrow diminishes although all bone marrow retains haemopoietic potential (see also Figs. 9.16 and 9.17).

The lineage of each blood cell type has been the subject of numerous theories but only one has gained substantial experimental support, the so-called *monophyletic theory*. This theory proposes that all blood cell types are derived from a single primitive stem cell type called a *multipotential stem cell*. The multipotential cells divide at a slow rate to replicate themselves and to give rise to five discrete cell types, each committed to a different developmental fate. Each of the five committed cell types is capable of giving rise to only one of the following cell types: erythrocytes, granulocytes, lymphocytes, monocytes and thrombocytes; thus such stem cells are referred to as *unipotential stem cells*. The unipotential stem cell divides at a rapid rate to provide histologically recognisable precursors of the mature cell type; however, there is no general agreement about the exact histological characteristics of multipotent or unipotent stem cells. The rate of division of these cells is thought to be modulated by hormones called *poietins*, although only *erythropoietin* has been positively identified.

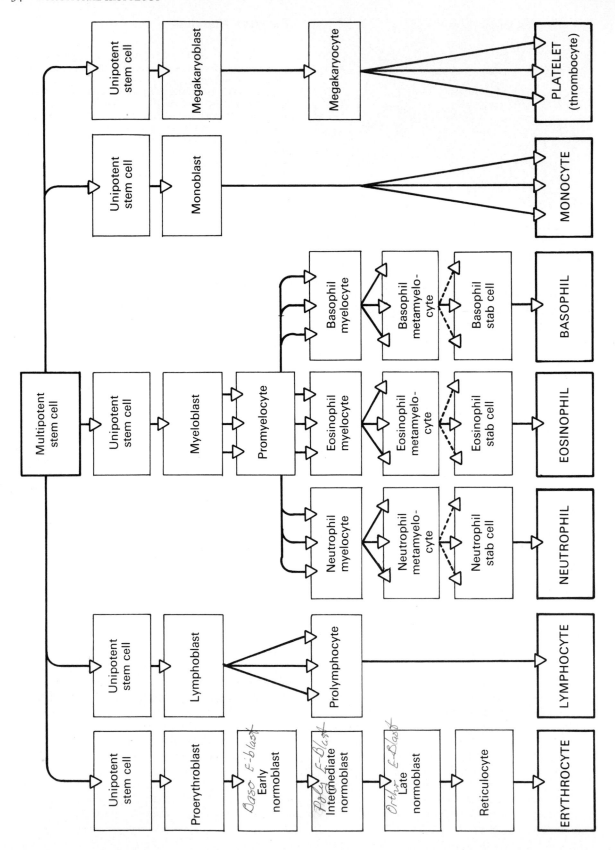

Fig. 2.18 Haemopoiesis *(illustration opposite)*

This diagram summarises the main recognisable developmental stages in blood cell formation; such a classification is somewhat arbitrary since the process of haemopoiesis is a continuum of proliferation and progressive differentiation from stem cell to the mature form found in circulating blood.

Red cell formation (erythropoiesis): the process of erythropoiesis is directed towards producing a cell devoid of organelles but packed with haemoglobin. The first recognisable erythrocyte precursor is known as the *proerythroblast*, a large cell with numerous cytoplasmic organelles and no haemoglobin. Further stages of differentiation are characterised by three main features:

(a) progressive decrease in cell size

(b) progressive loss of all organelles; the presence of numerous ribosomes at early stages accounts for the marked basophilic (blue) staining property of the cytoplasm which progressively decreases as the number of ribosomes (and rate of haemoglobin synthesis) falls

(c) progressive increase in the cytoplasmic content of haemoglobin; this accounts for the increasing eosinophilia (pink staining) of the cytoplasm towards maturity.

Haemoglobin synthesis begins during the *early normoblast (basophilic erythroblast)* stage and is complete by the end of the reticulocyte stage. Cell division ceases after the early normoblast stage, after which the nucleus progressively condenses and is finally extruded at the *late normoblast (orthochromatic erythroblast)* stage. The early normoblast stage also marks the beginning of the progressive loss of cytoplasmic organelles, only a few remnants of which remain by the reticulocyte stage. This process, accompanied by progressive haemoglobin synthesis, is represented morphologically by the transition from basophilia through polychromasia to the eosinophilia *(orthochromasia)* of the mature erythrocyte.

The process of erythropoiesis from stem cell to erythrocyte takes about one week. The rate of erythropoiesis is controlled by the hormone erythropoietin secreted by the kidney (see Fig. 13.25) and by the availability of red cell components particularly iron and protein precursors.

Granulocyte formation (granulopoiesis): the *myeloblast* is the earliest recognisable stage in granulopoiesis. The inappropriate name of myeloblast derives from an outdated view that granulocytes were the only white cells formed in *myeloid tissue* (bone marrow). Myeloblasts give rise to *promyelocytes* which are characterised by their content of azurophilic granules; since the azurophilic granules develop before the specific granules they were referred to as primary granules. As described earlier, the primary granules are merely large lysosomes and are present in all mature granulocytes.

From the promyelocyte stage onwards, the relative proportion of primary granules progressively decreases and the proportion of specific (secondary) granules progressively increases. From the *myelocyte* stage through the *metamyelocyte* stage to the mature granulocyte forms, the nucleus becomes increasingly more segmented. The immediate precursors of mature granulocytes tend to have an irregular horseshoe or sometimes ring-shaped nucleus and are termed *stab cells* or *band forms*.

Granulocytes are normally released from bone marrow only in the mature state but there is a large pool of metamyelocytes, stab cells and mature granulocytes in the marrow; this pool contains some 15 times more cells than are present in the peripheral circulation. Thus the bone marrow is able to respond to acute inflammation by release of both mature and nearly mature cells into the bloodstream. The immature forms may be distinguished from mature cells not only by their less segmented nuclei but also by their higher content of azurophilic granules.

Lymphocyte formation (lymphopoiesis): only two precursor stages, the *lymphoblast* and the *prolymphocyte*, are recognisable in the development of lymphocytes. The main feature of lymphopoiesis is a progressive diminution in cell size and an increase in the nuclear-cytoplasmic ratio.

Unlike all the blood cell types, lymphocytes also proliferate outside the bone marrow. This occurs in the tissues of the immune system in response to specific immunological stimulation (see Chapter 10).

Monocyte formation (monopoiesis): the *monoblast* is the only recognisable precursor of the monocyte. Monopoiesis is characterised by a reduction in cell size and progressive indentation of the nucleus. Mature monocytes circulate in blood for only one or two days before becoming sequestered in the tissues as tissue macrophages.

Platelet formation (thrombopoiesis): platelet formation begins with the development of a large binucleate cell, the *megakaryoblast*. After this stage, fusion of the nuclei occurs and successive duplication of the nuclear material takes place without the formation of separate nuclei and without cell division. The resulting polyploid cell, the *megakaryocyte*, has an enormous volume of cytoplasm and the cell may reach $100\,\mu m$ in diameter. Ultrastructural studies have shown that areas of cytoplasm representing the future platelets become demarcated by membranes and are eventually shed as platelets; whether the megakaryocyte synthesises further cytoplasm is uncertain.

In bone marrow smears, the earlier phases of haemopoiesis may be recognisable only with great difficulty. The characteristic, detailed features of each stage have been described using techniques of fixation and staining which are rarely applied in routine haematological practice. The recognition of such stages is of little practical value except in certain pathological conditions; under such circumstances the classical characteristics of each cell type are often distorted. Many of the later stages of haemopoiesis are readily recognisable in routine bone marrow smears, several of which are shown in the following micrographs.

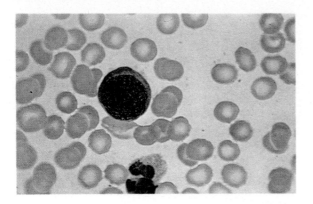

Fig. 2.19 Proerythroblast

(Giemsa × 800)

This bone marrow smear illustrates the typical appearance of a proerythroblast, the first recognisable stage in erythropoiesis. The cell at this stage has a large, intensely stained, granular nucleus containing one or more paler nucleoli. The sparse cytoplasm is strongly basophilic due to its high content of RNA and lack of haemoglobin. A narrow, pale zone of cytoplasm close to the nucleus represents the Golgi apparatus.

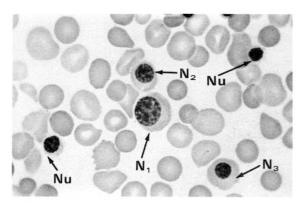

Fig. 2.20 Normoblasts

(Giemsa × 800)

This micrograph illustrates three normoblasts in various stages of development. The largest normoblast N_1 is of the intermediate form (polychromatic) since its cytoplasm exhibits both basophilia and eosinophilia. In the normoblasts N_2 and N_3 the process of haemoglobin synthesis has proceeded further, as evidenced by increased eosinophilia and more of the cytoplasmic organelles have degenerated. The nucleus becomes progressively condensed and is eventually extruded from the cell; two extruded nuclei **Nu** can be seen.

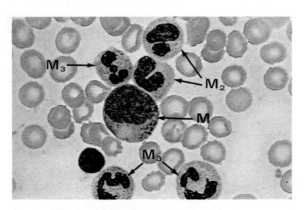

Fig. 2.21 Granulocyte precursors

(Giemsa × 800)

This micrograph illustrates three phases of neutrophil granulocyte development. A neutrophil myelocyte **M** is recognised by a large, eccentrically located nucleus, a prominent Golgi apparatus and cytoplasm containing many azurophilic (primary) granules. The next stage towards maturity, the metamyelocyte M_2 is a smaller cell characterised by indentation of the nucleus and loss of prominence of the azurophilic granules. The final stage before maturity, the stab M_3, has a more highly segmented nucleus approaching that of the mature neutrophil.

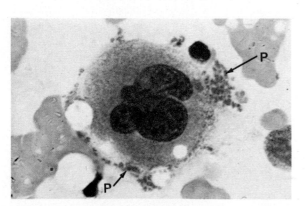

Fig. 2.22 Megakaryocyte

(Giemsa × 800)

Reflecting its name, the megakaryocyte is a huge cell with a single, highly irregular polyploid nucleus. The extensive cytoplasm appears finely granular and in parts of the periphery can be seen budding to form numerous platelets **P**.

Cell type	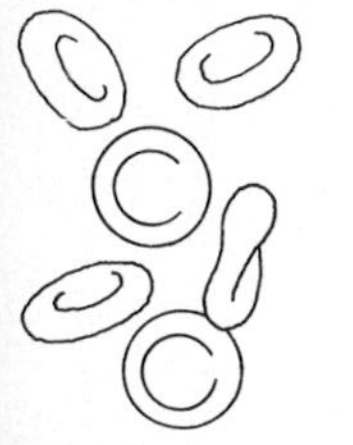 Erythro-cyte	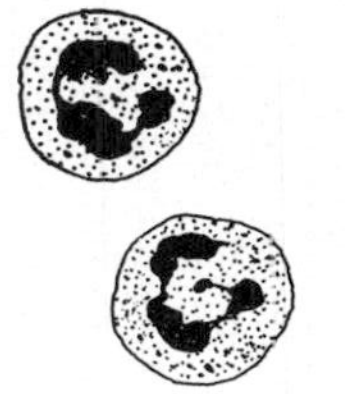 Neutro-phil	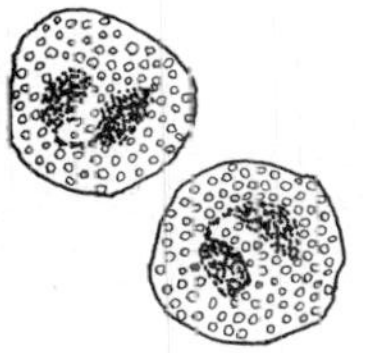 Eosino-phil	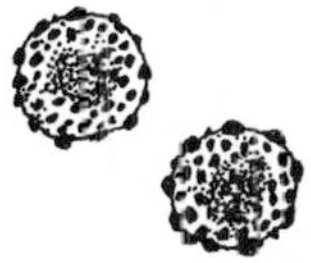 Basophil	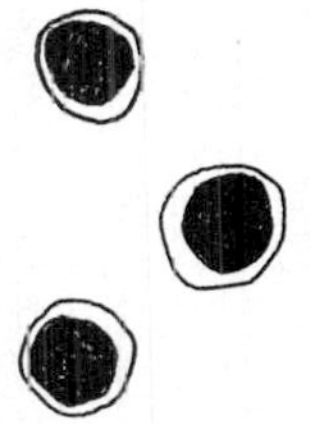 Lympho-cyte	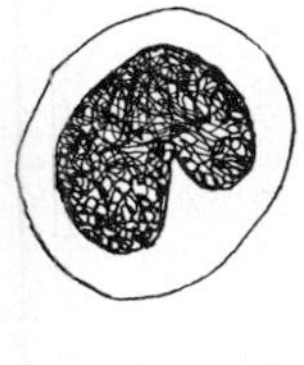 Monocyte	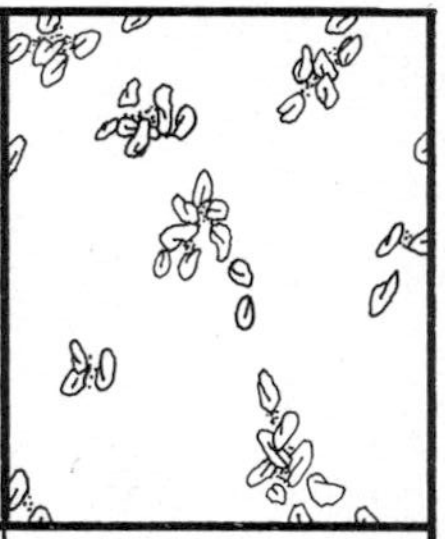 Platelets
size	6–8 μm _(7.5)_	10–12 μm _(12–14μ)_	10–12 μm _(12–17μ)_	9–10 μm _(10–14μ)_	7–8 μm → _(15–20μ)_	14–17 μm _(15–20)_	2–3 μm _(2–4)_
number per ml	4–6 million	2,800–5,250 _(4500)_	70–420	0–70	1,400–3,150 _(2500)_	140–700 _(460)_	150,000–400,000 _(200–400K)_
differential leucocyte count	—	40–75% _(55–65%)_	1–6%	<1% _(0.5–1.5)_	20–45% _(20–40%)_	2–6%	—
duration of development	5–7 days	6–9 days	6–9 days	3–7 days	1–2 days	2–3 days	4–5 days
lifespan of mature cell	120 days	6 hours to a few days	8–12 days	?	?	months to years	8–12 days

Fig. 2.23 Mature cell types in the circulating blood of human adults

3. Connective tissue

Introduction

Connective tissue is the term applied to a basic type of tissue of mesodermal origin which provides structural and metabolic support for other tissues and organs throughout the body. Connective tissues carry blood vessels and mediate the exchange of metabolites between tissues and the circulatory system. Rigid forms of connective tissue, particularly cartilage and bone, comprise the major tissues of the skeleton (see Chapter 9). Connective tissue has important metabolic roles such as the storage of fat, as in adipose tissue, whilst connective tissue elements constitute a major part of the body's defence mechanisms against pathogenic micro-organisms. The processes of tissue repair are largely a function of connective tissues. All connective tissues have two major constituents, *cells* and *extracellular material*.

The cells of connective tissue may be divided into three types according to their basic function:
(i) Cells responsible for synthesis and maintenance of the extracellular material. These cells are termed *fibroblasts*, and are derived from precursor cells in primitive connective tissue which is called *mesenchyme*.
(ii) Cells responsible for the storage and metabolism of fat. These cells are individually known as *adipocytes* and may collectively form *adipose connective tissue*.
(iii) Cells with defence and immune functions.

Extracellular material is the constituent which mainly determines the physical properties of each type of connective tissue. Extracellular material consists of a matrix of organic material called *ground substance* within which are embedded a variety of *fibres*. Ground substance is an amorphous, transparent material which has the properties of a semi-fluid gel. Tissue fluid is loosely bound to ground substance, thereby forming the medium for passage of materials throughout connective tissues and for the exchange of metabolites with the circulatory system. The molecular composition of ground substance is principally that of long, unbranched chains of large acidic polysaccharides bound to variable amounts of protein. These substances have been traditionally called *mucopolysaccharides* but this term is now being supplanted by the more precise term *glycosaminoglycan*. *Hyaluronic acid*, combined with approximately two per cent protein, is the predominant glycosaminoglycan in the ground substance of soft connective tissues. These large molecules are intimately entangled to confer the basic physical properties of connective tissue; the mechanical properties are reinforced by the presence of fibres. Ground substance, due to its physical nature, is an important barrier to the spread of micro-organisms; it is noteworthy that some pathogenic bacteria produce the enzyme *hyaluronidase* to facilitate their spread. In addition to the glycosaminoglycans, ground substance also contains soluble proteins and glycoproteins which may act as templates for the orientation and formation of the fibrous elements.

The fibrous components of connective tissue are of three main types: *collagenous, reticular* and *elastic*. These fibres are present in all connective tissues but occur in varying proportions. Classification of the basic connective tissues depends on the predominant fibre type. Collagenous connective tissue is the most common type; the density of collagen fibres varies greatly from loose to dense according to the mechanical supporting function. The regularity and arrangement of collagen fibres also varies according to function. Reticular connective tissue forms a delicate supporting framework for highly cellular organs such as liver, lymph nodes and endocrine glands. Elastic connective tissues contain, as their predominant fibre type, a highly elastic protein called *elastin*, which may be arranged into fibres or discontinuous sheets.

The growth and metabolism of all connective tissues are influenced by a variety of hormones, particularly growth hormone, corticosteroids and oestrogens.

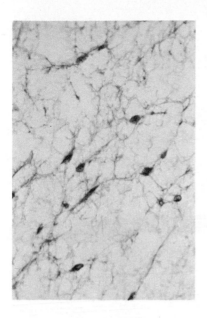

Fig. 3.1 Primitive mesenchyme
(H & E × 320)

Primitive mesenchyme is the embryological tissue from which all types of connective tissue, including that of the skeleton, are derived. Mesenchymal cells are relatively unspecialised and are believed to be capable of differentiation into all the cell types found in mature connective tissue. Some mesenchymal cells remain in fully mature connective tissue and provide a pluripotential source of cells as the need arises for replacement or repair of connective tissues.

Primitive mesenchymal cells have an irregular, stellate shape with delicate branching cytoplasmic extensions which form an interlacing network throughout the tissue. The oval nuclei have dispersed chromatin and prominent nucleoli. The extracellular material consists almost exclusively of ground substance and does not contain mature fibres. In this respect, mesenchyme forms a very loose variant of connective tissue which, in the well developed fetus, is referred to as *mucous connective tissue*. The circulatory system of the embryo is poorly developed until a late stage; mesenchyme thus constitutes an important medium for the diffusion of metabolites to and from developing tissues.

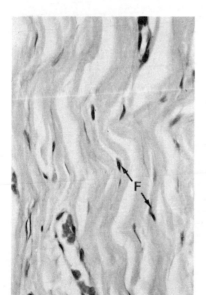

Fig. 3.2 Mature fibroblasts
(H & E × 320)

This micrograph demonstrates the typical histological appearance of mature fibroblasts in loose connective tissue; collagen fibres are stained pink in this preparation. The fibroblast nuclei **F** are condensed and elongated in the direction of the extracellular fibres. The cytoplasm is reduced and spindle-shaped, with long cytoplasmic processes extending into the matrix, to meet up with those of other fibroblasts; the cytoplasmic extensions are usually difficult to see with the light microscope. The main function of fibroblasts is to maintain the integrity of connective tissues by continuous slow turnover of the extracellular elements.

It is customary to describe a precursor or immature cell by the suffix 'blast' as in erythroblast (see Fig. 2.19) and the mature form by the suffix 'cyte' as in erythrocyte. This convention, however, is not commonly used to describe fibroblasts, where the term 'fibrocyte' might be more appropriate for the mature form.

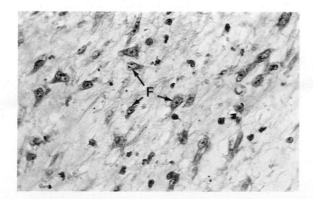

Fig. 3.3 Active fibroblasts: healing wound
(H & E × 320)

Active fibroblasts **F** are readily demonstrated in healing wounds, as in this micrograph. The nuclei are large and rounded in shape with prominent nucleoli suggesting active protein synthesis. The cytoplasm is extensive and its strongly stained, granular appearance is evidence of an extensive system of rough endoplasmic reticulum involved in protein synthesis. The relative absence of formed fibres in the extracellular matrix reveals the fine meshwork of cytoplasmic extensions between fibroblasts.

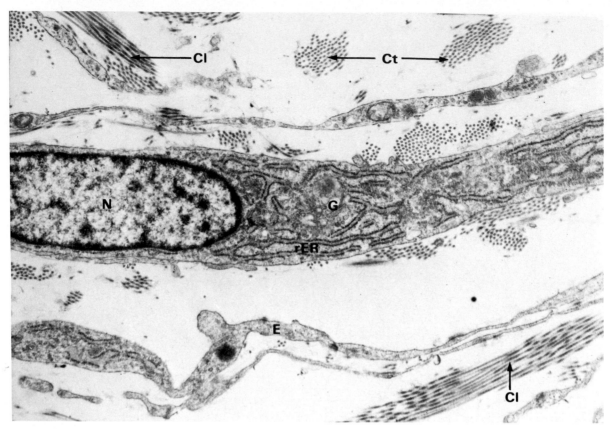

Fig. 3.4 Fibroblast

(EM × 12000)

This micrograph illustrates the body of a mature fibroblast within loose, collagenous connective tissue. Fine tapering cytoplasmic extensions **E** of adjacent fibroblasts can be seen on either side of the central fibroblast. Bundles of collagen fibres are seen in transverse **Ct** and longitudinal section **Cl** in the extracellular matrix. The nucleus **N** is moderately condensed, and nucleoli are not a prominent feature. The small quantity of cytoplasm contains a relatively sparse network of rough endoplasmic reticulum **rER**; the Golgi apparatus **G** is poorly developed and few mitochondria are present. During active synthesis of extracellular fibres, both the rough endoplasmic reticulum and Golgi apparatus become prominent features of a much more extensive cytoplasm. Fibroblasts synthesise and secrete the precursors of collagen, elastin, reticulin and the glycosaminoglycans of ground substance. In the mature, non-active fibroblast relatively few secretory vesicles are found within the cytoplasm.

Collagen is the principal fibre type found in the matrix of all connective tissues. Collagen is secreted into the extracellular matrix in the form of *tropocollagen*; each tropocollagen molecule consists of three peptide chains bound together to form a helical structure 1·5nm in diameter and 260nm long. In the extracellular matrix, tropocollagen molecules polymerise to form collagen fibres which are divided into four types, designated I, II, III and IV on the basis of morphology, amino-acid composition and physical properties. The exact physiological significance of these classes of collagen fibre is not fully understood at present.

Type I collagen is the most common form and is found in fibrous connective tissues, tendon and bone. Type II collagen is the form present in hyaline cartilage (see Chapter 9). Type III collagen is the form of collagen making up the fibres known as reticulin fibres (see Fig. 3.9). Type IV collagen is the form found in basement membranes (see Chapter 4).

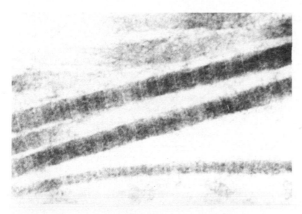

Fig. 3.5 Collagen

(EM ×124000)

The typical appearance of Type I collagen, the commonest variety, is seen in this electron micrograph. Type I collagen fibres have a prominent banded appearance with a regular periodicity of approximately 64nm. This periodicity results from the mode of polymerisation of tropocollagen molecules; it has been suggested that each molecule (260nm long) overlaps the adjacent molecule by approximately a quarter of its length.

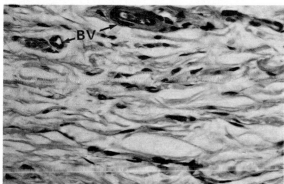

Fig. 3.6 Loose (areolar) connective tissue

(H & E ×320)

Loose collagenous connective tissue supports the epithelial linings of the gastro-intestinal, respiratory and urinary tracts, forms the deeper layers of the skin and occurs as a loose interstitial packing in many other organs. The collagen fibres are loosely arranged and have a wavy appearance in unstretched preparations. The open (*areolar*) spaces between collagen fibres are filled with ground substance which is not stained in this type of preparation since it is dissolved away during tissue processing.

The relatively inactive fibroblasts are recognised by their densely stained and elongated nuclei. Several small blood vessels **BV** are seen.

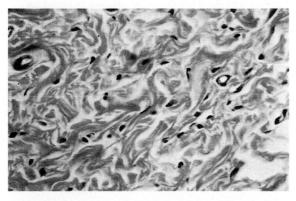

Fig. 3.7 Dense irregular connective tissue

(H & E ×320)

This micrograph illustrates collagen fibres in dense, irregular connective tissue, a type which is commonly encountered in the supporting tissues of the skin and many other sites. The fibres appear to be condensed into irregular masses. Note the absence of cellular detail in the fibroblasts and the presence of few blood vessels.

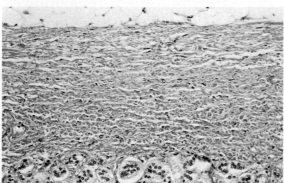

Fig. 3.8 Dense regular connective tissue

(H & E ×128)

This micrograph of the capsule of the adrenal gland shows the typical dense arrangement of collagen fibres where mechanical support is the primary function. The collagen fibres are elongated and arranged in a regular manner to provide a well organised and robust enveloping capsule. Fibroblast nuclei are elongated in the direction of the collagen fibres.

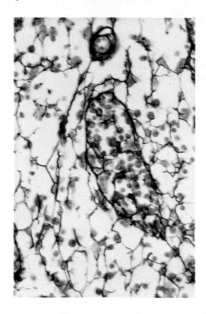

Fig. 3.9 Reticular connective tissue
(Silver method/haematoxylin × 800)

Reticular connective tissue forms a delicate supporting framework for many highly cellular organs such as endocrine glands, lymph nodes and the liver. Reticular tissue is made up of a fine network of branching reticulin fibres. Reticulin is a non-banded form of collagen designated collagen Type III (see Fig. 3.4). Reticulin fibres are usually poorly stained in common preparations but are able to adsorb metallic silver and are thus stained black with silver nitrate solutions under appropriate conditions. This phenomenon led early histologists to believe that reticulin had a completely different chemical composition from that of collagen. Reticulin is the earliest type of collagen fibre to be produced during the development of all connective tissues and is also present in varying quantities in most mature connective tissues.

This micrograph shows the fine reticular architecture of part of a lymph node; this framework provides a loose support for lymphoid cells, the nuclei of which have been counterstained blue.

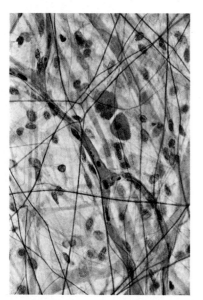

Fig. 3.10 Elastin fibres
(Areolar spread: elastin/H & E × 320)

Elastin is a protein found in varying proportions in most connective tissues where it confers elastic properties which enable recovery of tissue shape following normal physiological deformation or stretching. Elastin is thus present in large amounts in tissues such as lung, skin and bladder. In most tissues, elastin occurs as short branching fibres which form an irregular network throughout the tissue. This three-dimensional network is not easily seen in sections but is better demonstrated in spread preparations. In the spread of areolar connective tissue shown in this micrograph the elastin fibres are stained black. Collagen fibres are stained pink and nuclei are stained blue.

Elastin is synthesised and secreted by fibroblasts as the precursor form *tropoelastin* which polymerises in the extracellular matrix to form fibres. Elastin exists in an unusual form within blood vessels, particularly large arteries (see Chapter 6), where it forms discontinuous sheets rather than fibres.

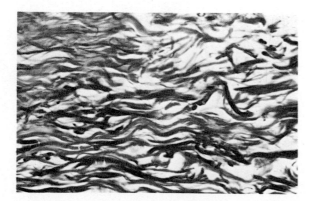

Fig. 3.11 Elastin fibres
(Elastic-van Gieson × 320)

This micrograph illustrates the appearance of elastin fibres in histological sections, when stained specifically; with this staining method elastin fibres appear black. Elastin fibres are a prominent feature of the connective tissue of skin, particularly that of the face and neck.

Adipose tissue

Most connective tissues contain cells which are adapted for the storage of fat; these cells, called *adipocytes*, are derived from primitive mesenchyme. Adipocytes are found in isolation or in clumps throughout loose connective tissue, or may constitute the main cell type as in adipose tissue.

Stored fat within adipocytes is derived from three main sources: dietary fat circulating in the blood stream as chylomicrons, triglycerides synthesised in the liver and transported in blood and triglycerides synthesised from glucose within adipocytes. Adipose tissue is often regarded as an inactive energy store, however, it is an extremely important participant in general metabolic processes in that it acts as a temporary store of substrate for the energy-deriving processes of almost all tissues. Adipose tissue, therefore, generally has a rich blood supply. The rate of fat deposition and utilisation within adipose tissue is largely determined by dietary intake and energy expenditure, but a number of hormones and the sympathetic nervous system profoundly influence the fat metabolism of adipocytes.

There are two main types of adipose tissue, *white* and *brown adipose tissue*:

(i) White adipose tissue: this type of adipose tissue comprises up to 20 per cent of total body weight in normal, well-nourished male adults and up to 25 per cent in females. It is distributed throughout the body particularly in the deep layers of the skin (see Chapter 8). In addition to being an important energy store, white adipose tissue acts as a thermal insulator under the skin and functions as a cushion against mechanical shock in such sites as around the kidneys.

(ii) Brown adipose tissue: this highly specialised type of adipose tissue is found in newborn mammals and some hibernating animals, where it plays an important part in body temperature regulation. Only small amounts of brown adipose tissue are found in human adults, where its function is thought to contribute little to thermoregulation. Brown adipose tissue is an important site of heat production in newborn humans, in whom heat loss is great, largely because of a high body surface area to volume ratio.

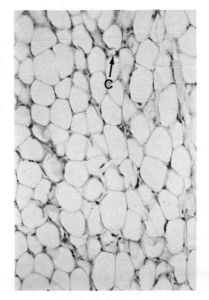

Fig. 3.12 White adipose tissue
(H & E × 128)

The typical appearance of white adipose tissue is illustrated in this micrograph. Fat stored in adipocytes accumulates as lipid droplets which fuse to form a single large droplet which distends and occupies most of the cytoplasm. The adipocyte nucleus is compressed and displaced to one side by the stored lipid droplet and the cytoplasm is reduced to a small rim around the periphery. In commonly used, routine histological sections, the lipid content of adipocytes is extracted during tissue processing leaving a large, unstained space within each cell.

Ultrastructural studies have shown that the cytoplasm of white adipocytes contains the usual organelles; the single lipid droplet is not bounded by a membrane and new lipid droplets entering the cell readily fuse with the major droplet which is highly accessible to the enzymes responsible for triglyceride breakdown when the need arises.

Note the minute dimensions of a capillary **C** compared with the size of the surrounding adipocytes.

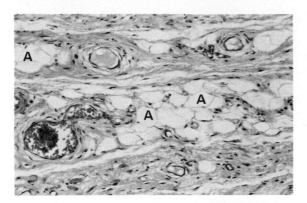

Fig. 3.13 Fibrofatty connective tissue
(H & E × 128)

This micrograph demonstrates the typical appearance of
adipocytes **A** distributed amongst loose, collagenous
connective tissue. Adipocytes occur either singly or in
groups in loose connective tissues, particularly those
supporting the gastro-intestinal tract lining. Like the
adipocytes of white adipose tissue, the size of adipocytes in
loose connective tissue depends on the equilibrium between
dietary fat intake and energy expenditure.

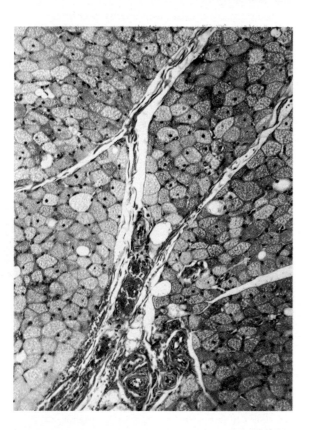

Fig. 3.14 Brown adipose tissue
(H & E × 120)

Brown adipose tissue may be differentiated from white
adipose tissue on the basis of the following features. Firstly,
lipid is stored in the form of multiple, small vesicles rather
than a single, large droplet; this gives the cytoplasm of
brown adipocytes a vacuolated appearance. Secondly,
brown adipocytes have a relatively large amount of
cytoplasm which is stained strongly due to a high content of
mitochondria. Thirdly, brown adipose tissue is extremely
vascular. These characteristics have led some histologists to
compare the appearance of brown adipose tissue to that of
steroid-secreting endocrine glands (see Chapter 14). The
discrete brown adipose tissue of hibernating mammals has
been inappropriately named the hibernating gland.

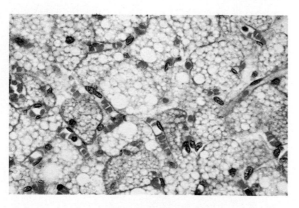

Fig. 3.15 Brown adipocytes
(H & E × 320)

At higher magnification, the nuclei of brown adipocytes are
seen to be eccentrically located within the cell, but unlike
the nuclei of white adipocytes, the nuclei are plump and
surrounded by a significant quantity of strongly
eosinophilic cytoplasm. The stored lipid is contained within
multiple droplets, all of which have been dissolved away
during tissue processing.

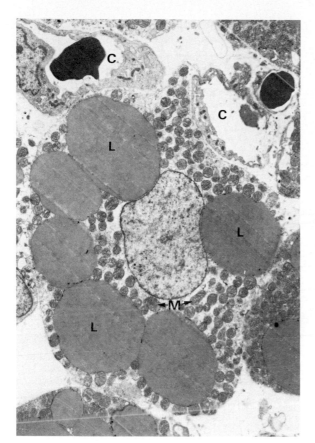

Fig. 3.16 Brown adipocyte
(Rabbit: EM ×4070)

The multilocular nature of stored lipid **L** within brown adipocytes is seen in this electron micrograph of brown adipose tissue taken from a newborn rabbit. The cytoplasm of brown adipocytes is crammed with mitochondria **M** which have numerous, closely packed cristae. These mitochondria are extremely rich in cytochromes, molecules involved in oxidative energy production; this accounts for the brown colour of brown adipose tissue when examined macroscopically. Unlike the metabolism of other tissues, in brown adipose cells the process of electron transport is readily uncoupled from the phosphorylation of ADP to form ATP. The energy derived from oxidation of lipids, and energy released by electron transport in the uncoupled state, is dissipated as heat; this is rapidly conducted to the rest of the body by the rich vascular network of brown adipose tissue. Note the intimate association of capillaries **C** with the brown adipocyte in this micrograph. Using these metabolic processes, neonatal humans and other mammals utilise brown adipose tissue to generate body heat during the vulnerable period after birth. Brown adipose tissue undergoes involution in early infancy and in adult humans is found only in odd sites such as around the adrenal gland and great vessels. The production of heat by brown adipose tissue is controlled directly by the sympathetic nervous system.

The defence cells of connective tissue

The basic connective tissues not only contain cells responsible for synthesis, maintenance and metabolic activity, but also contain a variety of cells with defence and immune functions. Traditionally, these cells have been divided into two categories: fixed (intrinsic) cells and wandering (extrinsic) cells. The fixed category included *tissue macrophages (histiocytes)* and *mast cells*. Tissue macrophages are now generally believed to be derived from circulating monocytes (see Chapter 2) which have become at least temporarily resident in connective tissues. Mast cells are functionally analogous to basophils (see Chapter 2) but there are structural differences which suggest that mast cells are not merely basophils resident in connective tissues. The wandering category of defence and immune cells includes all the remaining members of the white blood cell series (see Chapter 2). Although leucocytes are usually considered as a constituent of blood, their principal site of activity is outside the blood circulation, particularly within loose connective tissues. Leucocytes are normally found only in relatively small numbers within connective tissues but in response to inflammation and other disease processes their numbers increase greatly. The connective tissues of those regions of the body which are subject to the constant threat of pathogenic invasion, such as the gastro-intestinal and respiratory tracts, contain a large population of leucocytes, even in the absence of overt disease.

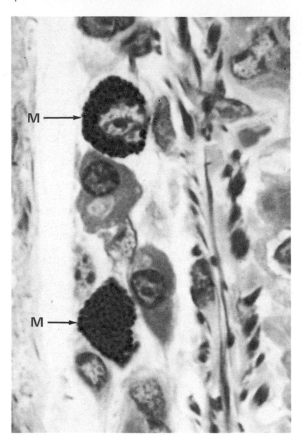

Fig. 3.17 Mast cells

(Resin embedded, one micron section: toluidine blue × 1200)

Mast cells are found in connective tissues, particularly in association with blood vessels. The function of these cells is poorly understood. They are not, however, considered to be responsible for synthesis and maintenance of connective tissue elements but possess features which suggest their involvement in defence and immune mechanisms.

Mast cells are not readily identified in routine histological preparations; with suitable staining, the characteristic feature of mast cells is an extensive cytoplasm packed with large granules. When stained with certain blue basic dyes, such as toluidine blue, the granules bind to the dye changing its colour to red. This property is known as *metachromasia*. Metachromasia is thought to be due to the presence of a highly acidic glycoprotein called *heparin*, which is a potent blood anticoagulant. Mast cell granules also contain histamine, one of the chemical mediators of inflammation, which causes dilatation of small vessels and increases capillary permeability. It is proposed, therefore, that mast cells are primarily involved in inflammatory and immune mechanisms.

Mast cell granules are similar in composition to basophil granules (see Fig. 2.12), but there is no evidence that mast cells are merely basophils resident in connective tissues, although both cell types appear to have similar actions and may degranulate in response to similar stimuli.

This micrograph of the connective tissue underlying the tracheal surface demonstrates two mast cells **M**. A pale nucleus can be seen in one cell but the plane of section is outside the nucleus of the other. Note the large, densely packed granules which exhibit metachromasia.

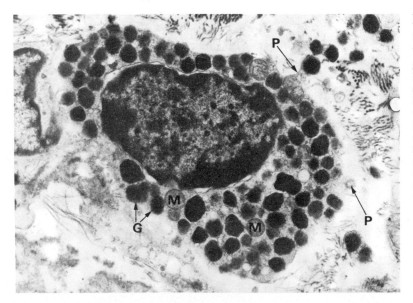

Fig. 3.18 Mast cell

(EM × 5250)

With electron microscopy, mast cell granules **G** are seen to be membrane-bound and to contain a dense amorphous material. The granules are liberated from the cell by exocytosis when stimulated during an inflammatory or allergic response. The cytoplasm contains several rounded mitochondria **M**, but little rough endoplasmic reticulum. Variable numbers of cytoplasmic processes **P** extend into the surrounding connective tissue matrix.

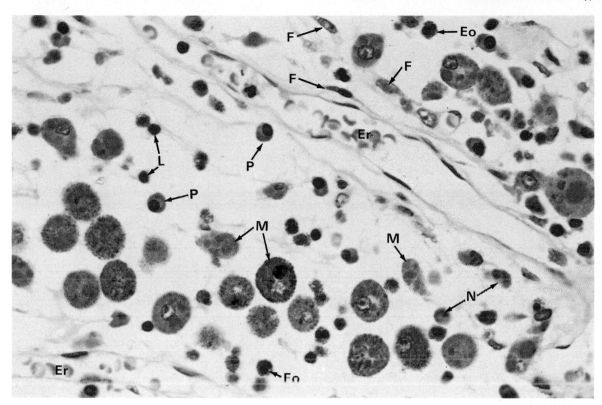

Fig. 3.19 Leucocytes in loose connective tissue

(H & E ×640)

The appearance of leucocytes within sections of connective and other tissues differs greatly from the appearance seen in blood smears (see Chapter 2). In this micrograph, a variety of leucocytes are seen in the loose connective tissue supporting the lining of the large intestine, a site which is normally rich in such cells even in the absence of inflammation.

Fibroblasts **F,** are identified by their relatively large, elongated nuclei. Erythrocytes **Er** within small blood vessels are intensely eosinophilic (red stained); the presence of erythrocytes (approximate diameter 7 μm) provides a reference for the size of other cells. Of the granulocyte series (see Chapter 2), neutrophils are only rarely seen in tissues except in acute or chronic inflammation. Neutrophils **N** are recognised by their multilobed nuclei and poorly stained cytoplasm. Eosinophils **Eo** are present in large numbers in normal connective tissues and are recognised by their bilobed nuclei and strongly eosinophilic cytoplasmic granules. Basophils, and their analogues mast cells, are poorly stained in H & E preparations and are therefore difficult to recognise.

Lymphocytes **L** are easily recognised as cells with small, densely stained nuclei and a thin halo of poorly stained cytoplasm. Plasma cells **P,** immunologically activated lymphocytes responsible for antibody synthesis (see Chapter 10), are recognised by their large granular nuclei and extensive basophilic (blue-stained) cytoplasm containing a pale stained peri-nuclear area which represents a well developed and active Golgi apparatus. The basophilia of plasma cells is largely attributable to profuse rough endoplasmic reticulum, involved in the synthesis of antibody molecules. Large mononuclear phagocytes, analogous to the monocytes of blood, are distributed throughout all connective tissues where they may exhibit intense phagocytic activity; these cells are also known as macrophages, tissue-fixed macrophages, and histiocytes when present in connective tissue. The macrophages of connective tissue drape themselves on the fibres of the matrix when inactive; actively phagocytic macrophages, however, may move in an amoeboid manner through the ground substance. Macrophages and monocytes have a common origin in primitive mesenchymal cells of bone marrow. Recent evidence suggests that monocytes and all macrophages should be considered as members of a single functional unit, *the macrophage-monocyte system.* Inactive macrophages are often difficult to visualise in histological sections, but when actively phagocytic, macrophages may be easily recognised by their large size and content of engulfed material; note, however, that active macrophages have an extremely variable appearance, depending on the nature of their phagocytic activity. Most of the cytoplasmic detail of the macrophages **M** shown in this preparation is obscured by engulfed material which appears brown. For comparison, a different example of the appearance of active macrophages is seen in Fig. 10.11.

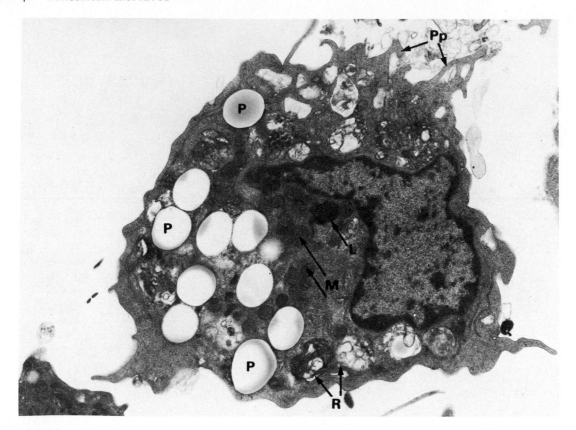

Fig. 3.20 Macrophage

(EM ×11600)

The ultrastructural features of macrophages vary widely according to their state of activity and tissue location. This micrograph shows an active macrophage obtained from the peritoneum of a rat which had previously been injected intra-peritoneally with latex particles; a number of particles **P** have been engulfed by the macrophage.

The macrophage nucleus is irregular with heterochromatin typically clumped around the nuclear envelope. The cytoplasm contains a few mitochondria **M** and a variable amount of free ribosomes and rough endoplasmic reticulum. In quiescent macrophages, lysosomes **L** are abundant but their number is much reduced in actively phagocytic cells; lysosomes are later regenerated by the Golgi apparatus. The macrophage cytoplasm contains an assortment of phagosomes and residual bodies **R**. Residual material may be released from the macrophage by exocytosis; such material may remain sequestered in the tissues, as occurs with the dyes used in tattooing of the skin, or the material may be returned to the circulation for excretion or re-use in biosynthetic processes.

Actively phagocytic cells exhibit irregular cytoplasmic projections or pseudopodia **Pp** which are involved in amoeboid movement and phagocytosis.

In addition to their role as tissue scavengers, macrophages play an important role in immune mechanisms (see Chapter 10) since they are often the first cells to make contact with antigens. Macrophages process antigenic material in some way before presenting it to lymphocytes; lymphocytes are then stimulated to undergo specific immune responses. As a result of various immune mechanisms, antigenic material may become combined or coated with substances such as antibodies and complement which are then collectively known as *opsonins*. Opsonins greatly enhance the phagocytic ability of macrophages and other phagocytes such as neutrophils (see Chapter 2), a process which is known as *opsonisation*. Other substances such as lymphokines, which are released during the immune response, act directly upon macrophages to increase greatly their metabolic and phagocytic activity.

4. Epithelial tissues

Introduction

The epithelia are a diverse group of tissues which, with rare exceptions, line all body surfaces, cavities and tubes. Epithelia thus function as interfaces between biological compartments. Epithelial interfaces are involved in a wide range of activities such as absorption, secretion and protection and all these major functions may be exhibited at a single epithelial surface. For example, the epithelial lining of the small intestine is primarily involved in absorption of the products of digestion, but the epithelium also protects itself from noxious intestinal contents by the secretion of a surface coating of mucus.

Surface epithelia consist of one or more layers of cells separated by a minute quantity of intercellular material which may represent the fused glycocalyces of adjacent cells (see Chapter 1); epithelial cells are closely bound to one another by a variety of specialisations of the cell membrane. All epithelia are supported by a *basement membrane* of variable thickness. Basement membranes separate epithelia from underlying connective tissues and are never penetrated by blood vessels; epithelia are thus dependent on the diffusion of oxygen and metabolites from underlying tissues. Basement membranes consist of a condensation of glycoprotein ground substance reinforced by reticular fibres which merge with those of the underlying connective tissue; both epithelial and connective tissue cells are thought to participate in the formation of basement membranes.

Epithelia are classified according to three morphological characteristics:

(i) The number of cell layers: a single layer of epithelial cells is termed *simple epithelium*, whereas epithelia composed of more than one layer are termed *stratified epithelia*.

(ii) The shape of the component cells when seen in sections taken at right angles to the epithelial surface: in stratified epithelia the shape of the outermost layer of cells determines the descriptive classification. Cellular outlines are often difficult to distinguish, but the shape of epithelial cells is usually reflected in the shape of their nuclei.

(iii) The presence of surface specialisations such as cilia and keratin: an example is the epithelial surface of skin which is classified as 'stratified squamous keratinising epithelium' since it consists of many layers of cells, the surface cells of which are flattened (squamous) in shape and covered by an outer layer of the proteinaceous material, keratin (see Fig. 4.14).

Epithelia may be derived from ectoderm, mesoderm or endoderm although in the past it was thought that true epithelia were only of ectodermal or endodermal origin; two types of epithelia derived from mesoderm, the lining of blood and lymphatic vessels and the linings of the serous body cavities, were not considered to be epithelia and were termed *endothelium* and *mesothelium* respectively. By both morphological and functional criteria, such distinction has little practical value, nevertheless, the terms endothelium and mesothelium are still used to describe these types of epithelium.

Epithelium which is primarily involved in secretion is often arranged into structures called *glands*. Glands are merely invaginations of epithelial surfaces which are formed during embryonic development by proliferation of epithelium into the underlying connective tissues. Those glands which maintain their continuity with the epithelial surface via a duct are called *exocrine glands* and secrete on to the free surface. In some cases, the duct degenerates during development to leave isolated islands of epithelial secretory tissue deep within other tissues. These glands, known as *endocrine* or *ductless glands*, secrete directly into the bloodstream and their secretions are known as hormones (see Chapter 14); in addition, some endocrine glands develop by migration of epithelial cells into connective tissues, without the formation of a duct.

Simple epithelia

Simple epithelia are defined as surface epithelia consisting of a single layer of cells. Simple epithelia are almost always found on absorptive or secretory surfaces; they provide little protection against mechanical abrasion and thus are almost never found on surfaces subject to such stresses. The cells comprising simple epithelia range in shape from extremely flattened to tall columnar, depending on their function. For example, flattened simple epithelia present little barrier to passive diffusion and are therefore found in sites such as the lung alveoli and the lining of blood vessels. In contrast, highly active epithelial cells, such as the cells lining the small intestine, are generally tall since they must accommodate the appropriate organelles. Simple epithelia may exhibit a variety of surface specialisations, such as microvilli and cilia, which facilitate their specific surface functions.

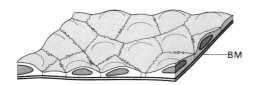

Fig. 4.1 Simple squamous epithelium

Simple squamous epithelium is composed of flattened, irregularly-shaped cells forming a continuous surface which is often referred to as *pavemented epithelium*. Like all epithelia, this delicate lining is supported by an underlying basement membrane **BM**.

Simple squamous epithelium is often found lining surfaces involved in passive transport of either gases, such as in the lungs, or fluids, such as the walls of blood capillaries. Simple squamous epithelium also forms a delicate lining to the pleural, pericardial and peritoneal cavities where it permits passage of tissue fluid into and out of these cavities; the simple squamous epithelium of these sites is traditionally known as mesothelium.

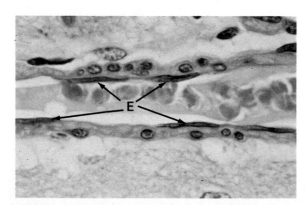

Fig. 4.2 Simple squamous epithelium
(H & E ×800)

This micrograph of a small blood vessel illustrates the typical appearance of simple squamous epithelium in section; the epithelial lining cells **E** (known as endothelium in the circulatory system) are so flattened that they can only be recognised by their nuclei which bulge into the vessel lumen. The supporting basement membrane is thin and, in haematoxylin and eosin stained preparations, has similar staining properties to the endothelial cell cytoplasm; hence the basement membrane cannot be seen in this micrograph.

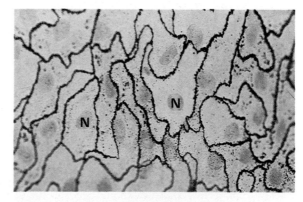

Fig. 4.3 Simple squamous epithelium
(Spread preparation: silver method ×320)

In this preparation, the mesothelial lining of the peritoneal cavity has been stripped from the underlying connective tissues and spread onto a slide thus permitting a surface view of simple squamous epithelium. The intercellular substance has been stained with silver thereby outlining the closely interdigitating cell boundaries; the nuclei **N** have been stained with the dye, neutral red.

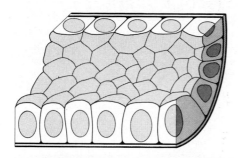

Fig. 4.4 Simple cuboidal epithelium

Simple cuboidal epithelium represents an intermediate form
between simple squamous and simple columnar epithelia;
the distinction between tall cuboidal and low columnar is
often arbitrary and is of descriptive value only. In section
perpendicular to the basement membrane, the epithelial
cells appear square, leading to its traditional description as
cuboidal epithelium; on surface view, however, the cells are
actually polygonal in shape.

Simple cuboidal epithelium usually lines small ducts and
tubules which may have excretory, secretory or absorptive
functions; examples are the small collecting ducts of the
kidney, salivary glands and pancreas.

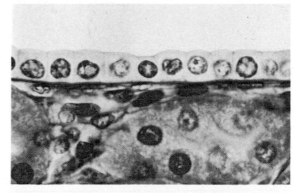

Fig. 4.5 Simple cuboidal epithelium
(Azan × 800)

This micrograph of the cells lining a small collecting tubule
in the kidney shows simple cuboidal epithelium in section.
Although the boundaries between individual cells are
indistinct, the nuclear shape provides an approximate
indication of the cell size and shape. The underlying
basement membrane appears as a prominent blue line with
this staining method.

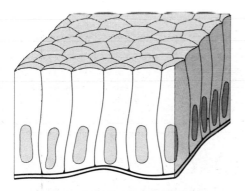

Fig. 4.6 Simple columnar epithelium

Simple columnar epithelium is similar to simple cuboidal
epithelium except that the cells are taller and appear
columnar in sections at right angles to the basement
membrane. The height of the cells may vary from low to tall
columnar depending on the site and/or degree of functional
activity. The nuclei are elongated and may be located
towards the base, the centre or occasionally the apex of the
cytoplasm. When the nucleus is eccentrically placed, the
cell is said to exhibit *polarity* which represents some
internal compartmentation of the cytoplasm related to the
specific function of the cell. Simple columnar epithelium is
most often found on highly absorptive surfaces such as in
the small intestine, although it may constitute the lining of
highly secretory surfaces such as that of the stomach.

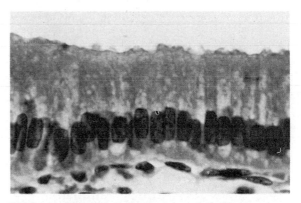

Fig. 4.7 Simple columnar epithelium
(H & E × 800)

This example of simple columnar epithelium is unusually
tall and is taken from the lining of the gall bladder where it
has the function of absorbing water, thus concentrating bile.
The luminal plasma membranes of highly absorptive
epithelial cells are often arranged into numerous, minute,
finger-like projections called *microvilli* which greatly
increase the surface area of the absorptive interface.
Microvilli are usually too small to be resolved individually
by light microscopy although they may collectively give the
appearance of a *striated* or *brush border* at the luminal
surface.

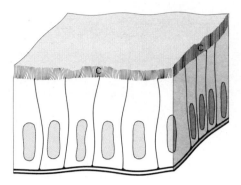

Fig. 4.8 Simple columnar ciliated epithelium

This type of simple columnar epithelium is traditionally described as a separate entity because of the presence of cilia **C**, surface specialisations which are readily visible with the light microscope. Cilia, which are much larger than microvilli, are motile projections from the luminal surface. The action of cilia generates a current which propels fluid or minute particles over the epithelial surface. *Simple columnar ciliated epithelium* is not common in humans except in the female reproductive tract.

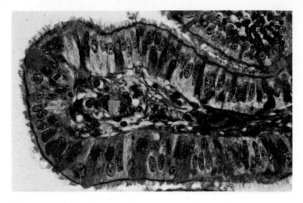

Fig. 4.9 Simple columnar ciliated epithelium

(Azan × 320)

This micrograph shows part of the highly folded epithelial lining of the oviduct. The predominant cell type in this epithelium is tall columnar and ciliated; the less numerous, blue-stained cells are not ciliated and have a secretory function. The cilia of the oviduct are believed to generate a current of fluid which helps to transport the ovum from the ovary to the uterus. As in this preparation, cilia are often stuck together in clumps by surface secretions or they may become flattened during tissue processing and therefore difficult to distinguish.

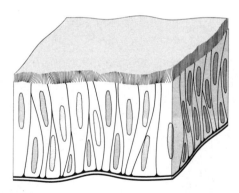

Fig. 4.10 Pseudostratified columnar ciliated epithelium

Another variant of simple columnar epithelium is described in which the cells are also usually ciliated. The term *pseudostratified* is derived from the appearance of this epithelium in section which conveys the erroneous impression that there is more than one layer of cells. This, however, is a true simple epithelium since all the cells rest on the basement membrane, although not all the cells extend to the luminal surface. The nuclei of these cells are disposed at different levels, thus creating the illusion of cellular stratification. Pseudostratified epithelium is almost exclusively confined to the larger airways of the respiratory system in mammals and is therefore often referred to as *respiratory epithelium*. The functional significance of pseudostratification has never been satisfactorily explained.

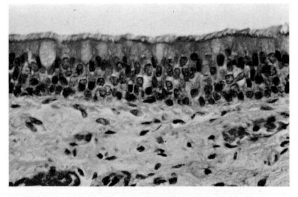

Fig. 4.11 Pseudostratified columnar ciliated epithelium

(H & E × 320)

The pseudostratified columnar ciliated epithelium shown in this micrograph is from the trachea. Pseudostratified columnar ciliated epithelium may be distinguished from true stratified epithelia by two characteristics. Firstly, the individual cells of the pseudostratified epithelium exhibit polarity, that is the apical cytoplasm does not contain nuclei. Secondly, cilia are never present on stratified epithelia. The cilia of respiratory epithelium continuously propel a surface coat of mucus containing entrapped particles towards the pharynx.

Stratified epithelia

Stratified epithelia are defined as epithelia consisting of two or more layers of cells. In contrast to simple epithelia, stratified epithelia primarily have a protective function and the degree and nature of the stratification is related to the kinds of physical stresses to which the surface is exposed. In general, stratified epithelia are poorly suited for the functions of absorption and secretion by virtue of their thickness, although some stratified surfaces are moderately permeable to water and other small molecules. The classification of the various stratified epithelia usually relates to the structure of the surface layer since cells of the basal layer are, in general, cuboidal in shape.

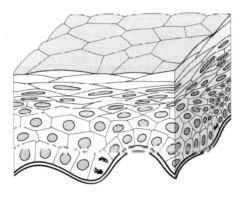

Fig. 4.12 Stratified squamous epithelium

Stratified squamous epithelium consists of a variable number of cell layers which undergo morphological and functional transition from the cuboidal basal layer to the extremely flattened surface layers. The basal cells undergo regular mitotic division giving rise to a succession of cells which are progressively pushed towards the free surface. During migration to the surface the cells undergo first maturation, then degeneration, as they become increasingly distant from the source of nutrition provided by the underlying connective tissue. Towards the surface, the cells show overt signs of degeneration particularly in the nuclei which become progressively condensed (*pyknotic*) and flattened, before ultimately disintegrating. The degenerate surface cells are continuously sloughed off and replaced from the deeper layers. The rate of mitosis in the basal layer normally approximates to the rate of surface loss.

Stratified squamous epithelium is well adapted to withstand moderate abrasion since loss of surface cells does not compromise the underlying connective tissue; stratified squamous epithelium is, however, poorly adapted to withstand desiccation. This type of epithelium constitutes the lining of the oral cavity, pharynx, oesophagus, anal canal and vagina; such sites are normally subject to moderate mechanical abrasion and are kept moist by local glandular secretions.

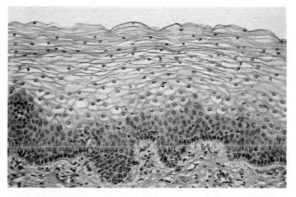

Fig. 4.13 Stratified squamous epithelium
(*H & E × 128*)

The vaginal epithelium demonstrated in this micrograph is a typical example of stratified squamous epithelium. Note the highly cellular basal layer and the transformation through the large polygonal cells of the intermediate layers to the degenerate superficial squamous cells. The junction between epithelium and underlying connective tissue is usually irregular, a feature which may enhance the adhesion of the epithelium to the underlying tissues. Note that, as in all epithelia, blood vessels do not extend beyond the basement membrane.

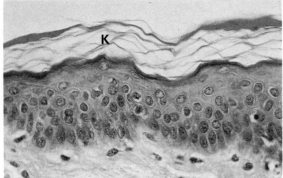

Fig. 4.14 Stratified squamous keratinising epithelium
(H & E × 320)

This specialised form of stratified squamous epithelium constitutes the epithelial surface of the skin and is adapted to withstand the constant abrasion and desiccation to which the body surface is exposed. During maturation, the epithelial cells undergo a process called *keratinisation* resulting in the formation of a tough, non-cellular surface layer consisting of the protein, *keratin* **K**, and the remnants of degenerate epithelial cells. Keratinisation may be induced in normally non-keratinising stratified squamous epithelium such as that of the oral cavity when exposed to excessive abrasion or desiccation.

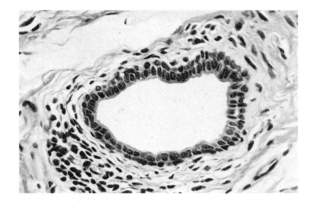

Fig. 4.15 Stratified cuboidal epithelium
(H & E × 320)

Stratified cuboidal epithelium is a thin, stratified epithelium which usually consists of only two or three layers of cuboidal or low columnar cells. This type of epithelium is usually confined to the lining of the larger excretory ducts of exocrine glands such as the salivary glands (as shown in this micrograph), the pancreas and sweat glands. Stratified cuboidal epithelium is probably not involved in significant absorptive or secretory activity but merely provides a more robust lining than would be afforded by a simple epithelium.

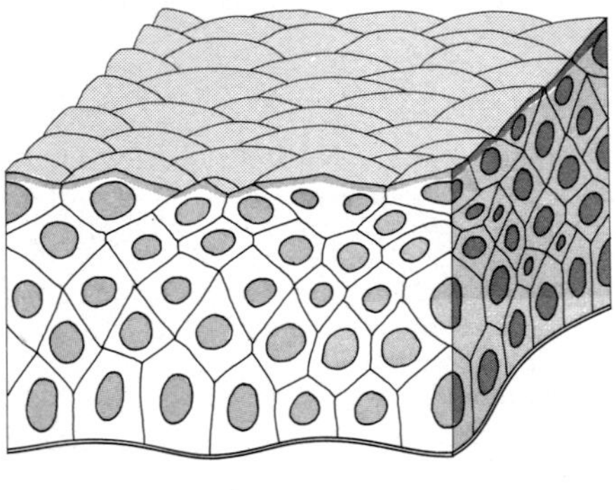

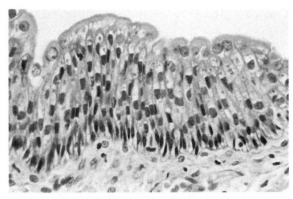

Fig. 4.16 Transitional epithelium

Transitional epithelium is a form of stratified epithelium almost exclusively confined to the urinary tract in mammals where it is highly specialised to accommodate a great degree of stretch and to withstand the toxicity of urine. This epithelial type is so named because it has some features which are intermediate between stratified cuboidal and stratified squamous epithelium. In the relaxed state, transitional epithelium appears to be about four to five cell layers thick; the basal cells are roughly cuboidal, the intermediate cells are polygonal and the surface cells are large and rounded and may contain two nuclei. In the stretched state, transitional epithelium often appears only two or three cells thick and the intermediate and surface layers are extremely flattened.

Fig. 4.17 Transitional epithelium
(H & E × 320)

This micrograph shows the appearance of transitional epithelium from the lining of a relaxed bladder. The shape and apparent size of the basal and intermediate cells vary considerably depending on the degree of distension, but the cells of the surface layer usually retain several characteristic features. Firstly, the surface cells are large and pale-stained and present a scalloped surface outline. Secondly, the luminal surface of the cells appears thickened and more densely stained. Thirdly, the nuclei of the surface cells are large and round, and often exhibit prominent nucleoli; some surface cells are binucleate.

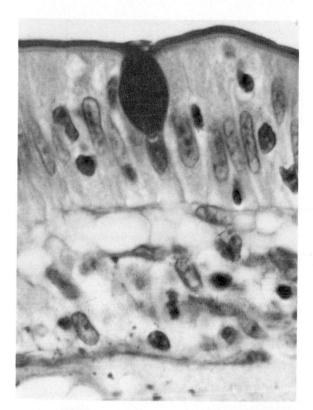

Fig. 4.18 Goblet cell

(PAS/haematoxylin × 800)

Goblet cells are modified columnar epithelial cells which synthesise and secrete mucus. In man, goblet cells are scattered amongst the cells of many simple epithelial linings, particularly those of the respiratory and gastro-intestinal tracts. Goblet cells are so named because of their resemblance to drinking goblets. The distended apical cytoplasm contains a dense aggregation of *mucigen* granules which, when released by exocytosis, combine with water to form the viscid secretion called mucus. Mucigen is composed of a mixture of neutral and acidic mucopolysaccharides (proteoglycans) and therefore can be readily demonstrated by the PAS method which stains carbohydrates magenta. The 'stem' of the goblet cell is occupied by a condensed, basal nucleus and is crammed with other organelles involved in mucigen synthesis. Note in this example from the lining of the small intestine, the tall columnar nature of the surrounding absorptive cells.

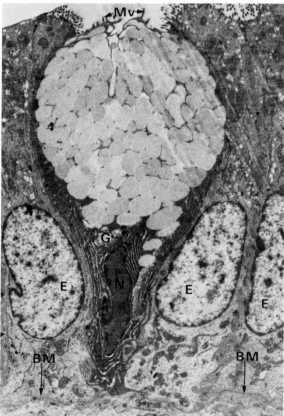

Fig. 4.19 Goblet cell

(EM × 3200)

This micrograph shows a goblet cell amongst columnar absorptive cells **E** of the small intestine. Although not always evident with light microscopy, goblet cells rest on the basement membrane **BM**. The base of the goblet cell contains an elongated nucleus **N** which has moderately condensed euchromatin. The surrounding cytoplasm is packed with rough endoplasmic reticulum and a few mitochondria are present; a prominent Golgi apparatus **G** is found in the supranuclear region. The protein component of mucigen is synthesised by the rough endoplasmic reticulum and passed to the Golgi apparatus where it is combined with carbohydrate and packaged into membrane-bound, secretory vacuoles called mucigen granules. Goblet cells secrete at a steady basal rate but they may be stimulated by local irritation to release their entire mucigen contents. Sparse microvilli **Mv** are seen at the surface of the goblet cell and may be associated with the secretory process.

Membrane specialisations of epithelia

The basal, luminal and intercellular surfaces of epithelial cells have a variety of specialisations.

(i) Basal surfaces: the interface between all epithelia and underlying connective tissues is marked by a non-cellular structure known as the *basement membrane* or *basal lamina*; these terms are often used synonymously but the term 'basal lamina' has a more specific meaning (see Fig. 4.20) and to avoid confusion, the term basement membrane is employed throughout this book. The basement membrane provides structural support for epithelia and may constitute an important barrier to the passage of materials between the epithelial and connective tissue compartments.

(ii) Luminal surfaces: the luminal surfaces of epithelial cells may exhibit three main types of specialisation: *cilia, microvilli* and *stereocilia*. Cilia are relatively long, motile structures which are easily resolved by light microscopy. In contrast, microvilli are short, often extremely numerous projections of the plasma membrane which cannot be individually resolved with the light microscope. Stereocilia are merely extremely long microvilli usually found only singly or in small numbers in odd sites such as the male reproductive tract; stereocilia are not motile and are thus inappropriately named.

(iii) Intercellular surfaces: epithelial cells are bound together by several types of specialisation of their apposed surfaces which permit epithelia to form cohesive, continuous layers and which may serve as points of metabolite or information transfer between cells. Analogous intercellular specialisations are found between cells in some non-epithelial tissues, particularly muscle, where they serve similar general functions.

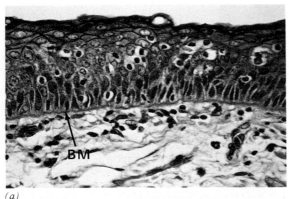

(a)

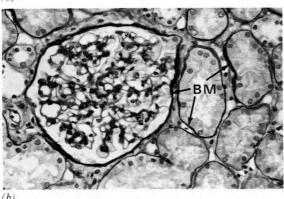

(b)

Fig. 4.20 Basement membranes

(a) Laryngeal epithelium (PAS × 320)
(b) Renal cortex (Jones' methenamine silver × 320)

These micrographs illustrate two methods for the demonstration of basement membranes **BM**. Basement membranes vary widely in thickness in different sites and even the thickest are often difficult to resolve in common haematoxylin and eosin stained preparations.

The structure of basement membranes is not well understood, but the current concept is that they consist of two basic layers. The layer in contact with the epithelial basal plasma membrane is composed of a fine feltwork of fibrils, biochemically similar to collagen and designated as collagen Type IV (see Fig. 3.4), embedded in an amorphous matrix of ground substance-like material; this layer is strictly described as the *basal lamina*. Deep to this layer, is a layer consisting mainly of fine reticulin fibres, also embedded in a ground substance-like matrix. This layer merges with underlying connective tissues.

The PAS staining method is thought to stain specifically the ground substance components and the silver method to stain the reticulin components of basement membranes; other common staining methods empirically differentiate basement membranes (see Fig. 4.5).

Which cells are responsible for elaborating basement membranes is in dispute. There is evidence that the true basal lamina is synthesised by epithelial cells and the reticular layer by the underlying connective tissue; in terms of this concept, the basal lamina may represent an extremely thickened epithelial glycocalyx (see Fig. 1.2).

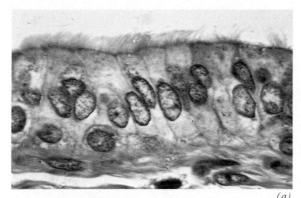

Fig. 4.21 Cilia

(a) Bronchiolar epithelium (resin embedded, one micron section: toluidine blue × 800)
(b) Bronchiolar epithelium (EM × 5600)
(c) Schematic diagram of a cilium

Cilia are motile structures which project in parallel rows from some epithelial surface cells. Cilia measure from about 7–10 μm in length and may therefore be of the order of half the length of the cell depending on cell size. A single epithelial cell may have up to 300 cilia and these are usually about the same length. Cilia beat with a wavelike, synchronous rhythm which tends to propel surface films of mucus or fluid in a consistent direction over the epithelial surface.

Each cilium, which is bounded by an evagination of the luminal plasma membrane, contains a central core called the *axoneme* consisting of twenty microtubules arranged as a central pair surrounded by nine peripheral doublets. Near the cytoplasmic surface, each axoneme inserts into a structure called a *basal body* **BB** which has a microtubular arrangement identical to that of a centriole; that is, nine triplets of microtubules forming a short cylinder (see Fig. 1.22). Each peripheral doublet of the cilium axoneme continues into the two inner microtubules of the corresponding triplet of the basal body. The central pair of axoneme microtubules terminates outside the basal body. Note that each axoneme doublet consists of one tubule, which is circular in cross section, closely applied to another incomplete tubule which is C-shaped in cross-section. From each complete tubule, pairs of 'arms' consisting of the protein *dynein*, which has ATP-ase activity, extend towards the incomplete tubule of the adjacent doublet. It is believed that ciliary action results from longitudinal movement of the doublets relative to one another, energy for the process being provided in the form of ATP probably by mitochondria which crowd the subjacent cytoplasm. It is not yet clear whether basal bodies arise *de novo* or by repeated division of centrioles. Note that evidence of basal bodies can be seen even with light microscopy. A three-dimensional surface view of cilia in the respiratory tract is shown in Fig. 11.5.

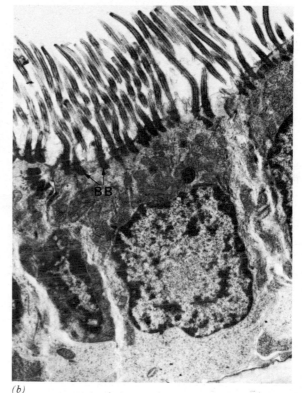

(b)

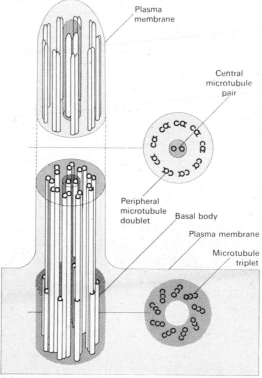

(c)

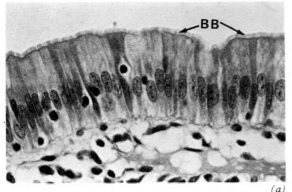

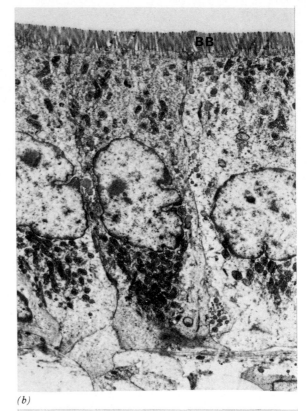

(a)

Fig. 4.22 Microvilli: small intestinal epithelium

(a) H & E × 320 (b) EM × 4750 (c) EM × 28 000

Microvilli are minute, finger-like projections of the luminal plasma membrane of many epithelia. Microvilli are only 0·5 to 1·0 μm in length and are thus very short in relation to the size of the cell, in marked contrast to cilia (see Fig. 4.21). Individual microvilli are too small to be resolved by light microscopy. Some epithelial cells have a small number of irregular microvilli whereas epithelia in such sites as the small intestine and renal tubules have up to 3000 regular microvilli per cell; collectively these can be seen with the light microscope as a *striated* or *brush border* **BB**. This surface specialisation may amplify the surface area for absorption by as much as thirty fold. Micrographs (a) and (b) illustrate the features of a typical striated border of columnar absorptive cells lining the small intestine.

The cytoplasmic core of each microvillus usually contains fine protein filaments which insert into the so-called *terminal web*, a specialisation of the cytoskeleton (see Chapter 1). The filaments are believed to maintain the stability of microvilli. This internal supporting structure is a particularly prominent feature of striated border microvilli as seen in (c) in which part of the terminal web **TW** is also shown.

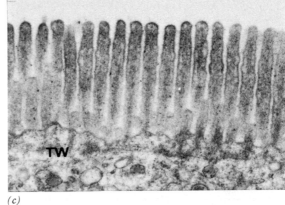

(c)

Fig. 4.23 Stereocilia

(H & E × 320)

Extremely long microvilli, readily visible with light microscopy, are found in small numbers in parts of the male reproductive tract such as the epididymis, shown in this micrograph, and other odd sites. Originally, these structures were thought to be an unusual form of cilia and were termed stereocilia; electron microscopy has shown that they do not have the internal structure of cilia but merely a filamentous skeleton like that of microvilli. Stereocilia **S** are thought to facilitate absorptive processes in the epididymis but the reason for their unusual form is not known.

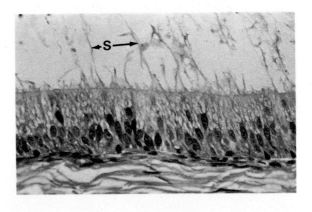

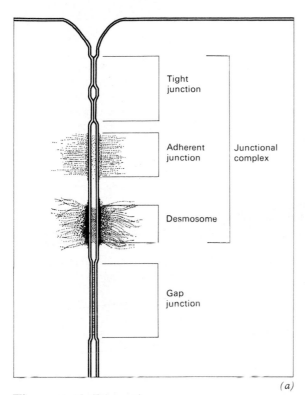

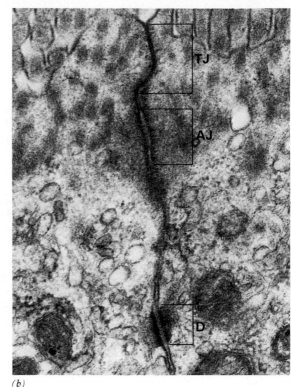

(a)   *(b)*

Fig. 4.24 Cell junctions
(a) Schematic diagram
(b) Junctional complex (EM × 59 400)

Before the advent of electron microscopy, epithelial cells were thought to be bound together by an intercellular adhesive which was called *intercellular cement*. It is now known that epithelial cells are bound together by several types of plasma membrane specialisations to which a variety of somewhat confusing names have been applied. The commonest type of cell junction is the *desmosome (macula adherens)*. Desmosomes are found scattered throughout intercellular interfaces where they provide strong points of cohesion between cells and act as anchorage points for the cytoskeleton of each cell. Another widely distributed type of cell junction is the *gap junction* or *nexus* which not only functions as an adherent zone but also permits transfer of information and metabolites between adjacent cells. Between the cells of simple cuboidal and simple columnar epithelia, the intercellular membranes exhibit specialisations called *junctional complexes* which prevent access of luminal contents to the intercellular spaces. Junctional complexes begin immediately below the luminal surface and are made up of three components, one of which is the desmosome; the other two components are called *tight junctions (zonula occludentes)* and *adherent junctions (zonula adherentes)*.

This electron micrograph of a typical junctional complex between two columnar intestinal epithelial cells illustrates tight and adherent junctions and a desmosome; the principal features of these junctions and of a gap junction are shown in the schematic diagram.

(i) Tight junctions: tight junctions **TJ** begin just below the luminal surface and consist of small areas where the outer lamina of opposing plasma membranes are fused with one another. Between these areas of fusion are areas which

are not fused. The tight junction forms a complete circumferential belt around each cell thus sealing the intercellular space from the lumen.

(ii) Adherent junction: adherent junctions **AJ** are found deep to the tight junctions and are areas where the opposing plasma membranes diverge; no structures are evident between the opposing cell membranes. On the cytoplasmic aspect of these junctions, there is a fine mat of filamentous material which merges with the filaments of the terminal web (see Fig. 4.22). Like tight junctions, adherent junctions also form a circumferential band around each cell.

(iii) Desmosomes: desmosomes **D** form the third component of junctional complexes but also occur singly at many other intercellular sites. At the desmosome, the opposing plasma membranes are separated by a gap in which many fine, transverse filaments or a dense, longitudinal lamina may be seen. At the cytoplasmic aspect of each plasma membrane there is a closely applied electron-dense layer into which fibrillar elements of the cytoskeleton appear to converge. Desmosomes always appear as the paired structures just described, except at the interface of stratified squamous epithelia and the basement membrane where half desmosomes (*hemi-desmosomes*) can be found.

(iv) Gap junctions: gap junctions are broad areas of closely opposed plasma membranes, but there is no fusion of the plasma membranes and a narrow gap remains. Although this type of junction is a site of intercellular adhesion, gap junctions also permit passage of ions and other molecules between adjacent cells; that is, they are sites of intercellular information exchange.

Glands

Exocrine glands are composed of epithelial cells which are specialised for secretion; they may be classified according to two major characteristics:

(i) The morphology of the gland: exocrine glands may be broadly divided into simple and compound glands. *Simple glands* are defined as those with a single, unbranched duct. The secretory portions of simple glands have two main forms, tubular or acinar, which may be coiled and/or branched. *Compound glands* have a branched duct system. The secretory portions of compound glands have similar morphological forms to those of the simple glands with the exception that both tubular and acinar forms may be found together draining into the same duct system. The morphology of the various exocrine gland types is summarised in Fig. 4.25 and examples are shown in Figs. 4.26 to 4.33.

(ii) The means of discharge of secretory products from the cells:

(a) *merocrine*. Merocrine secretion is an alternative name applied to the process of exocytosis (see Chapter 1) and is the most common form of secretion. It is also known as *eccrine* secretion.

(b) *apocrine*. Apocrine secretion involves the discharge of free, unbroken, membrane-bound vesicles containing secretory products and is an unusual means of secretion of lipid products in such glands as the breasts and some sweat glands.

(c) *holocrine*. This is another unusual form of secretion which involves the discharge of whole secretory cells with subsequent disintegration of the cells to release the secretory product. Holocrine secretion occurs principally in sebaceous glands.

Endocrine glands consist of clumps or cords of secretory cells surrounded by a rich network of blood capillaries. An unusual form of endocrine tissue is found in the thyroid gland where the epithelial cells are organised into spheroidal follicles which store hormone-precursor molecules. Figs. 4.34 to 4.37 illustrate these two endocrine gland conformations.

In general, all glands have a basal rate of secretion which is modulated by nervous and hormonal influences. The secretory portions of some exocrine glands are embraced by contractile cells which lie between the secretory cells and the basement membrane. The contractile mechanism of these cells is thought to be similar to that of muscle cells and has given rise to the term *myoepithelial cells*.

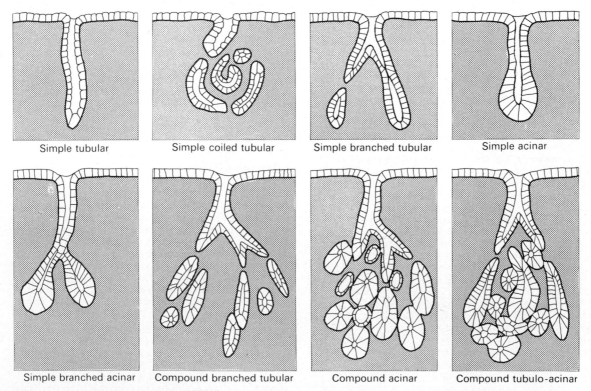

Simple tubular	Simple coiled tubular	Simple branched tubular	Simple acinar
Simple branched acinar	Compound branched tubular	Compound acinar	Compound tubulo-acinar

Fig. 4.25 Exocrine gland types

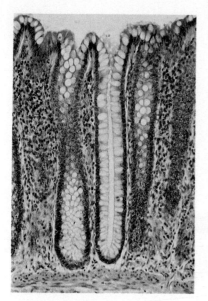

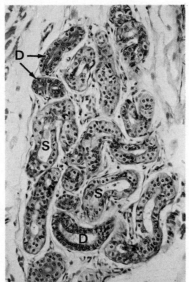

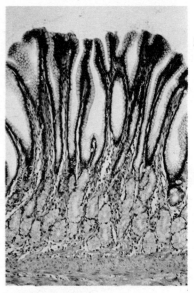

Fig. 4.26 Simple tubular glands

(H & E × 50)

This example of *simple tubular glands* is taken from the large intestine; this type of gland has a single, straight tubular lumen into which the secretory products are discharged. In this example, the entire duct is lined by secretory cells; the secretory cells are goblet cells. In other sites mucus is secreted by columnar cells which do not have the classical goblet shape but nonetheless function in a similar manner.

Fig. 4.27 Simple coiled tubular gland

(H & E × 80)

Sweat glands are almost the only example of *simple coiled tubular glands*. Each consists of a single tube which is tightly coiled in three dimensions; portions of the gland are thus seen in various planes of section. Sweat glands have a terminal secretory portion **S** lined by simple epithelium which gives way to a non-secretory (excretory) duct **D** lined by stratified cuboidal epithelium.

Fig. 4.28 Simple branched tubular glands

(H & E × 50)

Simple branched tubular glands are found mainly in the stomach; the mucous glands of the pyloric stomach are shown in this example. Each gland consists of several tubular secretory portions which converge on to a single, unbranched duct, which, in this case is also lined by mucus-secreting cells. Unlike those of the large intestine (see Fig. 4.26), these mucous cells do not have a goblet shape.

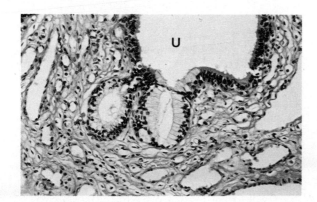

Fig. 4.29 Simple acinar glands

(H & E × 128)

Simple acinar glands occur as pockets in epithelial surfaces and are lined by secretory cells; in this example of the mucus-secreting glands of the penile urethra, the secretory cells are pale stained compared to the non-secretory cells lining the urethra **U**. Note that the term *acinus* can be used to describe any rounded exocrine secretory unit.

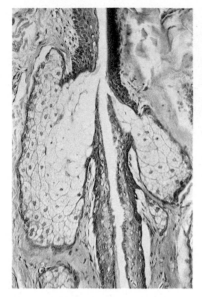

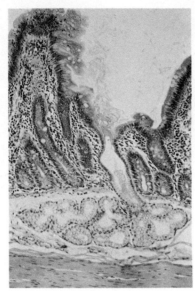

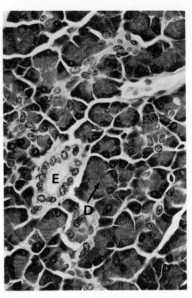

Fig. 4.30 Simple branched acinar gland

(Masson's trichrome × 80)

Sebaceous glands provide a good example of *simple branched acinar glands*. Each gland consists of several secretory acini which empty into a single excretory duct; the excretory duct is formed by the stratified epithelium surrounding the hair shaft. The mode of secretion of sebaceous glands is holocrine; the secretory product, sebum, accumulates within the secretory cells and is discharged by degeneration of the cells.

Fig. 4.31 Compound tubular gland

(H & E × 20)

Brunner's glands of the duodenum, as shown in this example, are described as *compound tubular glands*. The duct system is branched, thus defining the gland as a compound gland; the secretory portions have a tubular form which is branched and coiled.

Fig. 4.32 Compound acinar gland

(Chrome alum haematoxylin/phloxine × 320)

Compound acinar glands are those in which the secretory units are acinar in form and drain into a branched duct system. The pancreas shown in this micrograph consists of numerous acini, each of which drains into a minute duct. These minute ducts **D**, which are just discernible in the centre of some acini, drain into a system of branched excretory ducts of increasing diameter; a small excretory duct **E** lined by simple cuboidal epithelium is seen in the centre of the field.

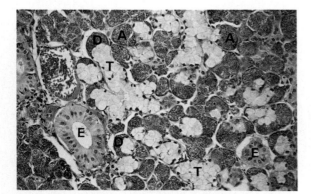

Fig. 4.33 Compound tubulo-acinar gland
(H & E × 128)

Compound tubulo-acinar glands have secretory units which consist of branched tubular components, branched acinar components, and branched tubular components with acinar end-pieces called *demilunes*. The submandibular salivary gland, which is the classical example and which is shown in this micrograph, has two types of secretory cells, mucous and serous. Generally, the mucous cells form tubular components **T** whereas the serous cells form acinar components **A** and demilunes **D**. Excretory ducts **E** of two different sizes are seen in this field.

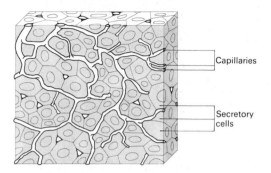

Fig. 4.34 Endocrine gland

Endocrine glands are ductless glands which secrete hormones into the circulatory system. Most endocrine glands consist of clumps or cords of secretory cells surrounded by a rich network of small blood vessels. Each clump of endocrine cells is surrounded by a basement membrane, reflecting its epithelial origin. Endocrine cells release hormones into intercellular spaces from which they diffuse rapidly into surrounding blood vessels.

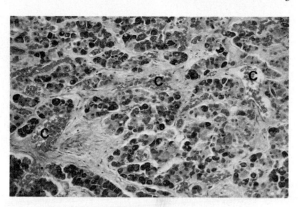

Fig. 4.35 Endocrine gland
(Isamine blue/eosin × 128)

This micrograph of the pituitary gland shows the features typical of most endocrine glands. The secretory cells are arranged in cords and clumps and are surrounded by a rich network of broad capillaries **C** in a fine supporting connective tissue. The basement membrane surrounding each clump of cells is not visible at this magnification. Like many other endocrine glands, the secretory cells of the pituitary are of several different types and thus may have different staining properties.

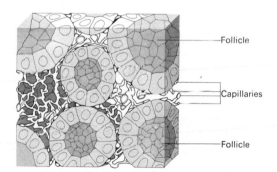

Fig. 4.36 Follicular endocrine gland

The thyroid gland is an unusual endocrine gland which stores hormone within spheroidal cavities enclosed by secretory cells; these spheroidal units are called follicles. The size of each follicle and the height of the cuboidal lining cells depends on the degree of secretory activity and quantity of hormone stored within the follicle. Secretion of stored hormone involves reabsorption of hormone from the follicular lumen, release into the surrounding interstitial spaces, and thence diffusion into the rich capillary network which embraces each follicle.

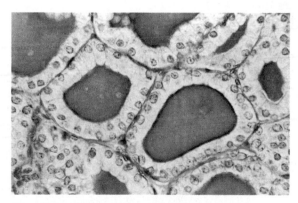

Fig. 4.37 Follicular endocrine gland
(PAS/haematoxylin × 320)

The follicular nature of the thyroid gland is evident from this micrograph. The secretory cells lining the follicles are cuboidal in shape and rest on a prominent basement membrane stained magenta by the PAS reaction. Stored thyroid hormone is bound to a glycoprotein which is also strongly PAS positive. The relatively sparse interfollicular connective tissue is mainly occupied by capillaries which are difficult to see in this preparation.

5. Muscle

Introduction

Contractility is an inherent property of all cells which is necessary for the performance of basic functions involving movement such as phagocytosis and cell division, and more specialised functions such as motility as in white blood cells. In multicellular organisms some cells are specialised to enable movement of tissues or organs. These cells may function as single contractile units, such as the myoepithelial cells surrounding the acini of some exocrine glands, or may be aggregated to form muscles for the movement of larger structures. Recent evidence, partly based on the study of the contractile mechanisms of some unicellular organisms, suggests that there is an homologous contractile mechanism in all cells. This mechanism consists of fibrillar proteins arranged in an organised manner in the cytoplasm, and linked by intermolecular bonds. Contraction results from the rearrangement of the intermolecular bonds with the utilisation of chemical energy.

There are three types of muscle tissue:

(i) Skeletal muscle: this is responsible for the movement of the skeleton and organs such as the globe of the eye and the tongue. Skeletal muscle is often referred to as *voluntary muscle* since it may be controlled voluntarily. The arrangement of the contractile proteins gives rise to the appearance of prominent cross-striations in some histological preparations and hence the name *striated muscle* is often applied to skeletal muscle.

(ii) Visceral muscle: this type of muscle forms the muscular component of diverse visceral structures, such as blood vessels, the gastro-intestinal tract, the uterus and the urinary bladder. Since visceral muscle is under inherent, autonomic and hormonal control it is described as *involuntary muscle*. As the arrangement of contractile proteins does not give the histological appearance of cross-striations, the name *smooth muscle* is commonly applied.

(iii) Cardiac muscle: cardiac muscle has many structural and functional characteristics intermediate between those of skeletal and visceral muscle; these provide for the continuous, rhythmic contractility of the heart. Although striated in appearance, cardiac muscle is readily distinguishable from skeletal muscle.

The highly specialised functions of the cytoplasmic organelles of muscle cells has led to the use of a special terminology: plasma membrane or plasmalemma=*sarcolemma*; cytoplasm=*sarcoplasm*; endoplasmic reticulum=*sarcoplasmic reticulum*; mitochondria=*sarcosomes*.

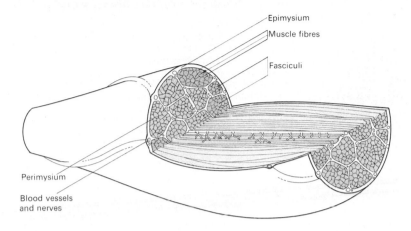

Epimysium
Muscle fibres
Fasciculi
Perimysium
Blood vessels
and nerves

Fig. 5.1 Skeletal muscle

This diagram illustrates the arrangement of the basic
components of skeletal muscle; a similar general
arrangement applies to visceral and cardiac muscle.

   Individual muscle cells, often referred to as *muscle fibres*
because of their elongated shape, are grouped together into
elongated bundles called *fasciculi*. Delicate connective tissue
called *endomysium*, composed mainly of reticulin fibres,
separates individual muscle fibres. The fasciculi are
surrounded by loose collagenous connective tissue called
perimysium. Most muscles are made up of many fasciculi
and are invested in a dense, outer connective tissue sheath
called the *epimysium*. Large blood vessels and nerves enter
the epimysium and divide to ramify throughout the muscle
in the perimysium.

   The size of the fasciculi reflects the function of the
muscle. Muscles responsible for fine, highly controlled
movements, e.g. the external muscles of the eye, have small
fasciculi and a relatively greater proportion of perimysial
connective tissue. In contrast, muscles responsible for gross
movements only, e.g. the muscles of the buttocks, have
large fasciculi and relatively little perimysial connective
tissue.

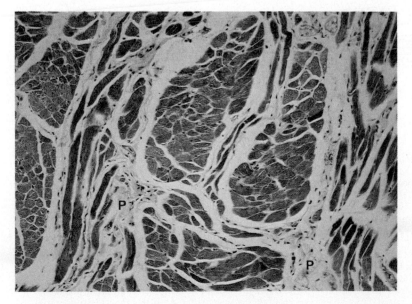

Fig. 5.2 Skeletal muscle
(Masson's trichrome × 198)

This preparation demonstrates the
contractile and connective tissue
elements of skeletal muscle. Fasciculi
of red-stained skeletal muscle fibres cut
in longitudinal and transverse section
can be seen separated by perimysium
P, containing blue-stained collagen
fibres. The endomysium, which
separates individual muscle fibres,
consists mainly of reticulin fibres and a
small amount of collagen. The
connective tissue of skeletal muscle also
contains elastin fibres which are most
common in muscles attached to soft
tissues, e.g., in the tongue and face.

   The connective tissue component of
skeletal muscle has the mechanical
function of controlling the degree of
extension and contraction of the
muscle.

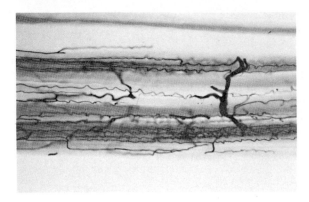

Fig. 5.3 Skeletal muscle: blood supply

(Perfusion method × 128)

This specimen was prepared by perfusing the blood supply of a skeletal muscle with a red dye; the muscle fibres were teased apart to reveal the endomysial capillary bed. Large blood vessels enter the epimysium and divide to ramify throughout the muscle in the perimysium. Fine branches arise from the perimysial arteries and pass between the muscle fibres transversely to their long axes. These give rise to numerous capillaries which run longitudinally through the endomysium. Frequent transverse anastomoses between capillaries result in a fine, elongated capillary network surrounding each muscle fibre.

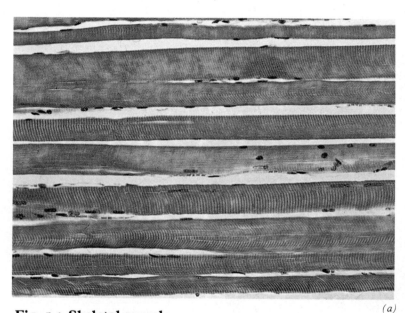

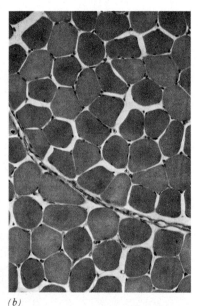

(a)   *(b)*

Fig. 5.4 Skeletal muscle

(a) LS (b) TS: H & E × 320

These micrographs demonstrate the characteristic histological features of skeletal muscle fibres in transverse and longitudinal section.

Skeletal muscle fibres are extremely elongated, unbranched cylindrical cells with numerous flattened nuclei located at fairly regular intervals just beneath the sarcolemma. These multinucleate cells are derived by fusion of mononuclear cells which cease mitotic division during embryonic development. Thus from birth, skeletal muscle growth results from enlargement of cells rather than from cell division; regeneration of muscle fibres does not occur after cell damage. The development of the organelles responsible for contraction mainly occurs after the formation of the multinucleate muscle cell. In short muscles, individual muscle fibres may extend the whole length of the muscle.

Regular cross-striations are a prominent characteristic of skeletal muscle fibres in some histological preparations. The contractile proteins of each muscle fibre are arranged in long cylindrical structures called *myofibrils* which lie parallel to one another in the sarcoplasm. The regular arrangement of the contractile proteins in each myofibril results in the myofibril appearing cross-striated with electron microscopy. The parallel myofibrils are arranged with their cross-striations in register so as to give rise to the appearance with light microscopy of regular cross-striations along the whole length of the muscle fibre.

In transverse sections, the peripheral location of the nuclei of skeletal muscle cells is readily seen. In some preparations the cut ends of myofibrils may be seen as dark dots regularly arranged within the cytoplasm. In transverse sections of unfixed skeletal muscle, fibres appear oval or round; however, in the more commonly seen fixed preparations such as this, the fibres appear artefactually irregular and polyhedral. Similarly the wide endomysial spaces seen between the muscle fibres result from shrinkage during tissue preparation.

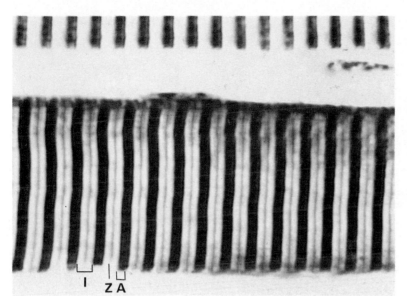

Fig. 5.5 Skeletal muscle
(LS: Heidenhain's haematoxylin × 1200)

This micrograph demonstrates the striations of a skeletal muscle fibre at a magnification close to the limit of resolution of the light microscope. The striations are composed of alternating broad, light I bands (isotropic in polarised light) and dark A bands (anisotropic in polarised light). Fine dark lines called Z bands (Zwischenscheiben) can be seen bisecting the light I bands.

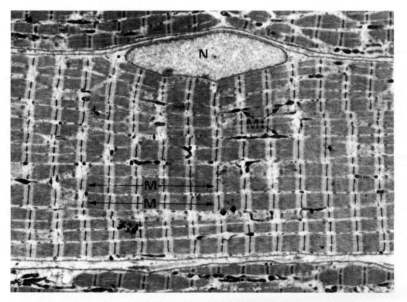

Fig. 5.6 Skeletal muscle
(LS: EM × 2860)

Electron microscopy reveals details of the structure of myofibrils. Many parallel myofibrils **M** separated by a small amount of sarcoplasm containing numerous mitochondria **Mt** which are oriented with their long axes parallel to the myofibrils. Note the manner in which the myofibrils are arranged with their cross-striations in register.

The Z bands are the most electron-dense bands in the myofibril and have been shown to divide each myofibril into numerous contractile units, called *sarcomeres*, arranged end to end. Note the nucleus **N** situated immediately beneath the sarcolemma.

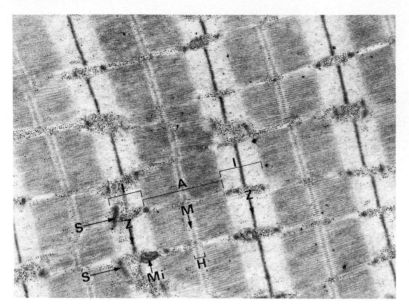

Fig. 5.7 Skeletal muscle: sarcomeres

(EM ×18700)

With further magnification, the arrangement of the contractile proteins or *myofilaments* may be seen in each sarcomere. Within the sarcomere, the dark A band is bisected by a broad lighter band, the H (heller) band, which is further bisected by a more dense M (Mittelscheibe) band. Irrespective of the degree of contraction of the muscle fibre, the A band remains constant in width. In contrast, the I bands and H bands narrow during contraction and the Z bands are drawn closer together. This led to the development of the *sliding filament theory* of muscle contraction.

Note the mitochondria **Mi** and numerous glycogen granules which provide a rich energy source in the scanty cytoplasm between the parallel myofibrils. The mature muscle cell contains little rough endoplasmic reticulum; it contains, however, a smooth membranous system **S** which conducts contractile stimuli to the myofibrils (see Figs. 5.9 and 5.10).

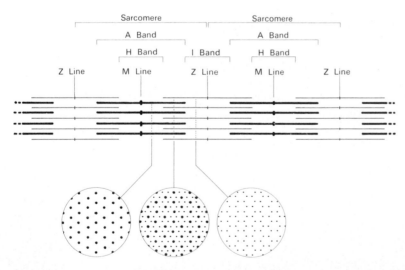

Fig. 5.8 The arrangement of myofilaments in the sarcomere

The sarcomere consists of two types of myofilaments, *thick filaments* and *thin filaments*. Each type remains constant in length irrespective of the state of contraction of the muscle. The filaments are arranged in a symmetrical interdigitating manner parallel to the long axis of the myofibril.

The thick filaments, which are composed mainly of the protein *myosin*, are maintained in parallel by their attachment to a disc-like zone represented by the M band. Similarly the thin filaments, which are composed mainly of

the protein *actin*, are united in a disc-like zone represented by the Z band. The I and H bands, both areas of low electron-density, represent areas where the thick and thin filaments do not overlap one another.

The widely accepted sliding filament theory proposes that under the influence of energy released from ATP, the thick and thin filaments slide over one another, thus causing contraction in the length of the sarcomere.

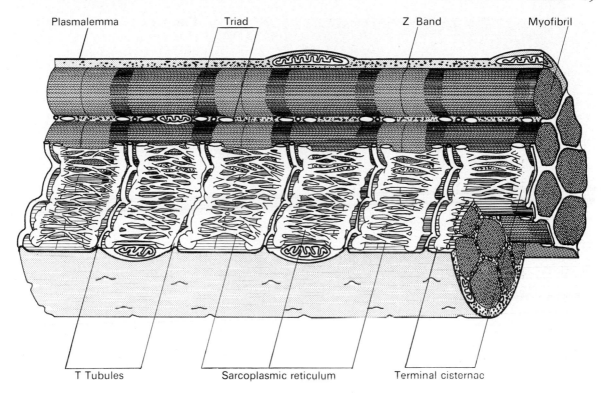

Plasmalemma Triad Z Band Myofibril

T Tubules Sarcoplasmic reticulum Terminal cisternae

Fig. 5.9 The conducting system for contractile stimuli

To permit the synchronous contraction of all sarcomeres in the muscle fibre, a system of tubular extensions of the muscle cell membrane or sarcolemma extends transversely into the muscle cell to surround each myofibril at the region of the junction of the A and I bands (in mammals). Thus, throughout the muscle fibre, there is a tubular system, the *T system*, the lumen of which is continuous with the extracellular space.

Closely associated with, but not interconnected with, each T tubule system there are two complementary membrane systems derived from smooth endoplasmic reticulum; these are called *sarcoplasmic reticulum*. The sarcoplasmic reticulum ramifies to form a membranous network which embraces each myofibril. Each T tubule, with its pair of associated sarcoplasmic reticulum elements called *terminal cisternae*, forms a *triad* near the junction of the I and A bands of each sarcomere.

Calcium ions are concentrated within the lumen of the sarcoplasmic reticulum. Excitation of the sarcolemma of the muscle fibre is rapidly disseminated throughout the sarcoplasm by the T tubule system. This promotes the release of calcium ions from the sarcoplasmic reticulum into the sarcoplasm surrounding the myofilaments. Calcium ions activate the sliding filament mechanism resulting in muscle contraction. The nervous control of muscle excitation is discussed in Chapter 7.

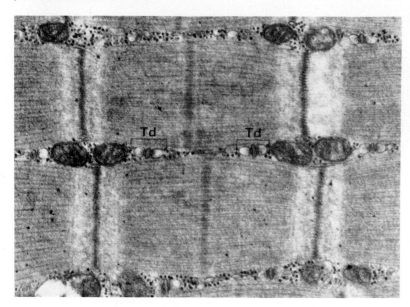

Fig. 5.10 Skeletal muscle
(EM × 38000)

This electron micrograph of mammalian skeletal muscle demonstrates triads **Td** of the conducting system, each comprising a tubule of the T system and a pair of terminal cisternae of the sarcoplasmic reticulum. In mammals the position of the triads approximates to the junction of the A and I bands; during contraction, these junctions move in relation to the triads.

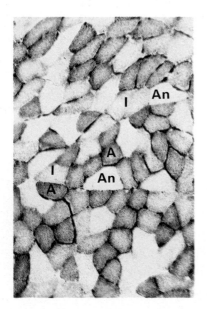

Fig. 5.11 Skeletal muscle
(TS: Histochemical technique for succinate dehydrogenase × 128)

With the naked eye, three types of skeletal muscle may be distinguished on the basis of colour: red, white and intermediate. In man, the three types of muscle are not readily obvious on gross examination. In domestic birds, the extremes are easily identified; flight muscles are white whereas leg muscles are red. The colour of any muscle depends on the characteristics of its constituent fibres. Skeletal muscle fibres are of three types, each differing in the mode of energy metabolism from aerobic through an intermediate type to anaerobic.

(a) Aerobic muscle fibres: these fibres are small in cross-section, contain abundant mitochondria, have a large content of *myoglobin* (an oxygen-storage molecule found in muscle) and a rich blood supply. These characteristics account for the red colour of such fibres and their predominant mode of metabolism which is aerobic. Aerobic muscle fibres are most abundant in muscles which contract almost continuously, such as the calf muscles of the legs.

(b) Anaerobic muscle fibres: these fibres are large in cross-section, contain few mitochondria and little myoglobin, and have a relatively poor blood supply. These muscle fibres are rich in glycogen and glycolytic enzymes. These characteristics account for the 'white' colour of such fibres and their predominant anaerobic mode of metabolism. Anaerobic fibres predominate in muscles responsible for intense but sporadic contraction such as the biceps and triceps of the arms.

(c) Intermediate muscle fibres: the morphological and functional characteristics of these fibres are intermediate between the aerobic and anaerobic fibre types.

This histochemical method for demonstrating the activity of the specific mitochondrial enzyme *succinate dehydrogenase*, which catalyses one of the stages of Krebs' cycle, demonstrates the relative proportions of mitochondria within the three fibre types. Note the presence of intensely staining, small-diameter aerobic fibres **A**, poorly stained, large-diameter anaerobic fibres **An** and intermediate fibres **I**.

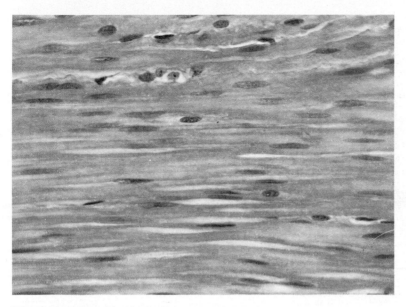

Fig. 5.12 Visceral muscle
(LS: H & E × 480)

The structure of visceral muscle reflects important functional characteristics:

(i) Continuous, inherent, rhythmic contractions which are modulated by the autonomic nervous system and a variety of hormones.

(ii) Relatively low force of contraction.

(iii) Relatively diffuse movements related to contraction of the whole muscle mass rather than finely controlled contraction of individual muscle fibres.

Visceral muscle fibres are elongated, spindle-shaped cells with pointed ends which may be occasionally bifurcated; the cell boundaries are usually indistinct in H & E stained preparations. Visceral muscle fibres are generally much shorter than skeletal muscle fibres and contain only one nucleus which is elongated and centrally located in the cytoplasm at the widest part of the cell. Depending on the contractile state of the fibres at fixation, the nuclei may appear to be spiral shaped.

Visceral muscle fibres are bound together in irregular, branching fasciculi and these fasciculi, rather than individual fibres, are the functional contractile units. Individual muscle fibres are arranged parallel to one another with the thickest part of one cell lying against the thin parts of adjacent cells.

The contractile proteins of visceral muscle are not arranged in myofibrils as in skeletal and cardiac muscle; thus visceral muscle cells are not striated, giving rise to the common name of smooth muscle.

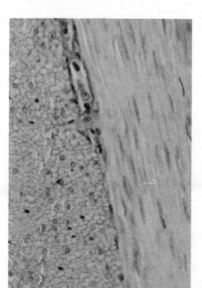

Fig. 5.13 Visceral muscle
(LS and TS: PAS/iron haematoxylin/orange G × 320)

This staining method demonstrates the thin layer of connective tissue (stained red) which separates visceral muscle fibres and which is analogous to the endomysium of skeletal muscle. This connective tissue consists of a glycoprotein matrix containing reticular and some elastic fibres.

Note the extreme elongation of the nuclei of muscle fibres seen in longitudinal section and the round, centrally located nuclei of the fibres cut in transverse section. The variable diameter of the fibres as seen in transverse section, and the apparent absence of nuclei from some fibres, is a function of the plane of section of each spindle-shaped cell.

In many tubular visceral structures, such as the oesophagus seen in this micrograph, smooth muscle is disposed in layers with the cells of one layer arranged at right angles to those of the adjacent layer. This arrangement permits a wave of contraction to pass down the tube propelling the contents forward; this action is called *peristalsis*.

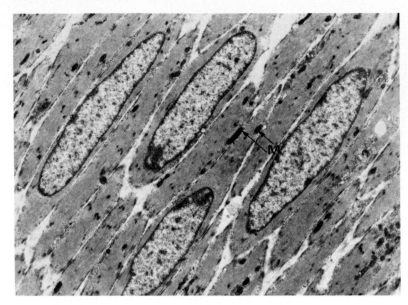

Fig. 5.14 Visceral muscle
(LS: EM × 5500)

At low magnification, electron microscopy demonstrates the spindle shape and elongated, central nuclei of visceral muscle cells. Note the relative sparsity of mitochondria **M** and other intracellular organelles. Most of the cytoplasm is occupied by fibrillar contractile protein, the organisation of which does not give rise to the appearance of cross-striations.

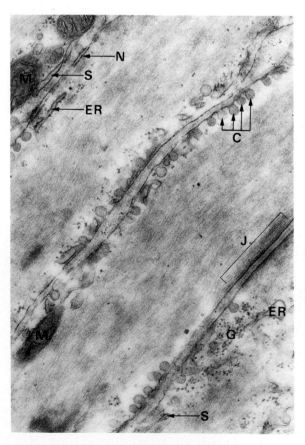

Fig. 5.15 Visceral muscle
(EM × 32400)

At high magnification, details of the plasma membrane and endomembrane system can be seen.

The plasma membrane contains numerous flask-shaped invaginations. In some areas these are irregular in shape and size and may be involved in pinocytosis. In other areas, the invaginations are regular in shape and distribution, and are called *caveolae* **C**.

The endomembrane system contains some elements which appear to represent a poorly developed Golgi and endoplasmic reticulum system **ER**. Other vesicular and tubular structures **S** are seen near the plasma membrane, often in association with caveolae. This has led to the theory that these structures constitute a system which is analogous to the sarcoplasmic reticulum of skeletal muscle and that the caveolae are analogous to the T tubule system.

At this magnification, parallel myofilaments are seen to occupy most of the cytoplasm. These are believed to be analogous to the thin (actin) filaments of skeletal muscle. Recently, thick (myosin) filaments have also been demonstrated in visceral muscle cells using special techniques. The mechanism of smooth muscle contractility is therefore believed to be basically similar to that of skeletal muscle. Note also mitochondria **M** and glycogen granules **G** throughout the cytoplasm.

The narrow intercellular spaces are of almost uniform width but at numerous sites the plasma membranes of adjacent cells closely approximate to each other. Some of these intercellular contact areas **N** are believed to facilitate spread of excitation throughout visceral muscle and may be considered as nexus-like junctions (see Fig. 4.24). Other contacts may bind adjacent cells and provide anchorage points for contractile proteins; such junctions **J** bear a resemblance to the desmosomes of epithelia (see Fig. 4.24).

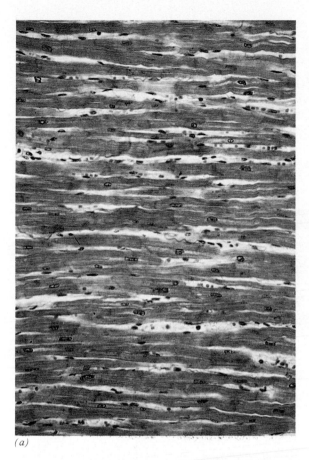

(a)

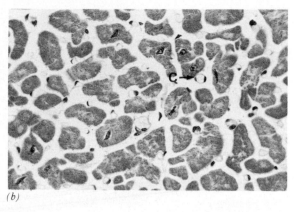

(b)

Fig. 5.16 Cardiac muscle
(H & E (a) LS × 198 (b) TS × 320)

Cardiac muscle exhibits structural and functional characteristics intermediate between those of skeletal and visceral muscle. In longitudinal section, cardiac muscle cells are seen to contain one or two nuclei and an extensive cytoplasm which branches to give the appearance of a continuous three-dimensional cytoplasmic network or *syncytium*. The elongated nuclei are mainly centrally located, a characteristic well demonstrated in transverse section. In H & E preparations, cross-striations are seldom seen in cardiac muscle.

Delicate connective tissue, extremely rich in blood capillaries **C**, fills the intercellular spaces. The great vascularity of cardiac muscle reflects the high metabolic demands of strong, continuous contractility.

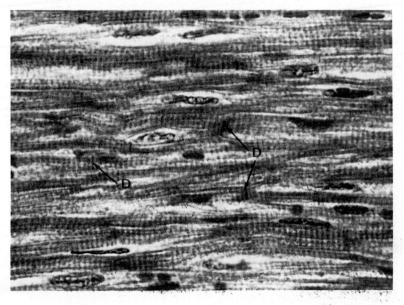

Fig. 5.17 Cardiac muscle
(Masson's trichrome × 480)

This staining method reveals cross-striations in cardiac muscle cells which reflect a similar arrangement of contractile proteins to that of skeletal muscle.

This technique also demonstrates the junctions between adjacent cardiac muscle cells known as *intercalated discs* **D**. Intercalated discs have areas of low electrical resistance which permit the rapid spread of contractile excitation throughout the muscle mass of the heart. Thus, though not a true cytoplasmic syncytium, cardiac muscle acts as a functional syncytium.

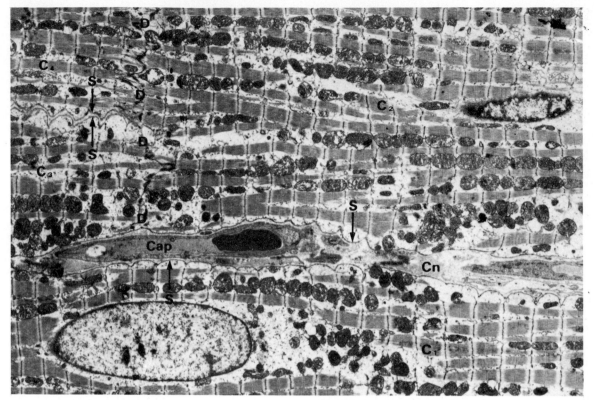

Fig. 5.18 Cardiac muscle

(EM × 4500)

This micrograph illustrates portions of four cardiac muscle cells C_1, C_2, C_3 and C_4. Note that the nuclei of cells C_1 and C_2 are characteristically located deep to the sarcolemma **S**. The intercellular space between cells C_1, C_2 and C_3 are occupied by capillaries **Cap** and collagen fibres **Cn**. The cell junctions between C_4 and C_2 and between C_3 and C_2 are defined by a single intercalated disc **D**.

The sarcomeres of cardiac muscle have an identical banding pattern to that of skeletal muscle. The sarcomeres are not, however, arranged into single columns making up cylindrical myofibrils as in skeletal muscle, but form a branching network continuous in three dimensions

throughout the cytoplasm. The branching columns of sarcomeres are separated by sarcoplasm containing rows of mitochondria and sarcoplasmic reticulum. The great abundance of mitochondria in cardiac muscle, compared with skeletal muscle, reflects the enormous metabolic demands of continuous cardiac muscle activity.

Conduction of excitatory stimuli to the sarcomeres of cardiac muscle is mediated by a system of T tubules and sarcoplasmic reticulum essentially similar in arrangement to that of skeletal muscle. The T tubules, however, ramify throughout the cardiac muscle cytoplasm at the Z lines; their origins are seen as indentations in the sarcolemma.

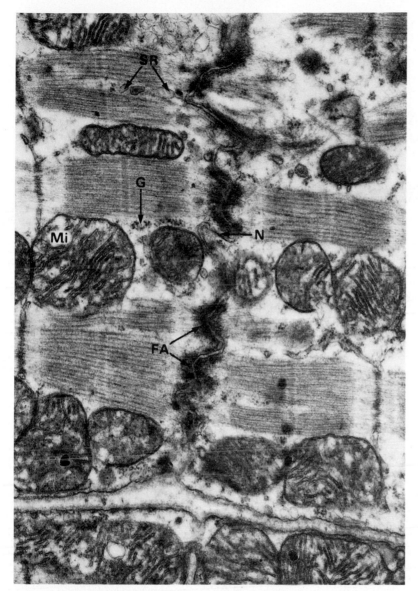

Fig. 5.19 Cardiac muscle: intercalated disc
(EM ×29000)

Intercalated discs are specialised transverse junctions between cardiac muscle cells at sites where they meet end to end. Intercalated discs always coincide with the Z lines. Intercalated discs bind the cells, transmit forces of contraction and provide areas of low electrical resistance for the rapid spread of excitation throughout the myocardium.

The intercalated disc is an interdigitating junction, the entire surface of which consists of three types of membrane to membrane contacts. The predominant type of contact, the *fascia adherens* **FA** resembles the zona adherens of epithelial junctional complexes (see Fig. 4.24) but is more extensive and less regular. The ends of terminal sarcomeres insert into fasciae adherentes and thereby transmit contractile forces from cell to cell. Desmosomes occur less frequently and provide additional intercellular adhesion.

Gap junctions or nexuses **N** occur in some longitudinal portions of the interdigitations and are believed to be sites of low electrical resistance through which excitation passes from cell to cell.

Note the similarity of the sarcomeres of cardiac and skeletal muscle (see Fig. 5.7). The mitochondria **Mi** of cardiac muscle are elongated or spheroidal and have abundant closely packed cristae rich in oxidative enzyme systems. The sarcoplasm within and between the sarcomeres is rich in glycogen granules **G**.

The T tubule and sarcoplasmic reticulum system form triads at the Z lines. The sarcoplasmic reticulum **SR** is less extensive than that of skeletal muscle and does not form dilated terminal cisternae.

6. Circulatory system

Introduction

The circulatory system mediates the continuous movement of all body fluids; its principal functions are the transport of oxygen and nutrients to the tissues and transport of carbon dioxide and other metabolic waste products from the tissues. The circulatory system is also involved in temperature regulation and the distribution of molecules such as hormones, and cells such as those of the immune system. The circulatory system has two functional components: the blood vascular system and the lymph vascular system. The *blood vascular system* constitutes a circuit of vessels through which a flow of blood is maintained by continuous pumping of the heart. The *arterial system* provides a distribution network to the *capillaries* which are the main sites of interchange between the tissues and blood. The *venous system* returns blood from the capillaries to the heart. In contrast, the *lymph vascular system* is merely a passive drainage system for returning excess extravascular fluid called *lymph* to the blood vascular system. The lymph vascular system has no intrinsic pumping mechanism.

The whole circulatory system has a common basic structure:

(i) An inner lining comprising a single layer of extremely flattened epithelial cells called *endothelium* supported by a basement membrane and connective tissue. This constitutes the *tunica intima*.

(ii) An intermediate muscular layer, the *tunica media*.

(iii) An outer connective tissue layer called the *tunica adventitia*. The tissues of the walls of larger vessels cannot be sustained by diffusion from their lumens. Thus they are supplied by small arteries called *vasa vasorum* (i.e. 'vessels of vessels') which are derived either from the main vessel itself or from adjacent arteries. The vasa vasorum give rise to a capillary network within the tunica adventitia which may extend into the tunica media.

The muscular layer exhibits the greatest variation throughout the system; for example, it is totally absent in capillaries but comprises almost the whole mass of the heart. Blood flow is predominantly influenced by variations in activity of the muscular layer.

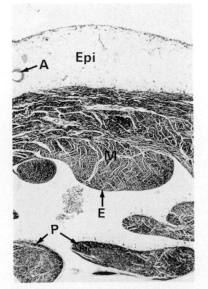

Fig. 6.1 Heart: wall of ventricle

(Masson's trichrome × 20)

This micrograph illustrates the three basic layers of the heart wall. The tunica intima of the heart is called the *endocardium* **E**, and is difficult to see at this magnification. The tunica media of the heart is called the *myocardium* **M** and is thickest in the ventricular walls. The myocardium is made up of cardiac muscle, the structure of which meets the unique functional requirements of the heart (see Chapter 5).

The tunica adventitia of the heart, the *epicardium* **Epi** (also called *visceral pericardium*), is surrounded by a space, the *pericardial cavity*, enclosed by a fibrous sac, the *pericardium* (the *parietal pericardium*) which is not shown in this micrograph. The parietal pericardium is loosely fixed to the surrounding mediastinal structures. The parietal and visceral layers of the pericardium move freely against one another thus permitting relatively unimpeded movement of the heart.

Note a branch **A** of the coronary arterial system; these arteries are the vasa vasorum of the heart. Note also papillary muscles **P** of the ventricle, extensions of the myocardium which, via the chordae tendinae, stabilise the cusps of the mitral and tricuspid valves.

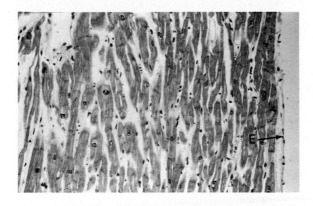

Fig. 6.2 Heart: myocardium and endocardium
(H & E × 128)

The endocardium, the innermost layer of the heart, consists of an endothelial lining and supporting connective tissue. The endothelium **E**, is a single layer of flattened epithelial cells, which is continuous with the endothelium of the vessels entering and leaving the heart. The endothelium is supported by a delicate layer of fibro-elastic connective tissue which accommodates gross movements of the myocardium without damage to the endothelium.

The subendothelial connective tissue becomes continuous with the perimysium of the cardiac muscle. The endocardium contains blood vessels, nerves and branches of the conducting system of the heart.

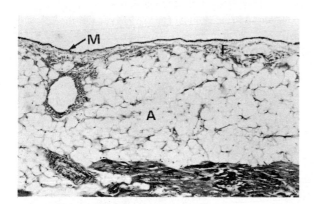

Fig. 6.3 Heart: epicardium
(H & E × 128)

The free surface of the epicardium is covered by a single layer of flattened epithelial cells, the mesothelium **M**; a similar mesothelial layer lines the opposing parietal pericardial surface. The mesothelial cells secrete a small amount of serous fluid which lubricates the movement of the epicardium on the parietal pericardium. A thin layer of fibro-elastic connective tissue **F** supports the mesothelium; this layer is connected to the myocardium by a broad layer of adipose connective tissue **A**. Branches of the coronary vessels and the nerves pass in the epicardium to supply the myocardium.

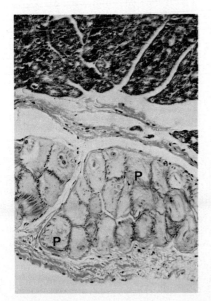

Fig. 6.4 Purkinje fibres
(Sheep: TS: Masson's trichrome × 128)

The co-ordinated contraction of the myocardium during each pumping cycle is mediated by a specialised conducting system of modified cardiac muscle fibres. With each cardiac cycle, a wave of excitation originates in the pacemaker region of the right atrium, the *sino-atrial node*. The excitatory stimuli arise spontaneously at regular intervals in the sino-atrial node and the rate is modulated by the autonomic nervous system. The wave of excitation spreads throughout the atria causing them to contract, thus forcing blood into the ventricles. The wave of excitation then spreads to the *atrioventricular node* from which an excitatory stimulus is passed rapidly throughout the whole ventricular myocardium via the *atrioventricular bundle* or *bundle of His*. This bundle divides within the interventricular septum to give rise to smaller branches called *Purkinje fibres* which course in the subendocardial connective tissue before penetrating the ventricular myocardium. This system permits almost simultaneous contraction of the entire ventricular myocardium.

The characteristics of the specialised muscle fibres of the conducting system are demonstrated in this micrograph of Purkinje fibres **P** in the subendocardium of a ventricle from a sheep; Purkinje fibres are similar but less readily identified in the human heart. The conducting cells are large, often binucleate, with extensive pale cytoplasm which contains few myofibrils. The myofibrils are arranged in an irregular manner immediately beneath the plasma membrane of the cell. The cytoplasm is rich in glycogen and mitochondria. The mechanism of impulse conduction in Purkinje fibres is poorly understood.

The arterial system

The function of the arterial system is to distribute blood from the heart to capillary beds throughout the body. The cyclic pumping action of the heart produces a pulsatile blood flow in the arterial system. With each stroke of the ventricles, blood is forced into the arterial system causing expansion of the arterial walls; subsequent recoil of the arterial walls assists in maintenance of arterial blood pressure between strokes of the ventricles. This expansion and recoil is facilitated by the presence of elastic tissue within the walls of the arterial system. The flow of blood to various organs and tissues may be regulated by varying the diameter of the distributing vessels. This function is performed by the smooth muscle component of vessel walls and is principally under the control of the sympathetic nervous system and adrenal medullary hormones.

Although the walls of the arterial system conform to the general structure of the circulatory system, they are characterised by the presence of variable amounts of elastic fibres and a smooth muscle wall which is thick relative to the diameter of the lumen. There are three main types of vessel in the arterial system:

(i) Elastic arteries: these comprise the major distribution vessels and include the aorta, the innominate, common carotid and subclavian arteries and most of the pulmonary arterial vessels.

(ii) Muscular arteries: these are the main distributing branches of the arterial tree, for example the radial arteries.

(iii) Arterioles: these are the terminal branches of the arterial tree which supply the capillary beds.

There is a gradual transition in structure and function between the three arterial types. In general, the amount of elastic tissue decreases as the vessels become smaller and the smooth muscle component assumes greater prominence.

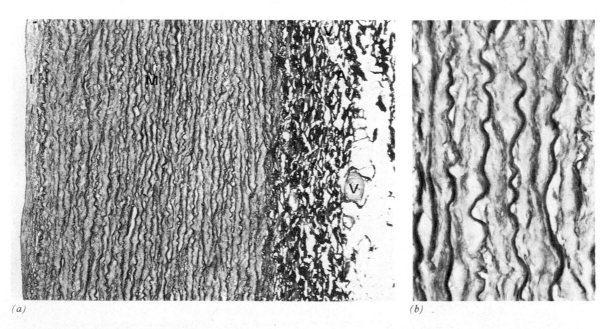

(a)   *(b)*

Fig. 6.5 Elastic artery: aorta

(Elastic van Gieson (a) × 33 (b) × 320)

The highly elastic nature of the aortic wall is demonstrated in these preparations in which the elastic fibres are specifically stained black. Note the three basic layers: the tunic intima **I**, the tunica media **M** and the tunica adventitia **A**.

The tunica intima is composed of collagenous connective tissue with few elastic fibres: the endothelial lining cannot be seen at this magnification. The tunica media is particularly broad and extremely elastic; at high

magnification it is seen to consist of fenestrated sheets of elastin separated by collagenous connective tissue and relatively few smooth muscle fibres. The collagenous tunica adventitia, stained red in this preparation, contains small vasa vasorum **V**.

Blood flow within elastic arteries is highly pulsatile; with advancing age the arterial system becomes less elastic thereby increasing peripheral resistance and thus arterial blood pressure.

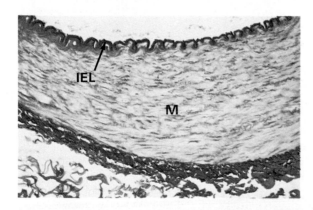

Fig. 6.6 Muscular artery

(TS: Elastic van Gieson × 80)

Muscular arteries have the same basic composition as elastic arteries but the elastic tissue is reduced to a well defined, fenestrated elastic sheet, the *internal elastic lamina* **IEL**, in the tunica intima, and a diffuse *external elastic lamina* in the tunica adventitia; elastin is stained black in this preparation. A few elastic fibres are scattered throughout the tunica media **M** which is mainly composed of a thick layer of smooth muscle, stained yellow in this preparation. Note the red-stained collagen fibres within each layer. The vasa vasorum are mainly confined to the adventitial layer, although small branches may extend into the tunica media.

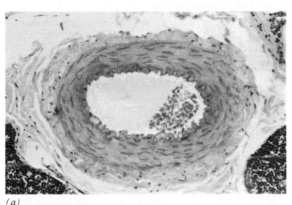

(a)

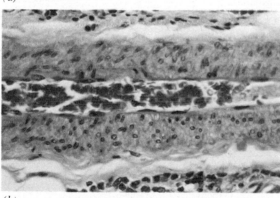

(b)

Fig. 6.7 Large arteriole

(H & E (a) TS × 128 (b) LS × 320)

Arterioles may be defined as those vessels of the arterial system with a lumen less than 0.3 mm in diameter, although the distinction between small muscular arteries and large arterioles is somewhat artificial. Arterioles are characterised by the following features which are seen in these micrographs:

(i) The tunica intima is very thin and comprises the endothelial lining, little collagenous connective tissue and a thin, but distinct, internal elastic lamina.

(ii) The tunica media is almost entirely composed of smooth muscle cells in six concentric layers or less.

(iii) The tunica adventitia may be almost as thick as the tunica media and merges with the surrounding connective tissues. There is no external elastic lamina.

The flow of blood through capillary beds is regulated mainly by the arterioles which supply them. Contraction of circularly arranged, smooth muscle fibres of the arteriolar wall reduces the diameter of the lumen and hence blood flow. Generalised constriction of arterioles throughout the body markedly increases peripheral resistance to blood flow and hence the arteriolar compartment of the circulatory system has an important role in the regulation of systemic blood pressure.

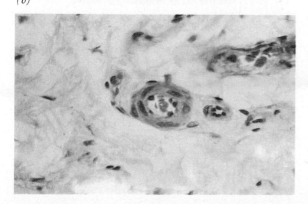

Fig. 6.8 Small arteriole

(TS: H & E × 480)

This micrograph illustrates the smallest type of vessel in the arterial system, an arteriole with only one layer of smooth muscle cells. Note the absence of elastic tissue. The adventitial layer is almost indistinguishable from the surrounding connective tissue.

The microcirculation

The microcirculation is that part of the circulatory system concerned with the exchange of gases, fluids, nutrients and metabolic waste products. Exchange occurs mainly within the capillaries. The arterioles, and muscular sphincters at the arteriolar-capillary junctions called *precapillary sphincters*, control blood flow within capillary networks. The capillary networks drain into a series of vessels of increasing diameter, *post-capillary venules*, *collecting venules* and small *muscular venules*; these vessels comprise the venous component of the microcirculation.

In different tissues, the structure of the microcirculation varies to meet specific functional requirements. There are four main structural variables:

(i) The diameter of the capillaries: capillary diameter varies between as little as 3 to 4μm (i.e. half the diameter of a red blood cell) and 30 to 40μm. Large diameter capillaries are called *sinusoids*.

(ii) The nature of the capillary endothelium: three types of capillary endothelium are found:

(a) *continuous capillaries:* the endothelial cells form an uninterrupted capillary lining; this is the most common type of capillary.

(b) *fenestrated capillaries:* the endothelial cells contain numerous large pores or fenestrations.

(c) *discontinuous endothelium:* the endothelial cells do not form a continuous interface between the lumen and surrounding tissues; this arrangement is found only within the sinusoids of the liver (see Fig. 12.71).

(iii) The presence of arterio-venous shunts, direct connections between the arterial and venous systems.

(iv) The abundance of the capillary network; for example, dense connective tissue has a poor capillary network in contrast to cardiac muscle.

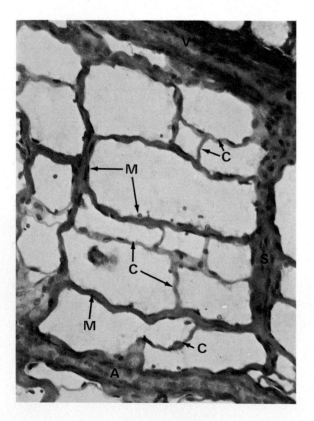

Fig. 6.9 The microcirculation
(Mesenteric spread: H & E × 120)

This micrograph demonstrates an anastomosing network of capillaries between an arteriole **A** and a venule **V**. The capillary network comprises small diameter capillaries **C** consisting only of a single layer of endothelial cells, and larger diameter capillaries with a discontinuous outer layer of smooth muscle cells, known as *metarterioles* **M**.

Note that small capillaries arise both from arterioles and metarterioles. At the origin of each capillary there is believed to be a sphincter mechanism which is involved in regulation of capillary blood flow. Note also a direct wide-diameter communication between the arteriole and venule, an arteriovenous shunt **S**. Metarterioles also form direct communications between arterioles and venules. Contraction of the smooth muscle of the shunts and metarterioles directs blood through the network of small capillaries. Thus regulation of blood flow in the microcirculation is mediated by arterioles, metarterioles, precapillary sphincters and arteriovenous shunts. The smooth muscle activity of these vessels is modulated by the autonomic nervous system and circulating hormones. In addition, the concentration of oxygen and metabolites, such as lactic acid, regulates the local flow of blood within tissues; this process is called *autoregulation*.

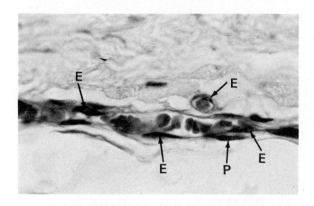

Fig. 6.10 Capillaries
(H & E × 800)

The vessels seen in longitudinal section and transverse section illustrate the characteristic features of capillaries:

(i) A single layer of flattened endothelial cells **E**, the cytoplasm of which is difficult to resolve by light microscopy. The flattened endothelial cell nuclei bulge into the capillary lumen; in longitudinal section the nuclei appear elongated whereas in transverse section they appear more rounded in shape.

(ii) The absence of muscular and adventitial layers.

(iii) The presence of occasional flattened cells embracing the capillary endothelial cells; these cells are called *pericytes* **P** and may have a contractile function.

(iv) The diameter of capillaries is similar to that of the red blood cells contained within them.

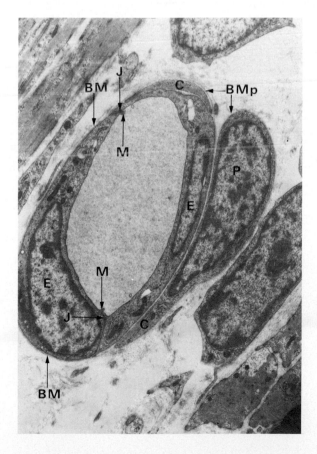

Fig. 6.11 Capillary (continuous type)
(TS: EM × 7500)

This electron micrograph illustrates the ultrastructure of a capillary of the continuous endothelium type, the usual type found in most tissues. Two endothelial cells **E** are seen to encircle the capillary lumen; their plasma membranes approximate to one another very closely and in places form discrete junctional complexes **J**. Small cytoplasmic flaps called *marginal folds* **M** extend across the intercellular junctions at the luminal surface. The capillary endothelium is supported by a thin basement membrane **BM** containing a few reticular fibres.

Exchange between the lumen of the continuous capillary and the surrounding tissues is believed to occur in three ways:

(i) Passive diffusion through the endothelial cell cytoplasm; exchange of gases, ions and small molecular weight metabolites occurs in this manner.

(ii) Transport by pinocytotic vesicles; proteins and some lipids may be transported in this manner.

(iii) Passage through the intercellular space between the endothelial cells; members of the white blood cell series are believed to migrate through the endothelial cell junctions by a process called *diapedesis*. Some workers maintain that the intercellular spaces also permit molecular transport. In capillaries of this type the basement membrane is thought to present little barrier to exchange between capillaries and the tissues.

Note the pericyte **P** with its cytoplasmic extensions **C** which embrace the capillary. The pericyte is supported by its own basement membrane **BMp**.

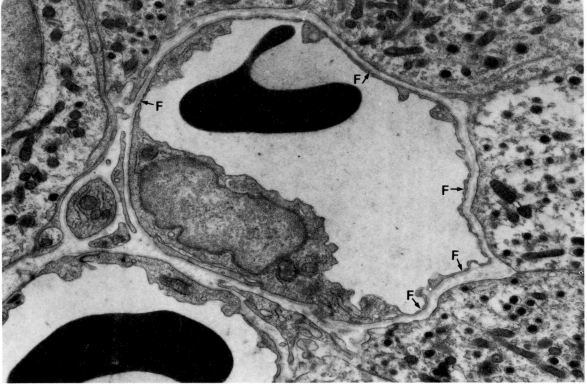

(a)

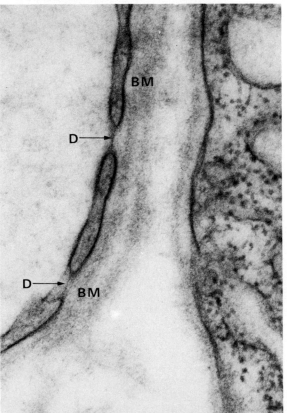

(b)

Fig. 6.12 Fenestrated capillary
(TS: EM (a) ×13000 (b) ×54000)

Fenestrated capillaries are found in some tissues where there is much molecular exchange with the blood; such tissues include the small intestine, endocrine glands and the kidney.

At low magnification, fenestrations **F** appear as pores through thin areas of the endothelial cytoplasm; however, only a small proportion of the thin areas are fenestrated. At high magnification, the fenestrations appear to be traversed by a thin electron-dense line which may constitute a diaphragm **D**, the biochemical and functional nature of which is in dispute. A diaphragm is not seen across the fenestrations of the glomerular capillaries of the kidney (see Fig. 13.15c).

The permeability of fenestrated capillaries is much greater than that of continuous capillaries; molecular labelling techniques have demonstrated that fenestrations permit the rapid passage of macromolecules smaller than plasma proteins.

Like continuous capillaries, all fenestrated capillaries are supported by a basement membrane **BM** which is continuous across the fenestrations. Pericytes are rarely found in association with fenestrated capillaries.

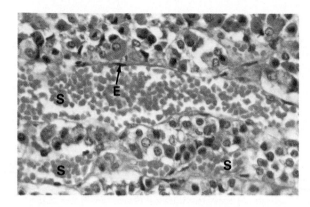

Fig. 6.13 Sinusoids
(H & E × 320)

Sinusoids are capillaries of wide diameter found in the liver, spleen, bone marrow and some endocrine glands. The endothelium of sinusoids may be fenestrated or discontinuous; the discontinuous type of endothelial lining is found only in the liver sinusoids (see Fig. 12.71). Sinusoids usually have an irregular outline which conforms to the cellular arrangement of the tissue in which they are found. This micrograph illustrates sinusoids **S** between cords of secretory cells in the anterior pituitary. Several endothelial cell nuclei **E** can be distinguished by their flattened shape.

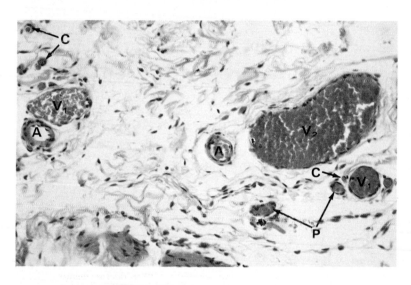

Fig. 6.14 Post-capillary and collecting venules
(H & E × 198)

This micrograph illustrates five types of vessel of the microcirculation; small arterioles **A**, capillaries **C**, post-capillary venules **P**, collecting venules V_1 and a small muscular venule V_2.

Post-capillary venules are formed by the union of several capillaries to produce a vessel similar in structure but of a wider diameter. Post-capillary venules perform molecular exchange functions in a similar manner to that of capillaries. Post-capillary venules drain into collecting venules which are characterised by their larger diameter and a greater number of enveloping pericytes. The function of the collecting venules is to conduct blood from the post-capillary venules to the larger muscular venules.

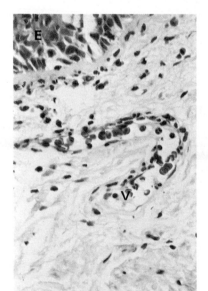

Fig. 6.15 Post-capillary venule
(H & E × 320)

This micrograph illustrates a post-capillary venule **V** in the connective tissue underlying an inflamed epithelial surface **E**. Blood flow in post-capillary venules is extremely sluggish, a phenomenon which may facilitate the exit of leucocytes from the microcirculation. During inflammatory responses, post-capillary venules are the major sites in the circulation from which leucocytes gain access to the tissues. In contrast to capillaries, intercellular junctional complexes are relatively uncommon between the endothelial cells of post-capillary venules; this may also facilitate leucocyte emigration. Note in this micrograph, leucocytes, mainly neutrophils, in the process of migrating towards the epithelial surface.

The venous system

With the exception of the venous components of the microcirculation, the venous system merely functions as a low-pressure collecting system for the return of blood from the capillary networks to the heart. Blood flow in veins occurs passively down a pressure gradient towards the heart. With each respiratory inspiration, a negative pressure is created within the thorax and hence within the right atrium of the heart. Venous return from the extremities is aided by the contraction of skeletal muscles which compress the veins contained within them. With each respiratory expiration, the pressure gradients are reversed and blood tends to flow in the opposite direction. This tendency is prevented by the presence of valves in veins of medium diameter.

The structure of the venous system conforms to the general structure of the whole circulatory system, but the elastic and muscular components are much less prominent features. A major part of the total blood volume is contained within the venous system. Variations in relative blood volume, for example, due to dilatation of capillary beds or haemorrhage, may be compensated for by changes in the capacity of the venous system. These changes are mediated by smooth muscle in the tunica media which controls the luminal diameter of muscular venules and veins.

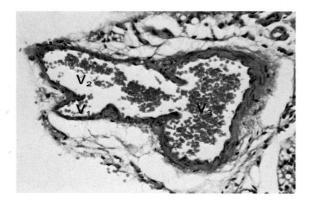

Fig. 6.16 Muscular venules and small vein
(H & E × 128)

This micrograph illustrates the confluence of a small muscular venule V_1 with a larger muscular venule V_2 which then joins a small vein V_3 cut in transverse section. Note the valve at the junction of the large venule and vein. Muscular venules are characterised by a clearly defined intimal layer devoid of elastic fibres and a tunica media consisting of one or two layers of smooth muscle fibres. Veins are characterised by a thicker muscular wall and a poorly developed internal elastic lamina. Note that the tunica adventitia of these vessels is continuous with the surrounding connective tissue.

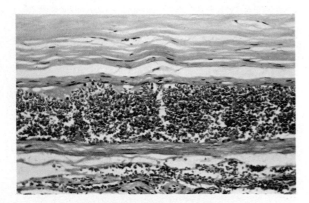

Fig. 6.17 Small vein
(LS: H & E × 128)

This micrograph illustrates a small vein cut in longitudinal section and fixed whilst still distended with blood. The wall of the vein consists of two to three layers of smooth muscle fibres. Note the wide diameter of the lumen relative to the thickness of the wall.

Fig. 6.18 Vein
(TS: H & E × 128)

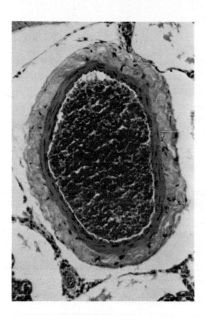

Small and medium size veins are characterised by the following features demonstrated in this micrograph of a medium size vein:

(i) The tunica intima consists of little more than the endothelial lining. In veins that are not distended with blood the endothelium may be thrown up into small folds.

(ii) The tunica media is thin compared with that of arteries and consists of two or more layers of circularly arranged smooth muscle fibres.

(iii) The tunica adventitia is the thickest layer of the vessel wall and is composed of longitudinally arranged thick collagen fibres which merge with the surrounding connective tissue.

Note that the wall of the vein is thin relative to the diameter of the lumen. In contrast, in most arteries, the thickness of the wall approaches the diameter of the lumen.

Fig. 6.19 Vein with valve
(LS: Masson's trichrome × 128)

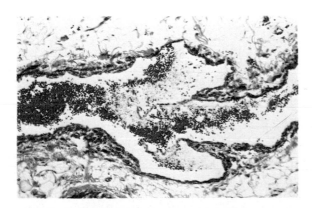

This micrograph demonstrates a valve in a small vein. The valve consists of delicate semilunar projections of the tunica intima of the vein wall; the projections are composed of fibro-elastic connective tissue lined on both sides by endothelium. Each valve usually consists of two leaflets, the free edges of which project in the direction of blood flow. Valves only occur in veins of more than 2mm in diameter, particularly those draining the extremities.

Fig. 6.20 Large muscular vein
(TS: Elastic van Gieson × 128)

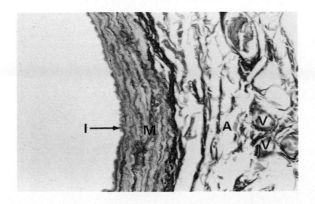

Large muscular veins, such as the renal vein, are characterised by the following features:

(i) A thin tunica intima **I** comprising endothelium and delicate supporting tissue containing occasional elastic fibres which do not form a distinct internal elastic lamina.

(ii) The tunica media **M** consists of several circular layers of smooth muscle (stained yellow) separated by layers of collagenous connective tissue (stained red) and containing a few elastic fibres (stained black).

(iii) A broad tunica adventitia **A** containing numerous vasa vasorum **V** which may extend into the tunica media. The many vasa vasorum present in veins reflects the need for arterial blood by the tissues of the vein wall.

The lymph vascular system

The lymph vascular system drains excess fluid called lymph from extracellular spaces and returns it to the blood vascular system. Lymph is formed in the following manner: at the arterial end of blood capillaries, the hydrostatic pressure of blood exceeds the colloidal osmotic pressure exerted by plasma proteins. Water and electrolytes therefore pass out of capillaries into the extracellular spaces; some plasma proteins also leak out through the endothelial wall. At the venous end of blood capillaries the pressure relationships are reversed and fluid tends to be drawn back into the blood vascular system. In this way, about two per cent of plasma passing through the capillary bed is exchanged with the extracellular tissue fluid. The rate of tissue fluid formation at the arterial end of capillaries generally exceeds the re-uptake of fluid at the venous end. The excess fluid, lymph, is drained by a system of lymph capillaries which converge to form progressively larger diameter lymphatic vessels. Lymph enters the venous system by a single vessel on each side of the body, the thoracic duct and the right lymphatic duct. Movement of lymph in the lymph vascular system is similar to movement of blood in the venous system but valves are more numerous in lymphatic vessels.

Along the course of the larger lymphatic vessels are aggregations of lymphoid tissue called lymph nodes where cells of the immune system and antibodies join the general circulation (see Chapter 10). Lymphatic vessels are found in all tissues except the central nervous system, cartilage, bone, bone marrow, thymus, placenta and teeth. The structure of lymphatic vessels conforms closely to that of vessels of similar diameter in the venous system. Lymphatic vessels may be distinguished from venous vessels by the absence of erythrocytes and the presence of small numbers of leucocytes mainly lymphocytes. Lymphatic capillaries differ from blood capillaries in several respects which reflect the greater permeability of lymphatic capillaries: the endothelial cell cytoplasm is extremely thin and a basement membrane and pericytes are absent.

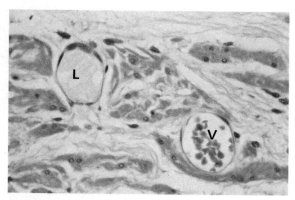

Fig. 6.21 Small lymphatic vessel
(H & E × 320)

This micrograph illustrates the characteristic histological differences between a small lymphatic **L** and a venule **V**. Lymphatics do not contain erythrocytes but often contain lymphocytes. The stained amorphous material seen in this lymphatic is the protein of lymph which becomes precipitated during tissue processing. The presence of such material is often a distinguishing feature of lymphatics in histological preparations.

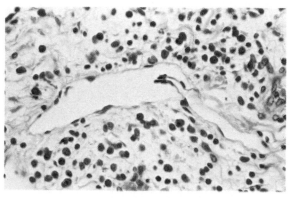

Fig. 6.22 Valve of a lymphatic vessel
(H & E × 320)

A characteristic feature of the lymphatic system is the numerous delicate valves in small and medium sized vessels. The structure of these valves is similar to that of valves in the venous system, but the connective tissue core consists merely of reticulin fibres and a little ground substance.

7. Nervous tissues

Introduction

The function of the nervous system is to receive stimuli from both the internal and external environments; these are then analysed and integrated to produce appropriate, co-ordinated responses in various effector organs. The nervous system is composed of an intercommunicating network of specialised cells called *neurones* which constitute most sensory receptors, the conducting pathways, and the sites of integration and analysis. The functions of the nervous system depend on a fundamental property of neurones called *excitability*. Like all cells, the resting neurone maintains an ionic gradient across its plasma membrane thereby creating an electrical potential. Excitability involves a change in membrane permeability in response to appropriate stimuli such that the ionic gradient is reversed and the plasma membrane becomes *depolarised*; a wave of depolarisation, known as an *action potential*, then spreads along the plasma membrane; this is followed by the process of *repolarisation* in which the membrane rapidly re-establishes its resting potential. At *synapses*, the sites of intercommunication between adjacent neurones, depolarisation of one neurone causes it to release chemical transmitter substances, *neurotransmitters*, which initiate an action potential in the adjacent neurone. Within the nervous system, neurones are arranged to form pathways for the conduction of action potentials from receptors to effector organs via integrating neurones. Neurotransmitters not only mediate neurone-to-neurone transmission but also act as chemical intermediates between the nervous system and effector organs which also exhibit the property of excitability. The effector organs of voluntary nervous pathways are generally skeletal muscle, and those of involuntary pathways are usually smooth muscle, cardiac muscle and muscle-like epithelial cells (myoepithelial cells) within some exocrine glands.

The nervous system is divided anatomically into the *central nervous system* (CNS) comprising the brain and spinal cord, and the *peripheral nervous system* (PNS) which constitutes all nervous tissue outside the CNS. Functionally, the nervous system is divided into the *somatic nervous system* which is involved in voluntary functions, and the *autonomic nervous system* which exerts control over many involuntary functions. Histologically, however, the entire nervous system merely consists of variations in the arrangement of neurones and their supporting tissues.

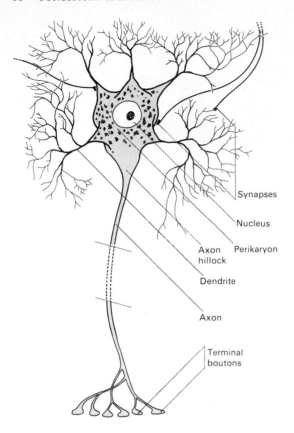

Synapses

Nucleus

Axon Perikaryon
hillock

Dendrite

Axon

Terminal
boutons

Fig. 7.1 The neurone

Despite great variation in size and shape in different parts of the nervous system, all neurones have the same basic structure as shown in this idealised diagram. The neurone consists of a large *cell body* containing the nucleus surrounded by cytoplasm known as the *perikaryon*. Processes of two types extend from the cell body: a single *axon* and one or more *dendrites*.

Dendrites are highly branched, tapering processes which either end in specialised sensory receptors, as in primary sensory neurones, or form synapses with neighbouring neurones from which they receive stimuli. In general, dendrites function as the major sites of information input into the neurone.

Each neurone has a single axon arising from a cone-shaped portion of the cell body called the *axon hillock*. The axon extends as a cylindrical process of variable length terminating on other neurones or effector organs by a variable number of small branches which end in small swellings called *terminal boutons*. Action potentials arise in the cell body as a result of integration of afferent stimuli; action potentials are then conducted along the axon to influence other neurones or effector organs. Axons are commonly referred to as *nerve fibres*. In general, the cell bodies of all neurones are located in the central nervous system with the exception of the cell bodies of most primary sensory neurones and the terminal effector neurones of the autonomic nervous system; such cell bodies lie in aggregations called *ganglia* in peripheral sites.

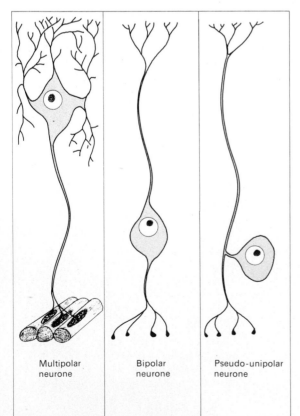

Multipolar
neurone

Bipolar
neurone

Pseudo-unipolar
neurone

Fig. 7.2 Basic neurone types

Throughout the nervous system, neurones have a wide variety of shapes which fall into three main patterns according to the arrangement of the axon and dendrites with respect to the cell body.

The most common form is the *multipolar neurone* in which numerous dendrites project from the cell body; the dendrites may all arise from one pole of the cell body or may extend from all parts of the cell body. In general, intermediate, integratory and motor neurones conform to this pattern.

Bipolar neurones have only a single dendrite which arises from the pole of the cell body opposite to the origin of the axon. These unusual neurones act as receptor neurones for the senses of smell, sight and balance. Most other primary sensory neurones are described as *pseudo-unipolar neurones* since a single dendrite and the axon arise from a common stem of the cell body; this stem is formed by the fusion of the first part of the dendrite and axon of a bipolar type of neurone during embryological development.

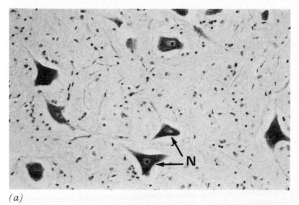

(a)

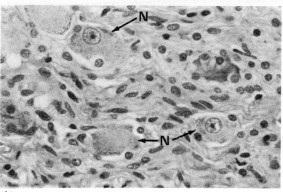

(b)

Fig. 7.3 Neurone cell bodies

(a) Grey matter (Nissl method × 128)
(b) Spinal ganglion (H & E × 320)

Since neurones have such extensive cytoplasmic processes, it is rarely possible to examine the whole structure of individual neurones in histological sections of nervous tissues. These micrographs show the typical histological appearance of neurones in two different sites. In the central nervous system as shown in (a), multipolar neurone cell bodies **N** are scattered in a mass of axons and dendrites of other neurones, supporting cells and small blood vessels. In somatic ganglia as in (b), the cell bodies of neurones **N** of the pseudo-unipolar type are closely aggregated with much less intervening tissue.

In histological sections, neurones are recognised as unusually large cells with pale-stained, centrally located nuclei which usually contain prominent nucleoli.

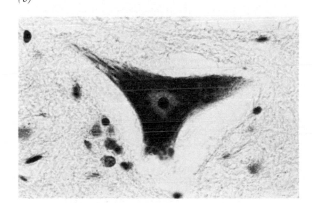

Fig. 7.4 Neurone: grey matter

(Nissl method × 800)

Nissl introduced a staining method which demonstrates, particularly in large neurones, the presence of numerous clumps of highly basophilic cytoplasmic material, called *Nissl substance*. Nissl substance is found in the perikaryon and dendrites but is not present in the axon hillock or axon. The Nissl staining method leaves the nucleus largely unstained although the nucleolus is very densely stained. Electron microscopy has subsequently revealed that Nissl substance represents the RNA of large aggregations of rough endoplasmic reticulum. This high concentration of rough endoplasmic reticulum is thought to be necessary for the production of the enzymes involved in neurotransmitter synthesis and in maintenance of the huge area of plasma membrane.

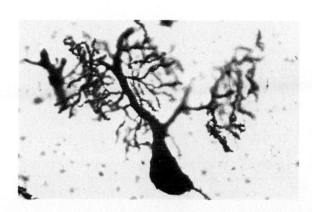

Fig. 7.5 Neurone: Purkinje cell of the cerebellum

(Golgi-Cox method × 320)

This method, used with thick sections, permits the study of the branched processes of neurones. This micrograph shows a most unusual variation of the multipolar neurone form which is characteristic of so-called Purkinje cells of the cerebellum. A common feature of most dendrites, as seen in this micrograph, is the presence of numerous minute *dendritic spines* projecting from each dendrite; the spines are sites where the dendrite forms synapses with the processes of other neurones.

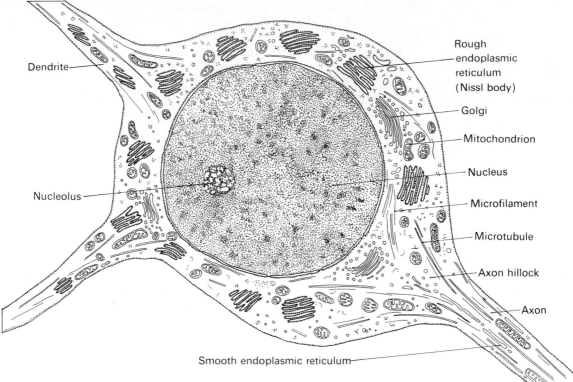

Dendrite

Nucleolus

Rough endoplasmic reticulum (Nissl body)

Golgi

Mitochondrion

Nucleus

Microfilament

Microtubule

Axon hillock

Axon

Smooth endoplasmic reticulum

Fig. 7.6 Ultrastructure of the neurone

This diagram illustrates the main ultrastructural features of the neurone. The nucleus is large, round or ovoid and usually centrally located within the perikaryon; reflecting intense activity of the neurone, the chromatin is completely dispersed and the nucleolus is a conspicuous feature.

The cytoplasm of the cell body contains large aggregations of rough endoplasmic reticulum which corresponds to the Nissl substance of light microscopy (see Fig. 7.4); the rough endoplasmic reticulum extends into the dendrites but not into the axon hillock or axon. Rough endoplasmic reticulum is a much more prominent feature in large neurones, such as somatic motor neurones, than in smaller neurones such as those of the autonomic nervous system. A diffuse Golgi apparatus is found adjacent to the nucleus; smooth endoplasmic reticulum is not a prominent

feature of the perikaryon but tubules, cisternae and vesicles are prominent in the axon and dendrites. The mitochondria of the perikaryon have the usual rod-like appearance, but those of the axon are extremely slender and elongated. Neurones are highly metabolically active cells and expend much energy in maintaining ionic gradients across the plasma membrane. Neurones synthesise neurotransmitter substances or their precursors in the perikaryon; these are then transported along the axon to the synapse where they are released when appropriately stimulated.

Numerous microfilaments and microtubules are arranged in parallel bundles throughout the perikaryon and along the length of the axon and dendrites. These elements form the neuronal cytoskeleton and may be involved in axonal transport of neurotransmitter substances.

Myelinated and non-myelinated nerve fibres

In the peripheral nervous system, all axons are enveloped by specialised cells called *Schwann cells* which provide both structural and metabolic support. In general, small diameter axons, for example those of the autonomic nervous system and small pain fibres, are simply enveloped by the cytoplasm of Schwann cells; these nerve fibres are said to be *non-myelinated*. Large-diameter fibres are wrapped by a variable number of concentric layers of the Schwann cell plasma membrane forming the so-called *myelin sheath*; such nerve fibres are said to be *myelinated*. Within the central nervous system, myelination is similar to that in the peripheral nervous system except that the myelin sheaths are formed by cells called *oligodendrocytes* (see Fig. 7.27). All non-myelinated fibres in the CNS have no specific cellular support but are indirectly supported by the mass of surrounding tissue.

In all nerve fibres, the rate of conduction of action potentials is proportional to the diameter of the axon; myelination greatly increases axon conduction velocity compared with a non-myelinated fibre of the same diameter.

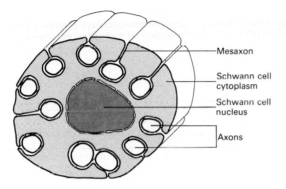

Fig. 7.7 Non-myelinated nerve fibres

The relationship of non-myelinated fibres and their supporting Schwann cell is illustrated in this diagram. One or more nerve fibres become longitudinally invaginated into the cytoplasm of a Schwann cell so that each fibre is embedded in a groove in the Schwann cell cytoplasm. The Schwann cell plasma membrane fuses along the opening of the groove, thus effectively sealing the nerve fibre within an extracellular compartment within the Schwann cell. The site of fusion of the Schwann cell membrane is called the *mesaxon*. Each Schwann cell extends for only a short distance along the nerve tract and at its termination its role is supplanted by another Schwann cell with which it interdigitates closely.

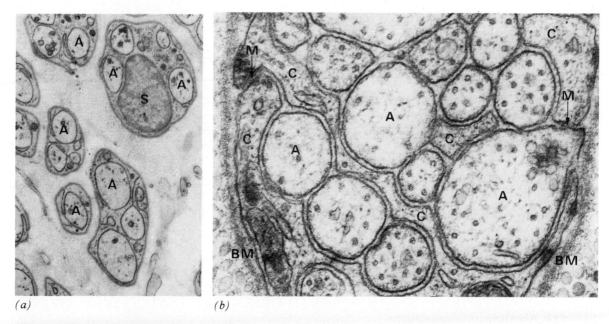

(a)   *(b)*

Fig. 7.8 Non-myelinated nerve fibres
(EM (a) ×9450 (b) ×75600)

At low magnification, non-myelinated axons **A** of various sizes are seen embedded in Schwann cells; one of the Schwann cells has been sectioned transversely through its nucleus **S**. Note the variable number of fibres enclosed by each Schwann cell.

At high magnification, part of the cytoplasm of a Schwann cell **C** is shown enveloping several axons **A**; axons are readily identified by their content of tubules of smooth endoplasmic reticulum and microtubules, seen in cross-section. Two mesaxons **M** can be seen. Note that more than one nerve fibre may occupy a single groove within the Schwann cell. The external surface of the Schwann cell is bounded by a condensation of extracellular material forming a basement membrane **BM**.

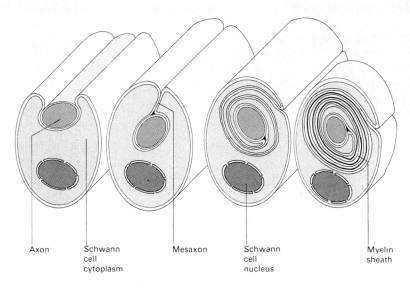

Axon   Schwann cell cytoplasm   Mesaxon   Schwann cell nucleus   Myelin sheath

Fig. 7.9 Myelin sheath formation in the peripheral nervous system

The process of myelination starts during fetal development and continues for a considerable time after birth. Myelination begins with the invagination of a single nerve fibre into a Schwann cell; a mesaxon, like that of unmyelinated fibres, is then formed (see Fig. 7.7). As myelination proceeds, the mesaxon wraps around the axon thereby enveloping the axon in a spiral layer of Schwann cell cytoplasm. As this process continues, the cytoplasm is excluded; by maturity, the inner layers of plasma membrane fuse with each other so that the axon becomes surrounded by several layers of modified membranes which together constitute the myelin sheath.

In the CNS, oligodendrocytes are responsible for the process of myelination which follows a similar pattern; a single oligodendrocyte, however, forms the myelin sheaths of several axons (see Fig. 7.27).

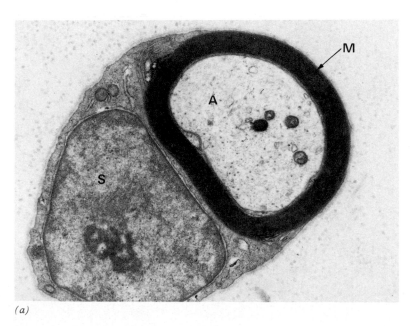

(a)

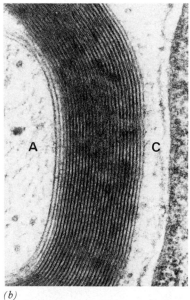

(b)

Fig. 7.10 Myelinated nerve fibre

(EM (a) ×17000 (b) ×75250)

At low magnification, a myelinated nerve fibre is seen sectioned transversly at the level of the nucleus of an associated Schwann cell **S**. A single large axon **A** is enveloped by many spiral layers of fused, Schwann cell plasma membrane forming a thick myelin sheath **M**. At higher magnification, it can be seen that Schwann cell cytoplasm is completely absent from the myelin sheath and

that the sheath consists merely of many regular layers of plasma membrane material. These successive layers of predominantly lipid material are thought to insulate the axon from the extracellular environment thus preventing ion fluxes across the plasma membrane of the nerve axon. The Schwann cell cytoplasm **C** encircles the myelin sheath and has no unusual ultrastructural features.

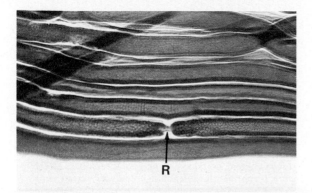

Fig. 7.11 Node of Ranvier
(Teased preparation: Sudan black × 320)

The myelin sheath of an individual axon is provided by many Schwann cells (oligodendrocytes in the CNS), each Schwann cell covering only a segment of the axon. Between the Schwann cells there are short intervals at which the axon is not covered by a myelin sheath; these points are known as *nodes of Ranvier*. In this teased preparation of myelinated axons, a node of Ranvier **R** is seen, representing a site where the continuity of the myelin sheath is interrupted. With this method, only the lipid of the myelin has been stained, thus Schwann cell nuclei are not seen.

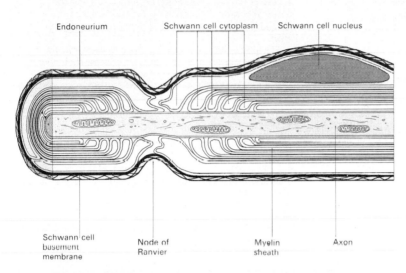

Endoneurium — Schwann cell cytoplasm — Schwann cell nucleus

Schwann cell basement membrane — Node of Ranvier — Myelin sheath — Axon

Fig. 7.12 Node of Ranvier

This diagram illustrates the manner in which Schwann cells terminate at the node of Ranvier, so exposing the axon to the external environment. It is believed that the myelin sheath prevents the nerve action potential from being propagated continuously along the axon and that the action potential travels by jumping from node to node. This mode of conduction, known as *saltatory conduction*, is thought to be the mechanism by which myelination greatly enhances the conduction velocity of axons. The internodal distance is proportional to the diameter of the fibre and may be up to one millimetre in the largest fibres.

Synapses and neuromuscular junctions

Synapses are highly specialised, intercellular junctions which link the neurones of each nervous pathway, and which link neurones and their effector cells such as muscle fibres; where neurones synapse with skeletal muscle they are referred to as *neuromuscular junctions* or *motor end plates*. Individual neurones intercommunicate via a widely variable number of synapses depending on their location within the nervous system. Classically, the axon of one neurone synapses with the dendrite of another neurone, but axons may synapse with the cell bodies or axons of other neurones; dendrite-to-dendrite and cell body-to-cell body synapses have also been described. For a given synapse, the conduction of an impulse is always in one direction only, but the response may be either excitatory or inhibitory depending on the specific nature of the synapse and its location within the nervous system.

The mechanism of conduction of the nerve impulse is thought to involve the release from one neurone of a chemical transmitter substance, or neurotransmitter, which then diffuses across a narrow intercellular space to induce excitation or inhibition in the other neurone or effector cell of that synapse. Neurotransmitters mediate their effects by interacting with specific receptors incorporated in the opposing plasma membrane.

The chemical nature of neurotransmitters and the morphology of synapses, is highly variable in different parts of the nervous system, but the principles of synaptic transmission and the basic structure of synapses is the same throughout the nervous system.

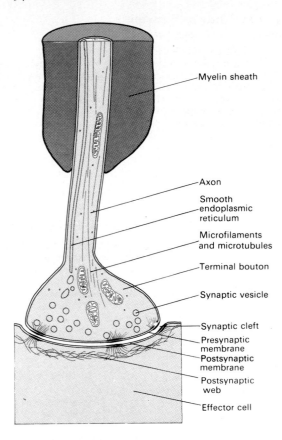

Myelin sheath

Axon

Smooth
endoplasmic
reticulum

Microfilaments
and microtubules

Terminal bouton

Synaptic vesicle

Synaptic cleft
Presynaptic
membrane
Postsynaptic
membrane
Postsynaptic
web

Effector cell

Fig. 7.13 Synapse

This diagram illustrates the general structure of the synapse. The neurone responsible for propagating the stimulus terminates at a swelling or terminal bouton; this is separated from the plasma membrane of the opposed neurone or effector cell by a narrow intercellular gap of uniform width (20 to 30nm) called the *synaptic cleft*. The terminal boutons are not myelinated. The boutons contain mitochondria and membrane-bound vesicles of neurotransmitter substance known as *synaptic vesicles*. Although many types of neurotransmitter substance occur in the CNS only two types are known in the peripheral nervous system: acetylcholine and noradrenaline (norepinephrine). Acetylcholine precursors, acetate and choline, are synthesised in the perikaryon and transported to the synapse where they are conjugated. Noradrenaline synthesis takes place in both the perikaryon and the terminal bouton. Synaptic vesicles are thought to be derived by budding from the smooth endoplasmic reticulum of the axon.

Synaptic vesicles tend to aggregate towards the *pre-synaptic membrane* and are thought to release their contents into the synaptic cleft by exocytosis on the arrival of an action potential. The neurotransmitter diffuses across the synaptic cleft to stimulate receptors in the *post-synaptic membrane*. Associated with synapses are a variety of biochemical mechanisms such as hydrolytic and oxidative enzymes which inactivate the released neurotransmitter between successive nerve impulses. The cytoplasm beneath the post-synaptic membrane often contains a feltwork of fine fibrils, the *post-synaptic web*, which may be associated with desmosome-like structures in maintaining the integrity of the synapse.

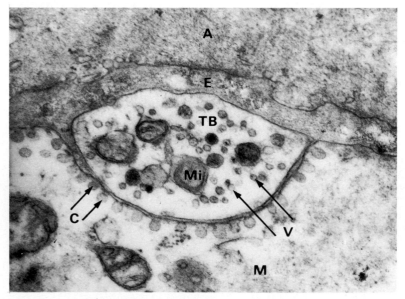

Fig. 7.14 Synapse
(EM ×45000)

This micrograph illustrates a synapse between a sympathetic nerve and a smooth muscle cell in the vas deferens. The terminal bouton **TB** is recessed into the surface of the effector muscle cell **M** in an area devoid of contractile filaments. Note the uniform width of the synaptic cleft between the pre- and post-synaptic membranes. The terminal bouton contains a few mitochondria **Mi** and numerous synaptic vesicles **V**. The post-synaptic membrane exhibits many flask-like invaginations **C** which may represent caveolae (see Fig. 5.15). Note an adjacent smooth muscle cell **A** and delicate intervening endomysial connective tissue **E**.

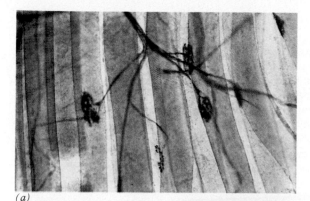

(a)

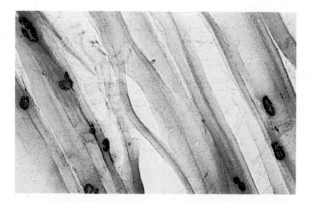

(b)

Fig. 7.15 Motor end plates

*(Teased preparations: gold impregnation method
(a) × 320 (b) × 800)*

These micrographs illustrate synapses between a motor neurone and skeletal muscle cells. One motor neurone may innervate from one to several hundred muscle fibres depending on the precision of movement of the muscle; a motor neurone and the muscle fibres which it supplies constitute a *motor unit*.

At low magnification the terminal part of the axon of a motor neurone is seen dividing into several branches, each terminating as a motor end plate on a different skeletal muscle fibre. At high magnification, a terminal branch is seen to lose its myelin sheath and divide to form a cluster of small swellings on the muscle fibre surface. The motor end plate occupies a recess in the muscle cell surface and is covered by an extension of the cytoplasm of the last Schwann cell surrounding the axon. The connective tissue covering the nerve (endoneurium) becomes continuous with the endomysium of the muscle fibre. Each of the terminal swellings of the cluster making up the motor end plate has the same basic structure as the synapse shown in Fig. 7.13. The post-synaptic membrane of the neuromuscular junction is highly folded, thus increasing the surface area exposed to the neurotransmitter.

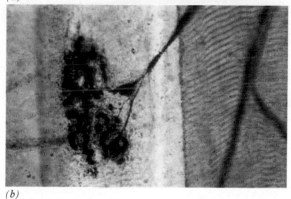

Fig. 7.16 Motor end plates

(Histochemical method for acetylcholinesterase × 320)

The neurotransmitter of somatic neuromuscular junctions is acetylcholine. The hydrolytic enzyme acetylcholinesterase is present at the synapse and is involved in deactivation of the neurotransmitter between successive nerve impulses. This histochemical method defines the location of motor end plates by demonstrating acetylcholinesterase activity which appears as a brown deposit.

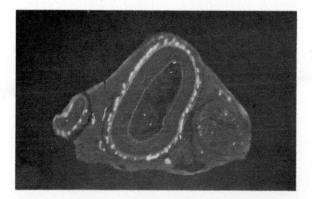

Fig. 7.17 Sympathetic nerve endings

(Formalin-induced fluorescence × 80)

Noradrenaline is the main post-ganglionic neurotransmitter in the sympathetic nervous system. When noradrenaline combines with formalin (and some other compounds) it becomes fluorescent and can be visualised by fluorescence microscopy.

This micrograph illustrates formalin-induced fluorescence in the adventitial layer of large and small arteries, corresponding to the presence of sympathetic, noradrenergic nerve endings. Background autofluorescence outlines the general tissue structure; note that the internal elastic lamina is particularly autofluorescent.

Peripheral nervous tissues

Peripheral nerves are anatomical structures which may contain any combination of afferent or efferent nerve fibres of either the somatic or autonomic nervous systems. The cell bodies of fibres coursing in peripheral nerves are either located in the CNS or in ganglia in peripheral sites.

Each peripheral nerve is composed of one or more bundles or *fascicles* of nerve fibres; within the fascicles, each individual nerve fibre, with its investing Schwann cell, is surrounded by a delicate packing of loose connective tissue called *endoneurium* which contains a few fibroblasts and blood capillaries. Each fascicle is surrounded by a condensed layer of collagenous connective tissue called the *perineurium*. In peripheral nerves consisting of more than one fascicle, a further layer of loose connective tissue called the *epineurium* binds the fascicles together and is condensed peripherally to form a cylindrical sheath. The larger blood vessels supplying the nerve are found within the epineurium. The fibres within a peripheral nerve derive considerable mechanical strength from these three layers of connective tissue.

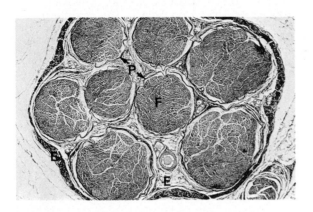

Fig. 7.18 Peripheral nerve
(TS: van Gieson × 20)

This micrograph illustrates the typical appearance of a medium sized peripheral nerve in transverse section. This nerve consists of eight fascicles **F**, each of which contains many nerve fibres. Each fascicle is invested by a condensed connective tissue layer, the perineurium **P**, and the nerve as a whole is encased in a loose connective tissue sheath, the epineurium **E**, which is condensed at its outermost aspect. Blood vessels of various sizes can be seen in the epineurium.

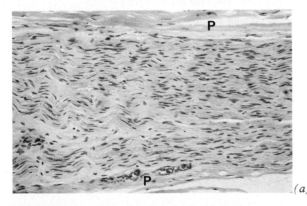

(a)

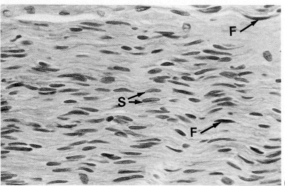

(b)

Fig. 7.19 Peripheral nerve
(LS: H & E (a) × 128 (b) × 320)

The peripheral nerves shown in these micrographs consist of a single fascicle invested by dense perineurium **P** containing small blood vessels; a separate epineurium cannot be distinguished. Most of the nuclei seen within the fascicle are those of Schwann cells which mark the course of individual axons; axons are not readily visible in this type of preparation. Fibroblasts of the endoneurium are scattered amongst the much more numerous Schwann cells. A striking feature of peripheral nerves is that the fibres follow a longitudinal zigzag course which permits stretching during movement.

At higher magnification, Schwann cell nuclei **S** are seen to be elongated in the long axis of the nerve. The relatively sparse fibroblasts **F** are distinguished by their more slender, condensed nuclei.

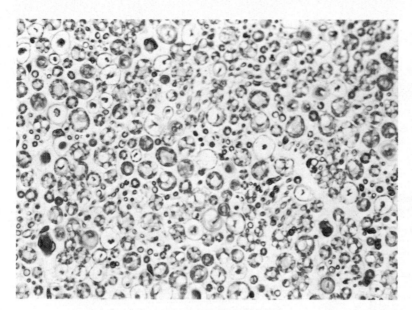

Fig. 7.20 Peripheral nerve

(TS: H & E ×640)

In routinely fixed and stained preparations, myelin is poorly preserved since it is largely composed of lipid material. In this preparation, Schwann cell cytoplasm is well preserved and appears as an eosinophilic band around unstained areas representing both myelinated and non-myelinated fibres. Several capillaries are seen within the endoneurium. Extreme variation in the diameter of the constituent nerve fibres reflects the functional heterogeneity typical of peripheral nerves.

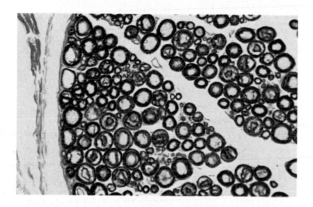

Fig. 7.21 Peripheral nerve

(TS: Osmium fixation: van Gieson ×800)

In osmium-fixed preparations, the lipid constituents of myelin are well preserved and are stained black. Note the wide variation in axon diameter. The collagen of the delicate endoneurium between the individual nerve fibres and in the condensed perineurium surrounding the fascicles is stained red by the van Gieson method.

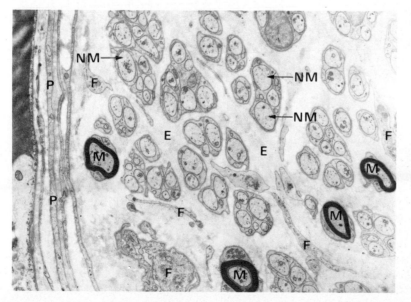

Fig. 7.22 Peripheral nerve

(TS: EM ×5200)

The ultrastructural features of peripheral nerves are seen in this example which contains both myelinated **M** and non-myelinated **NM** fibres. The endoneurium **E** consists of loosely arranged collagen fibres lying parallel to the nerve fibres. Strands of fibroblast cytoplasm **F** extend throughout the endoneurium. In contrast, the perineurium **P** consists of extremely flattened fibroblasts and more densely packed collagen fibres.

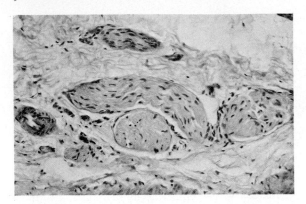

Fig. 7.23 Small peripheral nerves
(H & E × 320)

The typical appearance of small peripheral nerve branches is illustrated in this micrograph; such small nerves, in transverse, longitudinal and oblique section, are frequently encountered in the supporting tissues of many organs. The perineurium of very small peripheral nerves merges with the collagen fibres of surrounding connective tissues; such nerves are usually recognisable in longitudinal section as wavy bundles of Schwann cell nuclei.

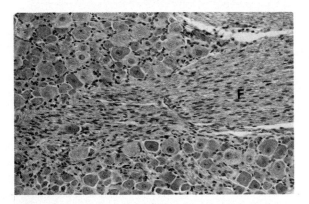

Fig. 7.24 Spinal ganglion
(H & E × 128)

Ganglia consist of discrete aggregations of neurone cell bodies located outside the CNS. Ganglia, such as the spinal sensory ganglia and sympathetic chain ganglia, are large and contain numerous nerve cell bodies. Each cell body is surrounded by a single layer of flattened support cells called *satellite cells*. The whole ganglion is encapsulated by condensed connective tissue which is continuous with the perineurial and epineurial sheaths of the associated peripheral nerve. This micrograph shows the large cell bodies of primary sensory neurones which are of the pseudounipolar form; note the fascicle **F** of nerve fibres derived from these cell bodies. A spinal ganglion is shown at higher magnification in Fig. 7.3 (b).

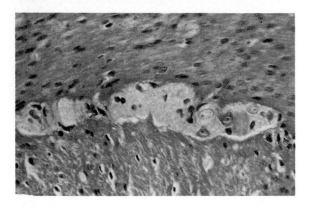

Fig. 7.25 Parasympathetic ganglion
(H & E × 320)

The cell bodies of the terminal effector neurones of the parasympathetic nervous system are usually located within the effector organs. The cell bodies may be aggregated as well-organised ganglia of moderate size, as in the otic ganglion; more usually, however, only a few cell bodies are clumped together to form minute, poorly organised ganglia scattered in the supporting connective tissue of the organs. This micrograph illustrates a minute ganglion in the supporting tissue between two smooth muscle layers in the wall of the gastro-intestinal tract.

Central nervous tissues

The central nervous system consists of the brain and spinal cord, each of which can be divided grossly into areas of so-called *grey matter* and *white matter*; grey matter contains almost all the neurone cell bodies and their associated fibres, whereas white matter consists merely of tracts of nerve fibres. Central nervous tissue consists of a vast number of neurones and their processes embedded in a mass of support cells, collectively known as *neuroglia*; there is little intercellular matrix.

Neuroglial cells are of four types: *astrocytes*, *oligodendrocytes*, *microglia* and *ependymal cells*. Astrocytes are extremely numerous, star-shaped cells which are thought to provide mechanical and metabolic support for neurones. Oligodendrocytes are functionally analogous to the Schwann cells of peripheral nervous tissues in that they are responsible for myelination in the CNS. Microglia are small phagocytic cells which are thought to be the CNS representatives of the macrophage-monocyte defence system. Ependymal cells form a simple epithelium which lines the ventricles of the brain and central canal of the spinal cord.

The outer surface of the brain and spinal cord is covered by three specialised connective tissue layers, collectively known as the *meninges*. Although each functional zone of the CNS has its own peculiar histological appearance, the basic organisation of grey and white matter remains consistent throughout; only the principles of organisation are discussed in this section.

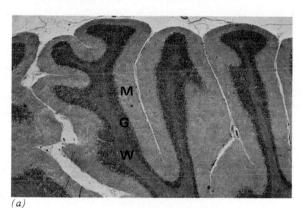

(a)

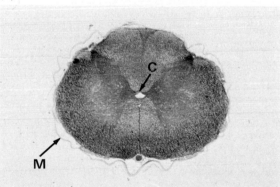

(b)

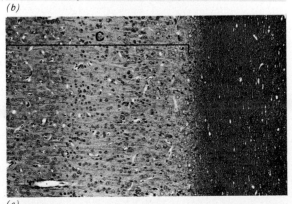

(c)

Fig. 7.26 Central nervous tissues

(a) Cerebellum (H & E × 8)
(b) Spinal cord (Gold method × 8)
(c) Cerebral cortex (Methylene blue × 20)

This series of micrographs illustrates the general features of three major regions of the CNS and three different staining methods useful in neurohistology. The cerebellar cortex comprises two zones, an outer so-called molecular layer **M** which is strongly eosinophilic, and an inner so-called granular layer **G** which is strongly basophilic. The unusual multipolar Purkinje cells shown in Fig. 7.5 are arranged at the junction of the two zones. The central core **W** of the cerebellum is white matter consisting of densely packed nerve fibres.

In transverse section, the spinal cord varies in appearance along its length, but it basically consists of a central butterfly-shaped region of grey matter, stained golden in this preparation, and an outer zone of white matter. Note the central canal **C** and the outer covering of meninges **M**.

The cerebrum, shown at higher magnification, has the opposite arrangement of grey and white matter to that of the spinal cord, the grey matter forming the outer cerebral cortex **C** and the white matter consisting of a mass of fibre tracts in the central core. The neurones of the cerebral cortex are arranged in a variable number of layers depending on the region, each layer containing neurones of a characteristic morphology; evidence of layering can be seen in this micrograph.

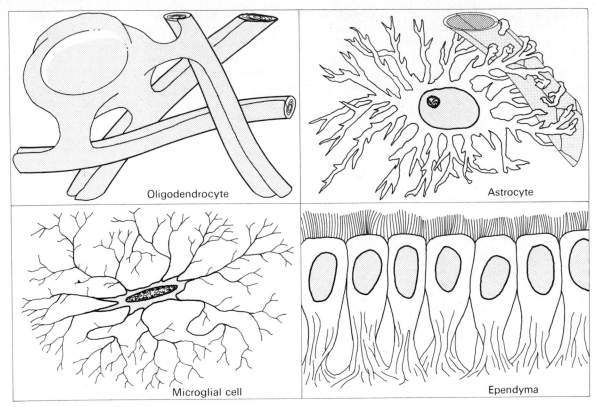

Fig. 7.27 Neuroglia

The neuroglia comprise all the non-neural cells of the CNS. These highly branched cells, which form almost half the total mass of the CNS, occupy the spaces between neurones; the CNS thus contains little extracellular material. The neuroglia have intimate and apparently essential functional relationships with neurones providing both mechanical and metabolic support.

Four principal types of neuroglia are recognised: oligodendrocytes, astrocytes, microglia and ependymal cells.

(i) Oligodendrocytes: oligodendrocytes (oligodendroglia) are cells of moderate size which were named for their appearance when stained by classical methods with which they appeared to have a small number of short, branched processes. It is now known that oligodendrocytes are the cells responsible for myelination of axons in the CNS and the dendrites previously described are the short pedicles that connect the cell body to the myelin sheaths. A single oligodendrocyte may be responsible for the myelination of up to fifty nerve fibres. Oligodendrocytes are the predominant type of neuroglia in white matter. Oligodendrocytes also aggregate closely around neurone cell bodies in the grey matter where they are thought to have a support function analogous to that of the satellite cells which surround neurone cell bodies in peripheral ganglia (see Fig. 7.24).

(ii) Astrocytes: classical impregnation methods (as in Fig. 7.29) identified the existence of star-shaped neuroglia subsequently called astrocytes. These cells, which are the most numerous glial cells in grey matter, have prolific, long,

highly branched processes which occupy most of the interneuronal spaces. In grey matter, many of the astrocyte processes end in terminal expansions upon the basement membranes of capillaries; these are thus called *perivascular feet*. Other processes of the same astrocytes terminate in close apposition to the non-synaptic regions of neurones. Perivascular feet cover most of the capillary basement membranes. On the basis of these observations it has been suggested that astrocytes in grey matter mediate some metabolic exchange between neurones and blood. All astrocytes contain bundles of intracellular microfilaments which are particularly prominent in the astrocytes of white matter. Thus astrocytes in white matter are called *fibrous astrocytes* whilst those of grey matter are called *protoplasmic astrocytes*.

(iii) Microglia: microglia are small cells, relatively few in number, derived from cells of mesenchymal origin which invade the CNS at a late stage of fetal development. Microglia have small, irregular nuclei and relatively little cytoplasm which extends as fine, highly branched processes. In response to tissue damage, microglia transform into large, amoeboid, phagocytic cells and are thus considered to be members of the macrophage-monocyte defence system (see Chapter 3).

(iv) Ependymal cells: ependymal cells form the simple, cuboidal, epithelial lining of the ventricles and spinal canal. Most ependymal cells are ciliated at their luminal surface and from their tapered bases give rise to a single branched process which intermingles with the cytoplasmic processes of underlying astrocytes.

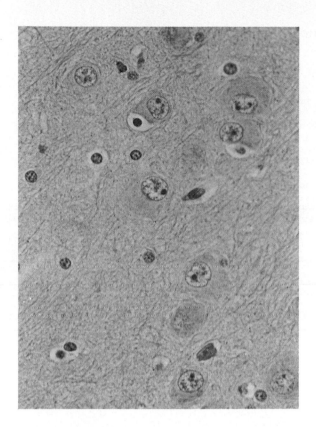

Fig. 7.28 Grey matter

(H & E × 480)

Common staining methods usually permit neurones to be readily distinguished from glial cells. Although the size and morphology of neurones varies greatly in different regions of the brain, they are usually recognisable by their basophilic, granular cytoplasm, one or more processes of which can often be seen. The nuclei of neurones are generally large and have prominent, dense nucleoli.

Neuroglia, particularly oligodendrocytes, have highly variable histological characteristics and are difficult to distinguish by common staining methods; they are best identified by metallic impregnation methods.

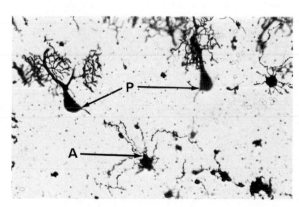

Fig. 7.29 Astrocyte

(Golgi-Cox × 128)

This impregnation method outlines the cytoplasmic processes of all the cellular elements of the CNS. In this preparation, taken from the cerebellar cortex, unusual neurones called Purkinje cells **P** and astrocytes **A** can be identified.

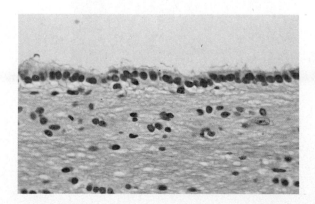

Fig. 7.30 Ependyma

(H & E × 320)

Ependymal cells form a simple epithelial lining to the ventricles and spinal canal. The cells are tightly bound together at their luminal surfaces by the usual epithelial junctional complexes (see Chapter 4). Unlike other epithelia, however, ependyma does not rest on a basement membrane but rather the tapering basal process of each ependymal cell extends as a fine branched process into a layer of processes derived from astrocytes. The role of the variable number of cilia present on the luminal surface in propelling cerebro-spinal fluid within the ventricles is unclear, as is the role of ependymal cells in absorption and secretion processes.

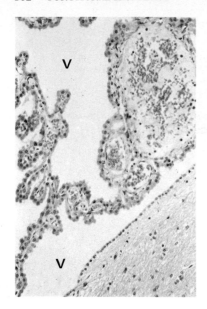

Fig. 7.31 Choroid plexus
(H & E × 128)

The choroid plexus is a vascular structure, arising from the wall of each of the four ventricles of the brain, responsible for the production of cerebro-spinal fluid (CSF). CSF drains from the interconnected ventricular cavities via three channels connecting the fourth ventricle with the subarachnoid space which surrounds the CNS (see Fig. 7.32). CSF is produced at a constant rate and is primarily reabsorbed from the subarachnoid space into the superior sagittal venous sinus via finger-like projections called *arachnoid villi*. Thus the CNS is suspended in a constantly circulating fluid medium which acts as a shock absorber.

Each choroid plexus consists of a mass of capillaries projecting into the ventricle **V** and invested by modified ependymal cells. The choroid epithelial cells are separated from the underlying capillaries and their supporting connective tissue by a basement membrane. Long, bulbous microvilli project from the luminal surfaces of the choroid epithelial cells and the cytoplasm contains numerous mitochondria. These features suggest that the elaboration of CSF is an active process. The capillaries of the choroid plexus are large, thin-walled and fenestrated. The mode of CSF secretion is thought to involve active secretion of sodium ions by choroid epithelial cells into the CSF, followed by passive movement of water from the choroid capillaries. Small amounts of protein, as well as glucose at the same concentration as that of plasma, are normal constituents of CSF but the mode of their passage into the CSF is unknown.

Fig. 7.32 Meninges

The brain and spinal cord are invested by three layers of connective tissue collectively called the meninges. The surface of the nervous tissue is covered by a delicate layer called the *pia mater* containing fibroblasts, collagenous fibres and the processes of underlying astrocytes. Overlying the pia mater is a thicker fibrous layer, the *arachnoid mater*, which derives its name from the presence of web-like strands which connect it to the underlying pia mater; since the pia and arachnoid are structurally continuous, they are often considered as a single unit, the *pia-arachnoid* or *leptomeninges*. The space between the pia and arachnoid layers is called the *subarachnoid space* and in places forms large cisterns. The subarachnoid space is connected with the ventricles by three foramina and CSF circulates continuously from the ventricles into the subarachnoid space. The apposed surfaces of the pia and arachnoid layers, and their interconnecting fibres, are lined by flattened mesothelial cells. The outer surface of the arachnoid mater is also lined by mesothelium.

The arteries and veins of the CNS pass in the subarachnoid space loosely attached to the pia mater. As the larger vessels extend into the nervous tissue they are surrounded by a delicate layer of pia mater. Between the penetrating vessels and the pia there is a *perivascular space* which is continuous with the subarachnoid space.

Beyond the arachnoid mater is a dense fibro-elastic layer called the *dura mater* which is lined on its internal surface by mesothelium. The dura is closely applied to, but not connected with, the arachnoid layer and a potential space, the *subdural space*, containing a minute amount of fluid separates the two layers. In the cranium, the dura mater merges with the periosteum of the skull whereas around the spinal cord the dura is suspended from the periosteum of the spinal canal by the so-called *denticulate ligaments*; the intervening *epidural space* is filled with loose, fibro-fatty connective tissue and a venous plexus.

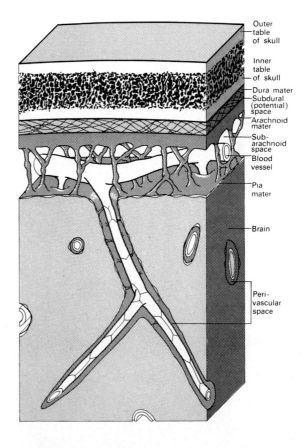

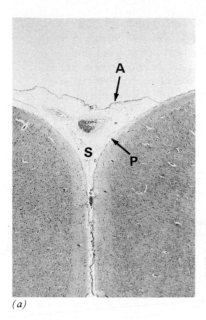

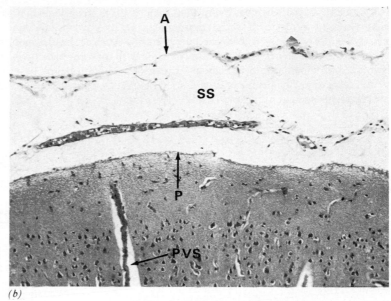

Fig. 7.33 Meninges

(H & E (a) ×20 (b) ×198)

These micrographs demonstrate the pia and arachnoid layers of the brain meninges; the dura mater remains adherent to the skull when the brain is removed from the cranial cavity.

The pia mater **P** is intimately attached to the surface of the brain and continues into the sulci **S** and around the penetrating vessels. The arachnoid mater **A** appears to be a completely separate layer and bridges the sulci. At higher magnification, delicate fibrous strands can be seen traversing the subarachnoid space **SS** to connect the pia and arachnoid layers. Both these layers consist of delicate connective tissue the surface of which is lined by flattened mesothelium.

The subarachnoid space contains arteries and veins; their branches dip into the brain substance, surrounded by a perivascular space **PVS** which is continuous with the subarachnoid space and is thus filled with CSF. The CNS contains no lymphatics, and interstitial fluid is thought to drain outwards from the brain substance to join the subarachnoid CSF via the perivascular spaces.

Many constituents of plasma are unable to pass from the circulatory system into the CNS and this has led to the theory that a *blood-brain barrier* exists. Although poorly understood, this barrier probably consists of the brain capillary endothelial cells, which are bound by tight junctions, and their supporting basement membrane. The perivascular feet of astrocytes (see Fig. 7.27) probably play a less important role.

Organs of sensory reception

Sensory receptors are nerve endings or specialised cells which convert (transduce) stimuli from the external or internal environments into afferent nerve impulses; the impulses pass into the CNS where they initiate appropriate voluntary or involuntary responses.

No classification system for sensory receptors has yet been devised which adequately incorporates either functional or morphological features. A widely used functional classification divides sensory receptors into three groups: *exteroceptors*, *proprioceptors* and *interoceptors*. Exteroceptors are those which respond to stimuli from outside the body, and include separate receptors for touch, light pressure, deep pressure, cutaneous pain, temperature, smell, taste, sight and hearing. Proprioceptors are located within the skeletal system and provide conscious and unconscious information about orientation, skeletal position, tension and movement; such receptors include the vestibular apparatus of the ear, tendon organs and neuromuscular spindles. Interoceptors respond to stimuli from the viscera and include the chemoreceptors of blood, vascular baroreceptors, the receptors for the state of distension of hollow viscera such as the gastro-intestinal tract and urinary bladder, and receptors for such nebulous senses as visceral pain, hunger, thirst, well-being and malaise.

The nature of the receptors involved in some of these sensory modalities is poorly understood; however, sensory receptors may be classified morphologically into two groups: *simple* and *compound*. Simple receptors are merely free, branched or unbranched nerve endings such as those responsible for cutaneous pain and temperature. Simple receptors are rarely visible with the light microscope unless special staining methods are employed. Compound receptors involve organisation of non-neural tissues to complement the function of neural receptors. The degree of organisation may range from mere encapsulation to highly sophisticated arrangements such as in the eye.

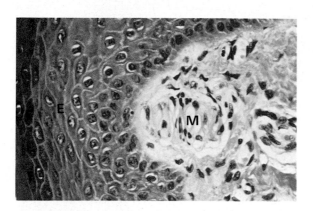

Fig. 7.34 Meissner's corpuscle
(*H & E × 320*)

Meissner's corpuscles are small, encapsulated, sensory organs found in the dermis of the skin, particularly of the fingertips, soles of the feet and erogenous areas. They are involved in the reception of light discriminatory touch; the degree of discrimination in a given area depends on the proximity of receptors to one another.

Meissner's corpuscles **M** are oval in shape and are usually located in the dermal papillae immediately beneath the skin epithelium **E**. The receptors consist of a delicate connective tissue capsule surrounding a mass of plump, oval cells arranged transversely; non-myelinated branches of large myelinated sensory fibres ramify throughout the cell mass.

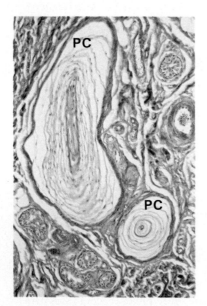

Fig. 7.35 Pacinian corpuscles
(*Masson's trichrome × 80*)

This micrograph illustrates Pacinian corpuscles **PC** in transverse and longitudinal section. These sensory organs are responsive to pressure or coarse touch, vibration and tension, and are found in the deeper layers of the skin, ligaments and joint capsules, serous membranes, mesenteries, some viscera and in some erogenous areas.

Pacinian corpuscles range from one to four millimetres in length and in section have the appearance of an onion. These organs consist of a delicate capsule enclosing many concentric lamellae of flattened cells separated by interstitial fluid spaces and connective tissue fibres. Towards the centre of the corpuscle the lamellae become closely packed and the core contains a single, large, unbranched, non-myelinated nerve fibre which becomes myelinated as it leaves the corpuscle. Distortion of the Pacinian corpuscle produces an amplified mechanical stimulus in the core which is transduced into an action potential in the sensory neurone.

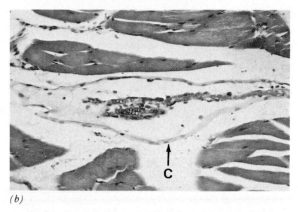

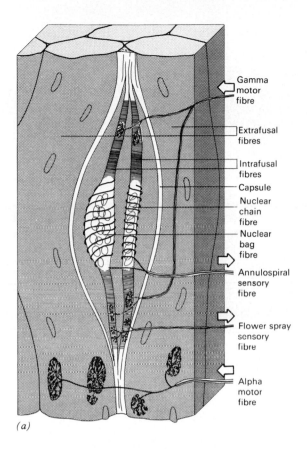

Gamma
motor
fibre

Extrafusal
fibres

Intrafusal
fibres

Capsule

Nuclear
chain
fibre

Nuclear
bag
fibre

Annulospiral
sensory
fibre

Flower spray
sensory
fibre

Alpha
motor
fibre

(a)

(b)

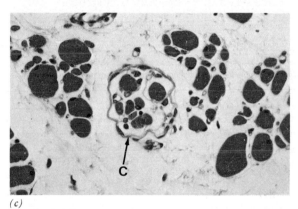

(c)

Fig. 7.36 Neuromuscular spindle

(a) Schematic diagram (b) LS (H & E × 320) (c) TS (Masson's trichrome × 320)

Neuromuscular spindles are stretch receptor organs within skeletal muscles which are responsible for the regulation of muscle tone via the spinal stretch reflex. The sensitivity of these receptors is modulated by higher centres via fibres passing in the extrapyramidal tracts. These receptors are particularly numerous in muscles involved in fine, precision movements such as the intrinsic muscles of the hand and the external muscles of the eye.

Neuromuscular spindles are encapsulated, lymph filled, fusiform structures up to six millimetres long but less than one millimetre in diameter. They lie parallel to the muscle fibres, embedded in endomysium or perimysium. Each spindle contains from two to ten modified skeletal muscle fibres called *intrafusal fibres* which are much smaller than the skeletal muscle fibres proper, the *extrafusal fibres*. The intrafusal fibres have a central non-striated area in which their nuclei tend to be concentrated. Two types of intrafusal fibres are recognised. In one type, the central nuclear area is dilated and these fibres are known as *nuclear bag fibres*. In the other type, there is no dilatation and the nuclei are arranged in a single row giving rise to the name *nuclear chain fibres*.

Associated with both types of intrafusal fibre are sensory receptors of two types. Firstly, branched, non-myelinated endings of large, myelinated sensory fibres are wrapped around the central non-striated area of the intrafusal fibres forming the so-called *annulo-spiral endings*. Secondly, so-called *flower-spray endings* of smaller, myelinated sensory fibres are located on the striated portions of the intrafusal fibres.

Together, these sensory receptors are stimulated by stretching of the intrafusal fibres which reflects stretching of the extrafusal muscle mass. This stimulus evokes reflex contraction of the extrafusal muscle fibres via large (alpha) motor neurons of a simple two-neurone spinal reflex arc. Contraction of the extrafusal muscle mass thus removes the stretch stimulus from the intrafusal stretch receptors and equilibrium is restored.

The sensitivity of the intrafusal fibres to stretching is modulated by higher centres via small (gamma) motor neurones arising from the extrapyramidal system. These gamma motor neurones innervate the striated portions of the intrafusal fibres thus controlling their state of contraction. Contraction of the intrafusal fibres increases the sensitivity of the intrafusal receptors to stretching of the extrafusal mass.

In any one histological section it is impossible to demonstrate all the structural features of a neuromuscular spindle, but many of the features of the organ are shown in these micrographs. The most easily recognisable features are the discrete capsule **C**, which is continuous with the endomysium of the surrounding muscle, and the small size of the intrafusal muscle fibres compared with the surrounding extrafusal fibres.

Fig. 7.37 Olfactory receptors

The receptors for the sense of smell are located in a modified form of respiratory epithelium (see Figs. 4.10 and 4.11), called *olfactory epithelium*, in the nasal cavity; although extensive in some mammals such as the dog, the olfactory epithelium is restricted to a small area in the roof of the nasal cavity in man. The olfactory epithelium is extremely tall, pseudostratified columnar in form and contains cells of three types: olfactory receptor cells, supporting epithelial (*sustentacular*) cells and basal epithelial cells.

The *olfactory receptor* cells are true bipolar neurones (see Fig. 7.2), the cell bodies of which are located in the middle stratum of the olfactory epithelium. A single dendritic process extends from the cell body to the free surface where it terminates as a small swelling which gives rise to about a dozen extremely long, modified cilia. These cilia are non-motile and lie flattened against the epithelial surface. The cilia are thought to be the sites of interaction between odiferous substances and the receptor cells. At the basal aspect, each receptor cell gives rise to a single fine, non-myelinated axon which penetrates the basement membrane to join the axons of other receptor cells. The bundles of axons pass via about twenty small holes on each side of the cribriform plate of the ethmoid bone to reach the olfactory bulbs of the forebrain where they synapse with second order sensory neurones.

The supporting or sustentacular cells are elongated cells with their tapered bases resting on the basement membrane. Many long microvilli extend from their luminal surfaces to form a tangled mat with the cilia of the receptor cells. At the luminal surface, the plasma membranes of the sustentacular and receptor cells are bound by typical junctional complexes. The functions of the sustentacular cells are poorly understood but they probably provide mechanical and physiological support for the receptor cells. The basal cells are small, conical cells which may represent epithelial stem cells.

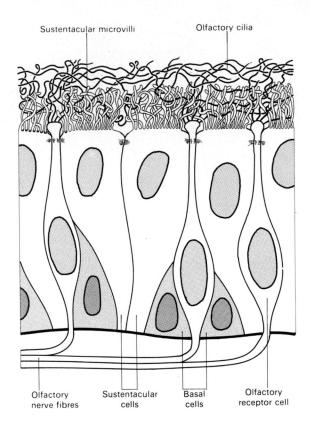

Fig. 7.38 Olfactory epithelium

(H & E × 480)

In histological section it is difficult to distinguish the different cell types of olfactory epithelial cells; the nuclei of sustentacular cells occupy the uppermost stratum, those of the receptor cells the middle stratum, and the basal cells lie close to the basement membrane. Note the terminal bar **B** at the luminal surface, representing junctional complexes; note also the tangled meshwork of microvilli and cilia on the surface.

The olfactory epithelium is supported by a vascular, loose connective tissue containing bundles of afferent nerve fibres **N** and numerous serous glands called *Bowman's glands* **G** which produce the watery surface secretions in which odiferous substances are dissolved.

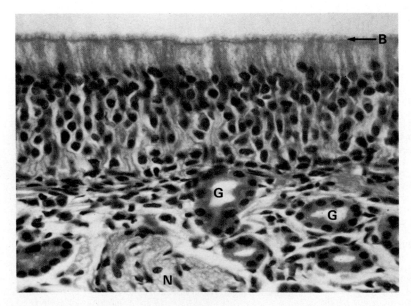

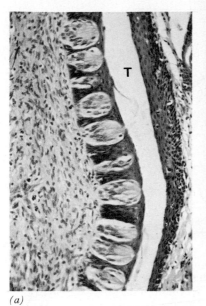

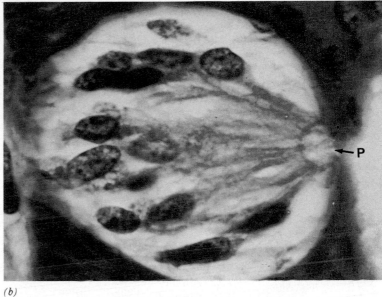

(a)   (b)

Fig. 7.39 Taste buds

(*H & E (a) × 128 (b) × 1200*)

Taste buds, the chemoreceptors for the sense of taste or *gustation*, are in man mainly located in the epithelium of the circumvallate papillae of the tongue (see Fig. 12.13), although they are also found scattered in other parts of the tongue, palate, pharynx and epiglottis. In the circumvallate papillae, taste buds face into the deep troughs **T** surrounding the papillae as shown in micrograph (a). Serous glands, called the glands of von Ebner (see Fig. 12.13), drain into the troughs where the serous secretion is thought to act as a solvent for taste-provoking substances.

The taste bud is a barrel-shaped organ extending the full thickness of the epithelium and opening at the surface via a pore known as the *taste pore* **P**. Each taste bud contains from twenty to thirty long, spindle-shaped cells which extend from the basement membrane to the taste pore. Classically, two types of cell are described in the taste bud: light *gustatory cells* and dark *supporting* or *sustentacular cells*. A third cell type, the *basal cell*, is now generally recognised and may constitute the precursor of one or both of the other cell types. Both gustatory and sustentacular cells have long microvilli which extend into the taste pore which contains a glycoprotein substance thought to be secreted by the sustentacular cells.

Ultrastructural studies have shown non-myelinated nerve fibres to be associated with both cell types, but there appears to be a more intimate, synapse-like relationship between the nerve fibres and the gustatory cells. Although the so-called gustatory cells are thought to be the taste receptors, the sustentacular cells may also serve some receptor function. Like the oral epithelium, all the cells of the taste bud are renewed continuously though the gustatory and sustentacular cells are replaced at different rates.

Four taste modalities are recognised: sweet, bitter, acid and salt. Each modality tends to be principally perceived in a specific region of the tongue; however, no structural differences have been demonstrated between taste buds from different areas. The sensations of taste and smell are closely associated and loss of olfactory sense is accompanied by diminished gustatory perception.

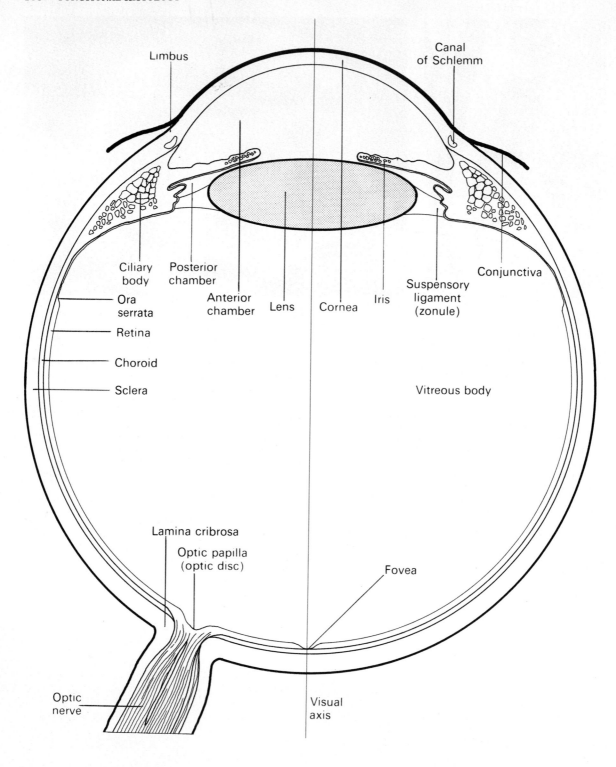

Limbus

Canal
of Schlemm

Ciliary
body

Posterior
chamber

Conjunctiva

Ora
serrata

Anterior
chamber

Lens

Cornea

Iris

Suspensory
ligament
(zonule)

Retina

Choroid

Sclera

Vitreous body

Lamina cribrosa

Optic papilla
(optic disc)

Fovea

Optic
nerve

Visual
axis

Fig. 7.40 The eye *(illustration opposite)*

The eye is a highly specialised organ of photoreception, a process which involves the conversion of different quanta of light energy into nerve action potentials. The photoreceptors are modified dendrites of two types of cells, *rod cells* and *cone cells*. The rods are integrated into a system which is receptive to light of differing intensity; this is perceived in a form analogous to a black and white photographic image. The cones are of three functional types receptive to one of the basic colours blue, green and red; they constitute a system by which coloured images may be perceived. The rod and cone receptors and a system of primary integrating neurones are located in the inner layer of the eye, the *retina*. All the remaining structures of the eye serve to support the retina or to focus images of the visual world upon the retina.

The eye is made up of three basic layers: the outer *corneo-scleral layer*, the intermediate *uveal layer* (*uveal tract*) and the inner *retinal layer*.

(i) Corneo-scleral layer: The corneo-scleral layer forms a tough, fibro-elastic capsule which supports the eye. The posterior five-sixths, the *sclera*, is opaque and provides insertion for the extra-ocular muscles. The anterior one-sixth, the *cornea*, is transparent and has a smaller radius of curvature than the sclera. The cornea is the principal refracting medium of the eye and roughly focuses an image on to the retina; the focusing power of the cornea depends mainly on the radius of curvature of its external surface. The corneo-scleral junction is known as the *limbus* and is marked internally and externally by a shallow depression.

(ii) Uveal layer: The middle layer, the uvea or uveal tract, is a highly vascular layer which is made up of three components: the *choroid*, *ciliary body* and the *iris*. The choroid lies between the sclera and retina in the posterior five-sixths of the eye. It provides nutritive support for the retina and is heavily pigmented, thus absorbing light which has passed through the retina. Anteriorly the choroid merges with the ciliary body which is a circumferential thickening of the uvea lying beneath the limbus. The ciliary body surrounds the coronal equator of the *lens* and is attached to it by the *suspensory ligament* or *zonule*. The lens is a biconvex transparent structure, the shape of which can be varied to provide fine focus of the corneal image upon the retina. The ciliary body contains smooth muscle, the tone of which controls the shape of the lens via the suspensory ligament. The lens, suspensory ligament and ciliary body partition the eye into a large posterior compartment and a smaller anterior compartment. The iris, the third component of the uvea, forms a diaphragm extending in front of the lens from the ciliary body so as to incompletely divide the anterior compartment into two chambers; these are known, somewhat confusingly, by the terms, *anterior* and *posterior chamber*. The highly pigmented iris acts as an adjustable diaphragm which regulates the amount of light reaching the retina. The aperture of the iris is called the *pupil*. The anterior and posterior chambers contain a watery fluid, the *aqueous humor*, which is secreted into the posterior chamber by the ciliary body and circulated through the pupil to drain into a canal at the angle of the anterior chamber, the *canal of Schlemm*. The aqueous humor is a source of nutrients for the non-vascular lens and cornea, and acts as an optical medium which is non-refractive with respect to the cornea. The pressure of aqueous humor maintains the shape of the cornea.

The large, posterior compartment of the eye contains a gelatinous mass known as the *vitreous body* consisting of so-called *vitreous humor*. The vitreous body supports the lens and retina from within as well as providing an optical medium which is non-refractive with respect to the lens. In life, the vitreous body contains a canal which extends from the exit of the optic nerve to the posterior surface of the lens; this so-called *hyaloid canal* represents the course of the degenerated hyaloid artery which supplied the vitreous body during embryological development. The vitreous body and hyaloid canal are rarely preserved in histological preparations.

(iii) Retinal layer: The photosensitive retina forms the inner lining of most of the posterior compartment of the eye and terminates along a scalloped line, the *ora serrata*, behind the ciliary body. Anterior to the ora serrata, the retinal layer continues as a non-photosensitive epithelial layer which lines the ciliary body and the posterior surface of the iris.

The visual axis of the eye passes through a depression in the retina called the *fovea* which is surrounded by a yellow pigmented zone, the *macula lutea*. The foveal retina is the area of greatest visual acuity and contains only cone photoreceptors.

Afferent nerve fibres from the retina converge to form the *optic nerve* which leaves the eye via numerous perforations through a part of the sclera known as the *lamina cribrosa*. The retina overlying the lamina cribrosa, the *optic papilla* (*optic disc*) is devoid of photoreceptors and is thus referred to as the *blind spot*.

The blood supply of the eye is derived from the ophthalmic artery via two separate systems, the retinal and uveal systems. The retina is supplied by a central artery passing in the substance of the optic nerve. This *central artery of the retina* branches from the centre of the optic papilla to give rise to end arteries which radiate over the surface of the retina; this system provides a unique view of the microcirculation when observed with an instrument called the ophthalmoscope. The uvea is supplied by branches of the ophthalmic artery which perforate the sclera.

Within the bony orbital cavity, the eye is supported by a loose packing of fatty connective tissue. The exposed surface of the eye is protected by the eyelids. The mucus-secreting epithelium lining the inner surface of the eyelids is reflected at the *superior* and *inferior fornices* on to the exposed surface of the sclera and is known as the *conjunctiva*. The conjunctiva and cornea are moistened and cleansed by watery secretions from the *lacrimal gland*, a small flattened gland located at the upper lateral aspect of the eye. Modified sebaceous glands and apocrine sweat glands (see Chapter 9) of the eyelid provide a superficial oily layer which inhibits evaporation. Tears drain to the inner aspect of the eye and thence into the nasal cavity via the *nasolacrimal duct*.

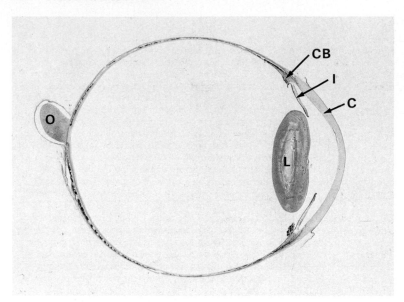

Fig. 7.41 Eye
(Monkey: H & E × 5)

This horizontal section shows the relative sizes of the components of the eye. At this magnification, the three layers comprising the wall of the globe are not readily distinguishable although in the wall of the posterior compartment, the middle layer of choroid is recognisable by its high content of pigment. The other uveal structures, the ciliary body **CB** and iris **I** are readily visible. The lens **L** has been artefactually distorted during preparation and the suspensory ligament is not preserved. Note the relative thickness of the cornea **C**. The optic nerve **O** is seen to penetrate the sclera medial to the visual axis; the fovea is not present in this section.

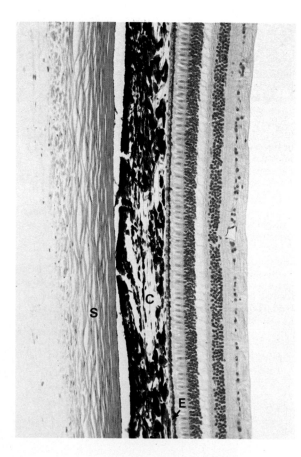

Fig. 7.42 Wall of the eye
(H & E × 198)

The three layers of the wall of the eye are illustrated in this micrograph. The inner, photosensitive retina is a multilayered structure, the outermost limit of which is defined by a layer of pigmented epithelial cells **E**. The choroid **C** is a highly vascular layer of loose connective tissue lying between the retina and the outer sclera **S**. The choroid blood vessels nourish the outer layers of the retina by diffusion.

The choroid contains numerous, large, heavily pigmented cells called *melanocytes* which confer the dense pigmentation characteristic of the choroid. The pigment absorbs light rays passing through the retina and prevents interference due to light reflection. The sclera consists of dense, fibro-elastic connective tissue, the fibres of which are arranged in bundles parallel to the surface. This layer contains little ground substance and few fibroblasts. The sclera varies in thickness, being thickest posteriorly and thinnest at the coronal equator of the globe.

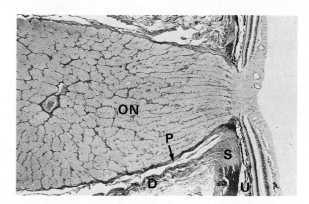

Fig. 7.43 Optic nerve

(Haematoxylin/van Gieson × 20)

The afferent fibres from the retina converge at a point medial to the fovea, the optic papilla or optic disc, and penetrate the sclera **S** through the lamina cribosa to form the optic nerve **ON**. Photoreceptor cells are absent from the optic papilla which is thus a blind spot in the retina.

The optic nerve and retina develop embryologically as an outgrowth of the primitive forebrain, thus the optic nerve is invested by meninges. The dura mater **D** becomes continuous with its developmental equivalent, the sclera, whilst the pia-arachnoid **P** continues into the eye as the uveal tract **U**.

Note the central artery and accompanying vein within the substance of the optic nerve and retinal branches of these vessels within the optic papilla.

Fig. 7.44 Ciliary body

(H & E (a) × 128 (b) × 320)

The ciliary body is continuous with the choroid and is located circumferentially between the ora serrata and the limbus. The ciliary body is lined by a double layer of cuboidal epithelium. The deep layer is highly pigmented and represents a forward continuation of the pigmented epithelial layer of the retina. The surface layer, which is not pigmented, is a non-photosensitive forward extension of the receptor layer of the retina.

The ciliary body is attached to the coronal equator of the lens **L** by the suspensory ligament **S** which consists of extremely fine collagenous strands which seldom remain intact after histological preparation; a few aggregated shreds of the suspensory ligament are seen in micrograph (a). Tension in the suspensory ligament tends to flatten the lens which, in the relaxed state, assumes a more globular shape. The bulk of the ciliary body consists of smooth muscle **M** arranged in such a manner that when it contracts, tension upon the suspensory ligament is reduced thus permitting the lens to assume a more convex shape. This mechanism permits fine focusing of images already roughly focused upon the retina by the cornea. The ciliary muscle is innervated by parasympathetic nerve fibres.

From that part of the ciliary body exposed to the angle of the posterior chamber **PC**, there project a number of epithelial folds called *ciliary processes* containing a connective tissue core rich in fenestrated capillaries. The ciliary processes are responsible for the continuous production of aqueous humor which then circulates into the anterior chamber via the pupil. Aqueous humor is continuously reabsorbed into the canal of Schlemm at the angle of the anterior chamber.

Aqueous humor is a clear, watery fluid somewhat similar in composition to CSF and hypotonic with respect to plasma. The mode of production of aqueous humor is presumed to be an active process mediated by the two epithelial layers lining the ciliary processes. Balanced rates of secretion and reabsorption of aqueous humor result in the maintenance of a constant intra-ocular pressure of about 15mm of mercury which stabilises the lens and cornea. The flow of aqueous humor also provides for a continuous exchange of metabolites with the cells of the avascular cornea and lens.

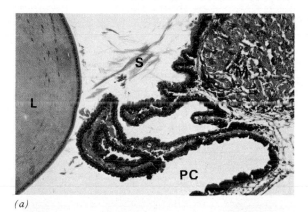

(a)

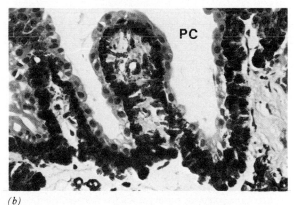

(b)

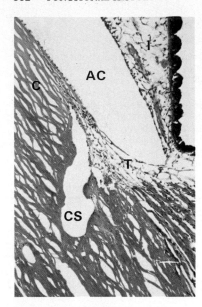

Fig. 7.45 Canal of Schlemm
(H & E ×50)

The canal of Schlemm **CS** is a circumferential canal lined by endothelium which is situated in the inner aspect of the corneal margin **C** immediately adjacent to the angle of the anterior chamber **AC**. At the angle of the anterior chamber there is a meshwork of fine connective tissue trabeculae **T** lined by endothelium; aqueous humor percolates through the spaces between the trabeculae before reaching the canal of Schlemm. There is no direct communication between the trabecular spaces and the canal of Schlemm thus reabsorption of aqueous humor involves passage across two layers of endothelium and intervening connective tissue. The mechanism of transport is not understood; disruption of this process leads to increased intraocular pressure as in the disease known as *glaucoma*. The canal of Schlemm drains via minute channels through the sclera into the episcleral venous system. Note the close relationship of the root of the iris **I** with the canal of Schlemm.

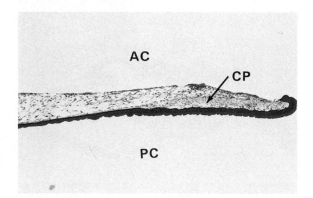

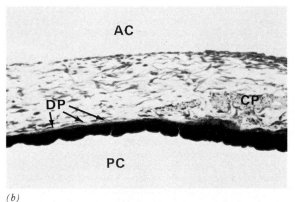

(a) *(b)*

Fig. 7.46 Iris
(H & E (a) ×20 (b) ×80)

The iris is the most anterior part of the uveal layer of the eye. It arises from the ciliary body and forms a diaphragm in front of the lens thus dividing the anterior compartment of the eye into posterior **PC** and anterior chambers **AC** which communicate via the pupil. The pupillary edge of the iris rests on the anterior edge of the lens in life.

The main mass of the iris consists of loose, highly vascular connective tissue which is pigmented due to the presence of numerous melanocytes scattered in the stroma. The anterior surface of the iris is irregular and consists of a discontinuous layer of fibroblasts and melanocytes. In contrast, the posterior surface is relatively smooth and is lined by epithelium which is derived embryologically as a continuation of the two layers which line the surface of the ciliary body (see Fig. 7.44). The surface layer, non-pigmented in the ciliary body, becomes heavily pigmented in the iris such that the individual cells are completely obscured. The deep layer, pigmented in the ciliary body, is transformed in the iris into non-pigmented myoepithelial cells which constitute the radially orientated *dilator pupillae* **DP** muscle of the iris. Even at high magnification, these myoepithelial cells are difficult to distinguish.

The *constrictor muscle of the pupil (constrictor pupillae)* **CP** consists of a band of circumferentially oriented smooth muscle fibres in the pupillary aspect of the stroma. Like the smooth muscle of the ciliary body, the constrictor pupillae is innervated by the parasympathetic nervous system whereas the myoepithelial cells of the dilator pupillae are innervated by the sympathetic nervous system.

The colour of the iris depends on the amount of pigment in the connective tissue stroma, the amount of pigment in the posterior epithelial layer being relatively constant between individuals. Blue eyes contain little stromal pigment whereas brown eyes have much stromal pigment.

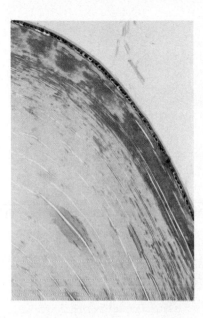

Fig. 7.47 Lens

(H & E × 50)

The lens is an elastic, biconvex body which, although transparent and apparently amorphous, is almost entirely composed of living cells. Embryologically, the lens is derived from ectodermal epithelium which becomes isolated from the surface during development. The mature lens is mainly composed of epithelial cells which have become extremely elongated and have lost their nuclei although their cytoplasmic metabolism continues at a low rate. These cells, which are known as *lens fibres*, contain a crystalline protein and the cell membranes of adjacent fibres are fused leaving little intervening extracellular substance. The cellular nature of the lens is not readily evident with conventional light microscopy and the lens is particularly prone to artefactual distortion during histological preparation.

The anterior aspect of the lens is marked by a single layer of cuboidal epithelial cells which retain their nuclei; some of the cells near the periphery of the equator of the lens also retain their nuclei although these degenerate with increasing age. The whole of the lens is enclosed by a homogenous capsule rich in glycoprotein which represents a specialised remnant of the epithelial basement membrane.

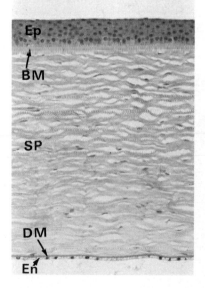

Fig. 7.48 Cornea

(H & E × 80)

The cornea is the thick, transparent portion of the corneo-scleral layer enclosing the anterior one-sixth of the eye. The relatively fixed convexity of the external surface provides the principal mechanism for focusing images upon the retina. The cornea is an avascular structure consisting of five layers. The outer surface is lined by stratified squamous epithelium **Ep** about five cells thick. This epithelium is supported by a specialised basement membrane known as *Bowman's membrane* **BM** which is particularly prominent in man. The bulk of the cornea, the *substantia propria* **SP**, consists of a highly regular form of dense collagenous connective tissues. Fibroblasts and occasional leucocytes are scattered in the corneal ground substance. The inner surface of the cornea is lined by a layer of flattened endothelial cells **En** which are supported by a very thick elastic basement membrane known as *Descemet's membrane* **DM**. The cornea is sustained by diffusion of metabolites from the aqueous humor and the blood vessels of the limbus; some oxygen is derived directly from the external environment.

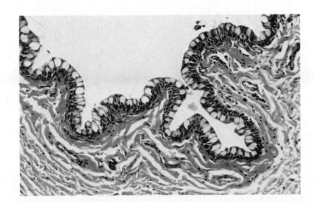

Fig. 7.49 Conjunctiva

(Haematoxylin/van Gieson × 128)

The conjunctiva, the lining of the exposed part of the sclera and inner surface of the eyelids, has a stratified columnar epithelium which is unusual in that it contains goblet cells in the surface layers. The conjunctival mucous secretions contribute to the protective layer on the exposed surface of the eye.

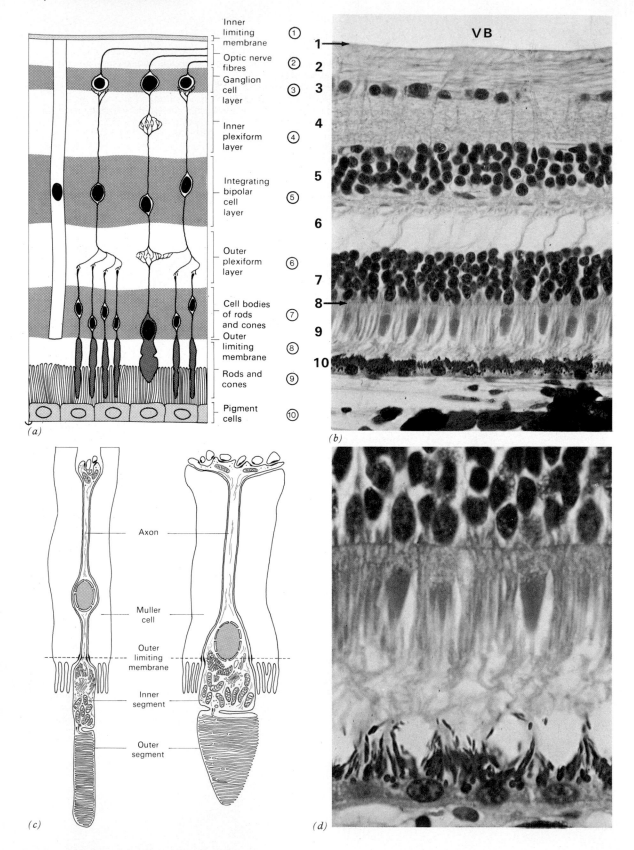

(a)

Inner limiting membrane	①
Optic nerve fibres	②
Ganglion cell layer	③
Inner plexiform layer	④
Integrating bipolar cell layer	⑤
Outer plexiform layer	⑥
Cell bodies of rods and cones	⑦
Outer limiting membrane	⑧
Rods and cones	⑨
Pigment cells	⑩

(b)

VB

(c)

Axon

Muller cell

Outer limiting membrane

Inner segment

Outer segment

(d)

Fig. 7.50 Retina *(illustrations opposite)*
(a) visual afferent pathways
(b) retina (H & E ×640)
(c) rod and cone receptors: ultrastructure
(d) rod and cone receptors (H & E × 1200)

Classically, the retina is divided into ten distinct histological zones as shown in (b); these layers represent the arrangement of five functional groups of neurones as shown diagramatically in (a). The outermost cell layer of the retina consists of pigmented epithelial cells resting on the choroid. Three functional layers of neurones extend to the inner limiting membrane of the retina: the outer layer (lying adjacent to the pigmented epithelium) consists of rod and cone receptor cells; the intermediate layer consists of a network of cells which integrate sensory inputs from the receptor cells before transmission to the CNS; the innermost layer comprises so-called *ganglion cells*, the cell bodies of afferent fibres passing to the CNS in the optic nerve. The fifth functional group of cells are support cells known as *Muller cells* which extend between the so-called *outer* and *inner limiting membranes*. The outer limiting membrane merely represents a dense zone of junctional complexes between Muller cells and the photoreceptor cells. The inner limiting membrane represents the basement membrane separating the bases of the Muller cells from the vitreous body **VB**.

The rod photoreceptors are long, slender, bipolar cells. As shown diagramatically in (c), the single dendrite of each cell extends beyond the outer limiting membrane as the rod proper. The rod proper consists of inner and outer segments connected by a thin, eccentric strand of cytoplasm containing nine microtubule doublets similar to those of cilia but without the inner pair of microtubules. The inner segment contains a prominent Golgi apparatus and many mitochondria. The outer segment has a regular, cylindrical shape and contains a stack of flattened membranous discs which incorporate the visual pigment *rhodopsin* (visual purple). The rods are ensheathed by cylindrical, cytoplasmic processes extending from the outer pigmented epithelial cells. The membranous discs of the rods are continuously shed from the end of each rod and phagocytised by the pigmented epithelial cells; the discs are continuously replaced from the inner segment of the rod. In essence, the transduction process involves the interaction of light with rhodopsin molecules which promotes a configurational change within the membrane thus initiating an action potential. The action potential then passes inwards along the dendrite and axon to the layer of integrating neurones.

Cone photoreceptors are similar in basic structure to the rod cells, but they differ in several important details. The outer segment of the receptor proper is a long, conical structure containing membranous discs; however, unlike the situation in the rods, the spaces between the discs are continuous with the extracellular environment as illustrated in (c). The discs are not shed although the tips of the cones

are invested by processes of pigmented epithelial cells. The cones contain pigments receptive to blue, green and red light rather than rhodopsin as in the rods; the mechanism of transduction is probably similar. The bodies of the cone cells are generally continuous with the inner segment of the cone proper without an intervening dendritic process. The nuclei of cone cells thus form a row of nuclei immediately inside the outer limiting membrane. The dimensions of the rods and cones differ in various parts of the retina as do the numerical proportions of rods and cones; the typical appearance of rods and cones at high magnification is shown in micrograph (d).

The photoreceptor cells are connected to the ganglion cells by a variety of bipolar neurones each of which may synapse with several receptor cells in the *outer plexiform layer*. Similarly, these interneurones may synapse with more than one ganglion cell in the *inner plexiform layer*. *Horizontal cells* (not shown in diagram (a)) with their cell bodies amongst those of the bipolar cells, make lateral connections in the outer plexiform layer between groups of rod and cone receptors. A variety of neurones, known as *amacrine cells*, which lack axons but have numerous dendrites, also have their cell bodies in the bipolar layers; these cells (also not illustrated diagramatically) form integrative connections in the inner plexiform layer.

All of the neurones of the retina are supported by extremely irregularly shaped Muller cells which radiate from the inner to outer limiting membranes. The nuclei of these cells are also located in the bipolar cell layer.

Fibres of the ganglion cells form the layer immediately adjacent to the inner limiting membrane; the fibres are interspersed with neuroglia similar to those of the CNS. This layer also contains the retinal vascular system derived from the central artery of the optic nerve.

In order to reach the photoreceptor units therefore, light rays must pass through blood vessels and several layers of cells and their processes. At the fovea, that part of the retina with the most visual acuity, the inner layers are flattened laterally so as to present less of a barrier to the light reaching the receptor units. In the fovea, the receptors are almost exclusively cones and there is an almost one to one ratio of optic nerve fibres to receptor units. The fovea and surrounding macula are not supplied by the retinal arteries but are dependant on diffusion from the underlying choroid vessels.

During histological preparation, the retina frequently becomes detached from the wall of the eye and the plane of cleavage is usually between the layer of rods and cones and the layer of pigmented epithelial cells. This is also the plane along which the retina cleaves in the living eye in the pathological condition known as *retinal detachment*.

8. Skin

Introduction

The skin, or integument, forms the continuous external surface of the body and in different regions of the body varies in thickness, colour and the presence of hairs, glands and nails. Despite these variations, which reflect different functional demands, all types of skin have the same basic structure. The external surface of skin consists of a keratinised squamous epithelium called the *epidermis*. The epidermis is supported and nourished by a thick underlying layer of dense, fibro-elastic connective tissue called the *dermis* which is highly vascular and contains many sensory receptors. The dermis is attached to underlying tissues by a layer of loose connective tissue called the *hypodermis* or *subcutaneous layer* which contains variable amounts of adipose tissue. Hair follicles, sweat glands, sebaceous glands and nails are epithelial structures termed *epidermal appendages* since they originate during embryological development from downgrowths of epidermal epithelium into the dermis and hypodermis.

The skin is the largest organ of the body, constituting almost one sixth of the total body weight; it has four major functions:

(i) Protection: the skin provides protection against ultraviolet light and mechanical, chemical and thermal insults; its relatively impermeable surface prevents excessive dehydration and acts as a physical barrier to invasion by micro-organisms.

(ii) Sensation: the skin is the largest sensory organ in the body and contains a variety of receptors for touch, pressure, pain and temperature.

(iii) Thermoregulation: in man, skin is a major organ of thermoregulation. The body is insulated against heat loss by the presence of hairs and subcutaneous adipose tissue. Heat loss is facilitated by evaporation of sweat from the skin surface and increased blood flow through the rich vascular network of the dermis.

(iv) Metabolic functions: subcutaneous adipose tissue constitutes a major store of energy, mainly in the form of triglycerides. Vitamin D is synthesised in the epidermis and supplements that derived from dietary sources.

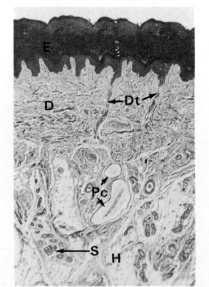

Fig. 8.1 Skin (fingertip)
(Masson's trichrome × 8)

The general structure of skin is illustrated in this preparation of thick skin from the fingertip. The epidermis **E** consists of a stratified squamous keratinising epithelium which, in this site, has an extremely thick keratinised surface layer. A prominent feature of the skin of the fingertips, palms and soles of the feet is a pattern of surface ridges formed by the epidermis; this pattern is unique to each individual.

The epidermis is supported by the dermis **D**, a layer of dense fibro-elastic tissue, the fibres of which are stained green in this preparation. The dermis merges with the loose connective tissue of the hypodermis **H** which consists largely of adipose tissue; in this site, adipose tissue acts as a soft, shock-absorbing layer. Numerous sweat glands **S** are located in the dermis and hypodermis and discharge their secretions on to the skin surface via long excretory ducts **Dt**. Pressure receptors, Pacinian corpuscles **Pc** (see Fig. 7.35) are located deep in the dermis and are a prominent feature of fingertip skin.

The junction between the epidermis and dermis is characterised by downward folds of the epidermis called *epidermal ridges* which interdigitate with upward projections of the dermis called *dermal papillae*. This arrangement enhances the adhesion of the epidermis to the dermis and is accentuated in skin subject to considerable frictional forces.

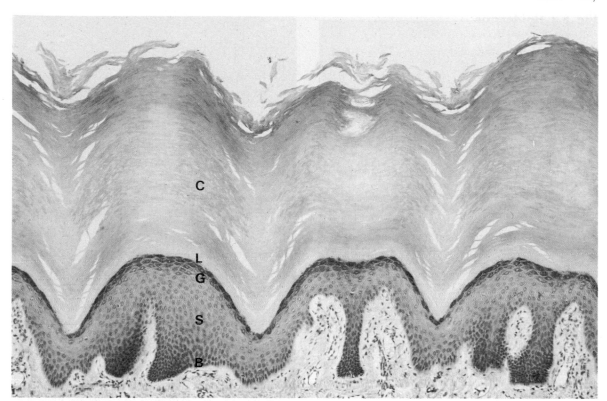

Fig. 8.2 Epidermis (fingertip)
(H & E × 104)

This section of thick skin, taken from the same specimen as Fig. 8.1, demonstrates the general features of the epidermis Cells produced by mitosis in the germinal layer adjacent to the dermis undergo maturational changes concerned with the production of keratin. The outer keratinised layer is shed continuously and is replaced by the progressive movement and maturation of cells from the germinal layer. The rate of mitosis in the germinal layer generally equals the rate of desquamation of keratin from the outer surface.

The phases of this dynamic process are represented in five morphological layers:

(i) The stratum germinativum or stratum basale B is the germinal layer of the epidermis.
(ii) The stratum spinosum or prickle cell layer S, so named for the 'prickly' appearance of the cells at high magnification (see Fig. 8.4), contains cells which are in the process of growth and early keratin synthesis.
(iii) The stratum granulosum or granular layer G is characterised by the presence within the cells of granules which contribute to the process of keratinisation.
(iv) The stratum lucidum L is only present in extremely thick skin, and appears as a homogeneous layer between the stratum granulosum and the keratinised layer.
(v) The stratum corneum or cornified layer C consists of flattened, fused cell remnants composed mainly of the fibrous protein, keratin.

The process of maturation of a basal cell through to desquamation takes approximately 27 days in man.

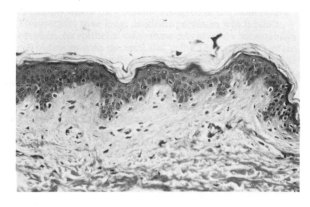

Fig. 8.3 Epidermis (abdomen)
(H & E × 128)

In this preparation of thin skin from the abdomen, the individual cellular layers are more difficult to discern and a stratum lucidum is not present. In comparison with thick skin, the stratum corneum is much reduced in thickness and the combined thickness of the other layers is reduced to a lesser extent.

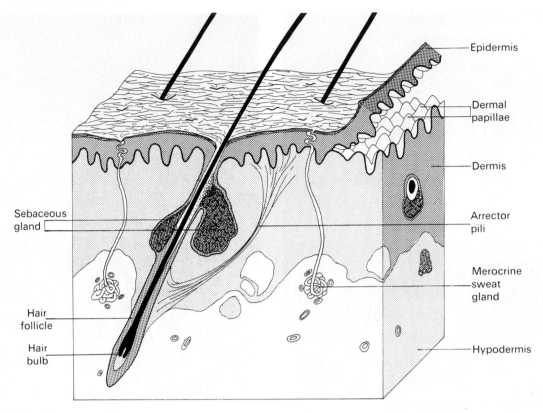

Epidermis

Dermal papillae

Dermis

Arrector pili

Merocrine sweat gland

Hypodermis

Sebaceous gland

Hair follicle

Hair bulb

Fig. 8.6 Skin appendages

Skin has a variety of appendages, principally hairs, sebaceous glands and sweat glands, which are derived embryonically from the surface epithelium. The distribution, arrangement and detailed structure of the appendages varies from one part of the skin to another but nevertheless the general structure conforms to a basic pattern. The three-dimensional arrangement shown in this diagram has been deduced from studies of serial sections of skin; individual sections of skin rarely demonstrate all these features.

Hairs: hairs are highly modified keratinised structures produced by *hair follicles* which are essentially cylindrical downgrowths of the surface epithelium ensheathed by connective tissue. Hair growth takes place within a terminal expansion of the follicle, the *hair bulb*, which consists of actively dividing epithelial cells surrounding a papilla of connective tissue, the *dermal papilla*. Hair follicles undergo periods of growth and quiescence and this is reflected in changes in their structure. Actively growing follicles penetrate deeply into the hypodermis and the hair bulb is prominent, whereas quiescent follicles are shorter and the hair bulb is smaller and lacking in a dermal papilla; quiescent follicles are known as *club hairs*. In addition, the structure of hair follicles depends on the type of hair being produced. For example, the follicles of the scalp tend to be long and straight, whereas those of the trunk, which produce fine, downy hair, are relatively short and plump; curly hair may be produced by curved follicles or follicles in which the hair bulb lies at an angle to the hair shaft.

A bundle of smooth muscle, the *arrector pili* muscle, is attached to the connective tissue sheath of each follicle and is inserted into the dermal papillary zone. Contraction of the arrector pili erects the hair and pulls down its point of

insertion, producing the effect known as 'goose-flesh'.

The arrector pili muscles are innervated by the sympathetic nervous system and pilo-erection is activated by cold or fear. In furry animals, hair erection traps a thicker layer of air over the skin surface thus increasing insulation against heat loss; hair erection also makes the animal appear larger and is thus a protective mechanism in aggressive circumstances. These functions are probably of little physiological significance in man.

Sebaceous glands: one or more sebaceous glands are associated with each hair follicle; these glands secrete an oily substance called *sebum* on to the skin surface in the upper part of the follicle. Sebum acts as a waterproofing agent on the hair and skin surface. In regions of transition from the skin to the body tracts such as the lips, eyelids, glans penis, labia minora and nipples, sebaceous glands are independent of hair follicles and secrete directly on to the skin surface.

Sweat glands: in most areas of the skin, sweat glands are simple, coiled tubular glands which secrete a watery fluid on to the skin surface by the process of merocrine secretion (see Chapter 4). The coiled, secretory portions of these glands are found in the dermis and hypodermis where they are surrounded by a rich plexus of capillaries.

Sweat glands are an important component of the thermoregulatory mechanism in man. When the body requires to lose heat, skin blood flow and sweat production are increased; evaporation of sweat causes cooling of the skin surface and loss of heat from the underlying vascular bed. Merocrine sweat glands are innervated by cholinergic fibres of the sympathetic nervous system; sweating is stimulated not only by excessive body heat but also by fear-provoking stimuli.

A different type of sweat gland is found in the skin of the axilla and genital regions of humans. These glands are analogous to the odiferous glands of many mammals and do not begin to function until puberty. In contrast to the merocrine sweat glands, these glands are believed to secrete by the apocrine process (see Chapter 4) and are thus called *apocrine sweat glands*. They also differ in that they produce a viscid secretion which is discharged into hair follicles rather than directly on to the surface. Apocrine sweat glands are innervated by adrenergic fibres of the sympathetic nervous system.

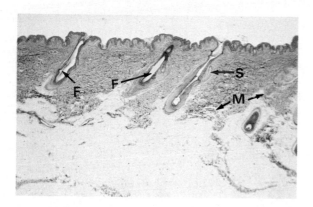

Fig. 8.7 Abdominal skin
(Masson's trichrome × 8)

This micrograph illustrates the typical histological appearance of the skin which covers most of the body. The hair follicles **F** with associated sebaceous glands **S** are sparse. Merocrine sweat glands **M** are relatively abundant.

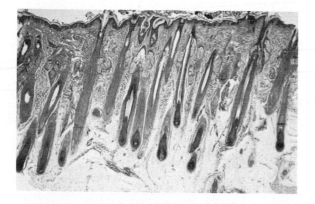

Fig. 8.8 Scalp skin
(H & E × 8)

This specimen from a young, dark-haired, caucasian male illustrates the high density of hair follicles characteristic of the scalp; in older people, and those with fair hair, the follicles are less dense. The follicles of the scalp are particularly long and have more numerous sebaceous glands than those of other areas; merocrine sweat glands are less prominent than in the skin of the trunk and limbs.

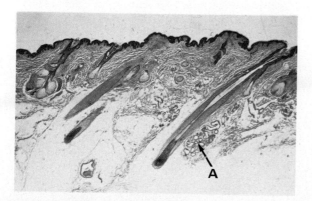

Fig. 8.9 Pubic skin
(H & E × 8)

The skin of the pubic region contains a moderate density of hair follicles which, unlike those of the scalp, tend to be orientated obliquely to the skin surface and are often curved rather than straight. Apocrine sweat glands **A** are a common feature of this type of skin and are seen typically associated with hair follicles.

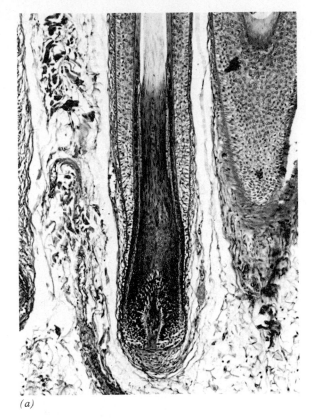

(a)

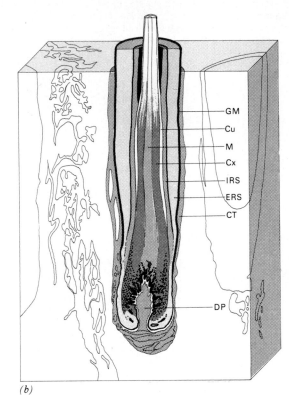

(b)

Fig. 8.10 Hair follicle

(a) LS: H & E × 120
(b) Explanatory diagram for (a)

The hair follicle is a tubular structure consisting of five concentric layers of epithelial cells. As they are pushed towards the skin surface from the hair bulb, the inner three layers undergo keratinisation to form the hair shaft whilst the outer two layers form an epithelial sheath. At the hair bulb, all the layers merge to become indistinguishable from one another.

During active hair growth, the epithelial cells surrounding the dermal papilla **DP** proliferate to form the innermost four layers of the follicle whilst the outermost layer merely represents a downward continuation of the stratum germinativum of the surface epithelium. The whole epithelial mass surrounding the dermal papilla constitutes the *hair root*.

The cells of the innermost layer of the follicle undergo moderate keratinisation to form the *medulla* **M** or core of the hair shaft; the medullary layer is often not distinguishable in fine hairs. The medulla is surrounded by a broad, highly keratinised layer, the *cortex* **Cx** which forms

the bulk of the hair. The third cell layer of the follicle undergoes keratinisation to form a hard, thin *cuticle* **Cu** on the surface of the hair. The cuticle consists of overlapping keratin plates, an arrangement which is said to prevent matting of the hair.

The fourth layer of the follicle constitutes the *internal root sheath* **IRS**; the cells of this layer become only lightly keratinised and disintegrate at the level of the sebaceous gland ducts leaving a space into which sebum is secreted around the maturing hair. The outermost layer, the *external root sheath* **ERS**, does not take part in hair formation; this layer is separated from the sheath of connective tissue **CT** surrounding the follicle by a thick, specialised basement membrane known as the *glassy membrane* **GM**.

In the growing follicle, large active melanocytes (see Fig. 8.5) are scattered amongst the proliferating cells of the hair root. Melanin is transferred mainly to the cells forming the cortex of the hair shaft thereby determining hair colour.

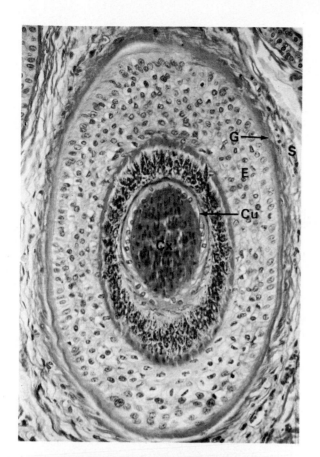

Fig. 8.11 Hair follicle

(H & E × 198)

This is a slightly oblique, transverse section through the lower part of a hair follicle. The broad external root sheath **E** is separated from the connective tissue sheath **S** by the glassy membrane **G**. Passing inwards, the internal root sheath **I** is recognised by its content of eosinophilic (keratohyaline) granules; the outermost cells of the internal root sheath have a more homogeneous appearance. Deep to the internal root sheath is the thin, pale-stained cuticle layer **Cu** which surrounds the strongly stained cortex **Cx**. A medulla is not present in this specimen.

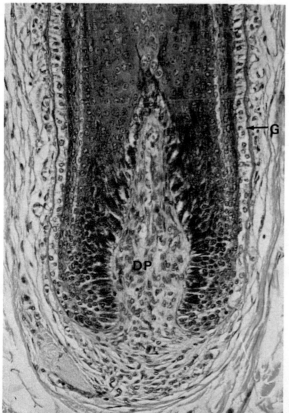

Fig. 8.12 Hair bulb

(Masson's trichrome × 198)

This staining method permits clear delineation of the epithelial and connective tissue elements of the hair follicle. The dermal papilla **DP** is highly vascular and is separated from the epithelial cells by a basement membrane which is continuous with the glassy membrane **G** surrounding the follicle externally. The connective tissue sheath of the follicle is also richly vascular and contains a delicate plexus of sensory nerve endings which are receptive to minute movements of the hair follicle and thus act as highly sensitive touch receptors.

Note the five cell layers of the hair follicle merging with the proliferating cells of the hair root. Note also the large, heavily pigmented melanocytes scattered along the basement membrane of the hair root.

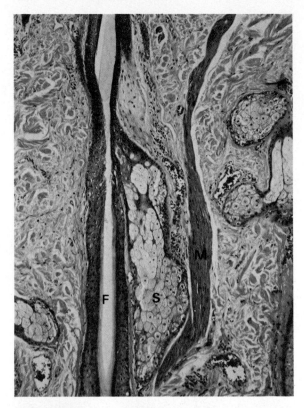

Fig. 8.13 Sebaceous gland and arrector pili muscle
(H & E × 33)

This micrograph illustrates the relationship of a sebaceous gland **S** and an arrector pili muscle **M** to a hair follicle **F**. At a point about one-third of its length from the surface, each hair follicle is surrounded by one or more sebaceous glands which discharge their secretions on to the hair shaft and thence on to the skin surface. Sebaceous glands lie within the connective tissue sheath surrounding the hair follicle and the glandular epithelium represents an outgrowth of the external root sheath.

The arrector pili muscle of each follicle consists of a bundle of smooth muscle fibres. The muscle inserts at one end into the connective tissue sheath of the follicle, at a point below the sebaceous glands, and at the other end into the dermal papillary area beneath the epidermis.

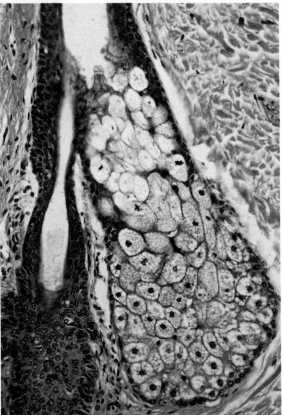

Fig. 8.14 Sebaceous gland
(H & E × 198)

Each sebaceous gland has a branched acinar form, the acini converging upon a short duct which empties into the hair follicle beside the maturing hair; a single acinus is illustrated in this micrograph.

Each acinus consists of a mass of rounded cells which are packed with lipid-filled vacuoles; during tissue preparation the lipid is largely removed, thus the cytoplasm of these cells is poorly stained. Towards the duct, the lipid content of the acinar cells increases greatly and the distended cells degenerate, so releasing their contents, sebum, into the duct by the process known as *holocrine secretion* (see Chapter 4). Cells lost by holocrine secretion are replaced by mitosis in the basal layer of the acinus.

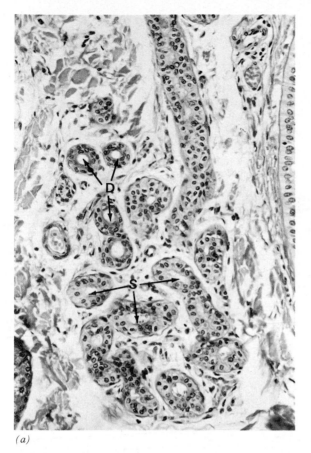

(a)

(b)

Fig. 8.15 Merocrine sweat gland

(H & E (a) ×198 (b) ×480)

Merocrine sweat glands are distributed in the skin of most parts of the body with the exception of areas such as the margins of the lips and the glans penis. Merocrine sweat glands secrete a watery fluid, hypotonic with respect to plasma, the evaporation of which plays an important role in thermoregulation. Sweat contains significant quantities of sodium and chloride ions, some other ions, urea and small molecular weight metabolites; thus sweating may be considered as a minor mode of excretion.

Merocrine sweat glands are unbranched, tubular glands, the secretory portion of which forms a compact coil deep in the dermis. In histological section, the glands appear as a mass of tubules cut in various planes; secretory portions are interspersed with sections of the first part of the excretory duct. The secretory portion **S** consists of a single layer of large cuboidal or columnar cells, whereas the excretory duct **D** is lined by two layers of smaller cuboidal cells. The surrounding dermal connective tissue contains a rich capillary plexus.

At higher magnification, the secretory portions **S** of merocrine sweat glands are seen to be mainly composed of pale-stained, pyramidal-shaped cells which rest on a prominent basement membrane. These cells are believed to pump sodium ions into the gland lumen; this is followed by passive diffusion of water. A second, darkly-stained cell type which is difficult to identify with light microscopy is described; this cell type has ultrastructural features typical of protein secreting cells. The dark cells are believed to secrete a glycoprotein, nevertheless the content of such in sweat is very low. Myoepithelial cells **M** form a discontinuous layer between the secretory cells and the basement membrane; contraction of these cells expels sweat into the excretory ducts.

Sections of the excretory duct **D** are readily distinguishable from sections of the secretory portion. The excretory duct has a narrower lumen, a double layer of small cuboidal cells, no underlying myoepithelial cells and a characteristically eosinophilic luminal aspect which may result from adsorption of the glycoprotein product of the dark secretory cells. The duct epithelium is thought to reabsorb sodium ions from the basic secretion thus making it hypotonic with respect to plasma.

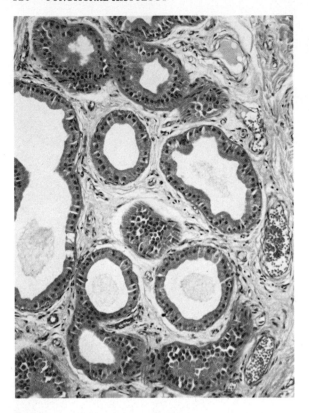

Fig. 8.16 Apocrine sweat gland
(H & E × 128)

Apocrine sweat glands are mainly confined to the axillae
and genital regions where they produce a viscid, milky
secretion which becomes odorous after the action of skin
commensal bacteria.

Apocrine sweat glands are large glands which always
secrete into an adjacent hair follicle via a duct which is
histologically similar to that of merocrine sweat glands. The
secretory portion of the gland is of the coiled, tubular type
with a widely dilated lumen. The secretory cells are usually
low cuboidal and have an eosinophilic cytoplasm. The
budding appearance of the apical cytoplasm of some cells
gave rise to the belief that the mode of secretion was of the
apocrine type but recent evidence suggests that this
appearance may be due to a fixation artefact and that the
original interpretations were erroneous. Like merocrine
sweat glands, apocrine glands have a discontinuous layer of
myoepithelial cells between the base of the secretory cells
and the prominent basement membrane.

Apocrine sweat glands do not become functional until
puberty and in women undergo cyclical changes under the
influence of the hormones of the menstrual cycle (see
Chapter 16). The biological significance of apocrine sweat
glands in humans is probably underestimated.

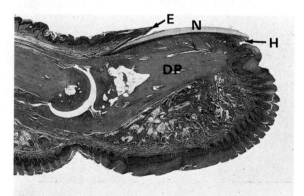

(a)

(b)

Fig. 8.17 Fingernail
(Monkey: H & E (a) × 5 (b) × 20)

The dorsal skin surface of the tip of each finger and toe
forms a highly specialised appendage, the nail. Each nail **N**
is a dense, keratinised plate which rests on a stratified
squamous epithelium called the *nail bed*. The proximal end
of the nail, the *nail root* **R**, and the underlying nail bed
extend deeply into the dermis to lie in close apposition to
the distal interphalangeal joint, and the dermis beneath the
nail plate is firmly attached to the periosteum of the distal
phalanx **DP**.

Nail growth occurs by proliferation and differentiation of
the epithelium surrounding the nail root, and the nail plate
slides distally over the rest of the nail bed which does not
actively contribute to nail growth. Reflecting its
proliferative activity, the epithelium beneath the nail root is
thicker than that of the rest of the nail bed and exhibits
pronounced epidermal ridges.

The skin overlying the root of the nail is known as the
nail fold **F** and its highly keratinised free edge is known as
the *eponychium* **E**. The skin beneath the free end of the nail
is known as the *hyponychium* **H**.

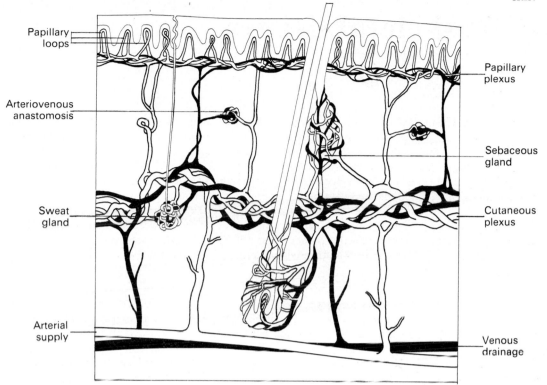

Papillary loops

Papillary plexus

Arteriovenous anastomosis

Sebaceous gland

Sweat gland

Cutaneous plexus

Arterial supply

Venous drainage

Fig. 8.18 The skin circulation

The circulation of the skin has an unusual arrangement which accommodates several different, sometimes conflicting, functional requirements: nutrition of the skin and appendages, increased blood flow to facilitate heat loss in hot conditions *and* decreased blood flow to minimise heat loss in cold conditions whilst maintaining adequate nutritional flow.

The arteries supplying the skin are located deep in the hypodermis from which they give rise to branches passing upwards to form two plexuses of anastomosing vessels. The deeper plexus lies at the junction of the hypodermis and dermis and is known as the *cutaneous plexus*; the more superficial plexus lies just beneath the dermal papillae and is known as the *papillary plexus*. Branches of the cutaneous plexus supply the fatty tissue of the hypodermis, the connective tissues of the deeper aspect of the dermis and capillary networks which envelop the hair follicles and deep

sebaceous glands and sweat glands. The papillary plexus supplies the upper aspect of the dermis and the capillary networks around the superficial appendages. The papillary plexus also gives rise to a capillary loop in each dermal papilla. The venous drainage of the skin is arranged into plexuses broadly corresponding to the arterial supply.

Numerous shunts provide direct arterio-venous communications which play an important role in thermoregulation by controlling blood flow to the appropriate part of the dermis. In the dermis of the finger tips, and other odd peripheral sites prone to excessive cold such as the external ear, the flow in arteriovenous shunts appears to be controlled by curious structures called *glomus bodies* (see Fig. 8.19).

The skin has a rich lymphatic drainage which forms plexuses corresponding to those of the blood vascular system.

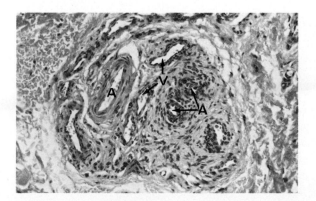

Fig. 8.19 Glomus body
(H & E × 128)

This micrograph illustrates a glomus body in the dermis of the finger tip. The glomus consists of a highly convoluted segment of an arteriovenous shunt enveloped by condensed connective tissue. In histological section, one or more convolutions of the arterial **A** and venous **V** elements of the shunt are usually seen. Just before the arteriovenous junction, the wall of the artery becomes greatly thickened and its smooth muscle cells assume an epithelial appearance. Glomus bodies are richly innervated by the sympathetic nervous system which controls their local thermoregulatory activity.

9. The skeletal tissues

Introduction

The skeletal system is composed of a variety of specialised forms of connective tissue. Bone provides a rigid protective and supporting framework for most of the soft tissues of the body, whereas cartilage provides semi-rigid support in limited sites such as the respiratory tree and external ear. Joints are composite structures which unite the bones of the skeleton and, depending on their structure, permit varying degrees of movement of the skeleton. Ligaments are flexible bands which contribute to the stability of joints. Tendons provide strong, flexible connections between muscles and their points of insertion into bones.

The functional differences between the various tissues of the skeletal system relate principally to the different nature and proportion of the ground substance and fibrous elements of the extracellular matrix. The cells of all the skeletal tissues, like the cells of connective tissues in general, have close structural and functional relationships and a common origin from primitive mesenchymal cells (see Chapter 3).

Cartilage

Cartilage is a semi-rigid form of connective tissue, the characteristics of which mainly stem from the nature and predominance of ground substance in the extracellular matrix. Glycoproteins, containing a high proportion of sulphated polysaccharide units, make up the ground substance and account for the solid, yet flexible, property of cartilage.

Within the ground substance are embedded varying proportions of collagen and elastic fibres giving rise to three main types of cartilage: *hyaline cartilage*, *fibro-cartilage* and *elastic cartilage*.

Cartilage formation commences with the differentiation of stellate-shaped, primitive mesenchymal cells (see Fig. 3.1) to form rounded cartilage precursor cells called *chondroblasts*. Subsequent mitotic divisions give rise to aggregations of closely packed chondroblasts which grow and begin synthesis of ground substance and fibrous extracellular material. Secretion of extracellular material traps each chondroblast in a space or *lacuna* within the cartilagenous matrix thereby separating the chondroblasts from one another. Each chondroblast then undergoes one or two further mitotic divisions to form a small group of mature cells separated by a small amount of extracellular material. Mature cartilage cells, known as *chondrocytes*, maintain the integrity of the cartilage matrix. This differentiation and maturation sequence is most advanced in the centre of a mass of growing cartilage. Towards the periphery of the cartilage, chondroblasts, at progressively earlier stages of differentiation, merge with the surrounding loose connective tissue. On completion of growth, the cartilage mass consists of chondrocytes embedded in a large amount of extracellular matrix. At the periphery of mature cartilage is a zone of condensed connective tissue called *perichondrium*, containing chondroblasts with cartilage-forming potential. Growth of cartilage occurs by *interstitial growth* from within and *appositional growth* at the periphery.

Cartilage is characterised by the absence of blood vessels, lymphatics and nerves. Consequently the exchange of metabolites between chondrocytes and surrounding tissues depends on diffusion through the water of solvation of the ground substance; this limits the thickness to which cartilage may develop, whilst maintaining viability of the innermost cells.

In mature mammals, cartilage has a limited distribution, whereas in immature mammals cartilage occurs more extensively since it forms a template for most of the developing bony skeleton.

Fig. 9.1 Hyaline cartilage: trachea

(H & E × 78)

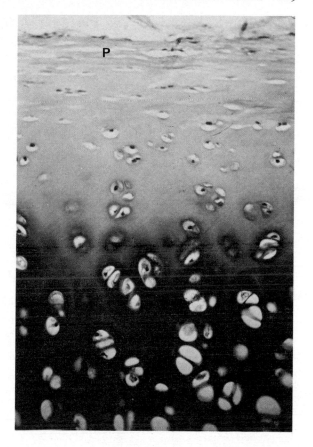

Hyaline cartilage is the most common type of cartilage and is found in the nasal septum, larynx, tracheal rings, most articular surfaces and the sternal ends of the ribs. Mature hyaline cartilage is characterised by small aggregations of chondrocytes embedded in an amorphous matrix of ground substance reinforced by collagen fibres.

In this preparation of mature hyaline cartilage, two distinct zones are evident: an inner, strongly basophilic zone and an outer, pale-stained zone which merges with adjacent connective tissue. The chondrocytes of the inner zone are arranged in characteristic clusters usually consisting of two or four fully differentiated cells. The clusters are separated by a large mass of amorphous cartilage matrix; the cells of each cluster are separated by only a thin zone of extracellular matrix. In standard histological preparations, considerable shrinkage distorts the cellular detail of the chondrocytes and thus they appear not to fully occupy their lacunae.

Extending from the inner zone towards the outer surface of the cartilage, cartilage cells are progressively less differentiated so that the cells of the outer surface, in the *perichondrium* **P**, resemble mature fibroblasts. Note that the cells of the outer zone have not divided to form clusters. The morphological gradation of cartilage cells from the perichondrium to the most mature chondrocytes of the inner zone represents the progressive changes that occur during the development of cartilage. In adult cartilage, cell differentiation in the perichondrium and outer zone is suspended unless growth is stimulated. When growth is stimulated, isolated chondrocytes divide to form clusters thereby promoting interstitial growth, and chondroblasts of the perichondrium differentiate into chondrocytes resulting in appositional growth.

The matrix of hyaline cartilage appears amorphous since the ground substance and collagen have similar refractive indices. With the exception of articular cartilage, the collagen of hyaline cartilage, designated as collagen Type II (see Fig. 3.4), is not cross-banded and is arranged in an interlacing network of fine fibrils; this collagen cannot be demonstrated by light microscopy. The variable staining intensity of the cartilage matrix reflects the concentration of acidic, sulphated glycoproteins; this is greatest around the clusters of fully differentiated cells and least in the perichondrium.

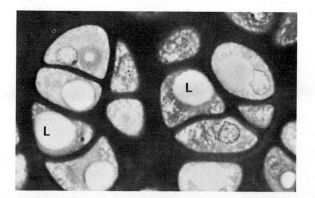

Fig. 9.2 Hyaline cartilage

(Resin embedded, one micron section: toluidine blue × 800)

With this technique the cellular detail of chondrocytes is preserved. Note that the chondrocytes fully occupy the lacunae in the matrix. Mature chondrocytes are characterised by small nuclei with dispersed chromatin and basophilic, granular cytoplasm reflecting a well developed rough endoplasmic reticulum. Lipid droplets **L**, often larger than the nuclei, are a prominent feature of chondrocytes; the cytoplasm is also rich in glycogen. These characteristics reflect the active role of chondrocytes in synthesis of both the ground substance and fibrous elements of cartilage matrix. In fully formed cartilage, the constituents of the extracellular matrix are continuously turned over; the integrity of the matrix is thus dependent on the viability of the chondrocytes.

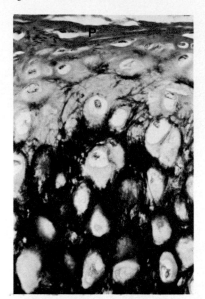

Fig. 9.3 Elastic cartilage
(Elastic van Gieson × 128)

Elastic cartilage occurs in the external ear and external auditory canal, the epiglottis, parts of the laryngeal cartilages and the walls of the Eustachian tubes. The histological structure of elastic cartilage is similar to that of hyaline cartilage; its elasticity, however, derives from the presence of numerous bundles of branching elastic fibres in the cartilage matrix. This network of elastic fibres, stained black in this preparation, is so dense as to obscure the ground substance in the inner zone. Note that a few elastic fibres extend to mingle with the red-stained collagen fibres of the perichondrium **P**. Development of elastic cartilage occurs by both interstitial and appositional growth in the same manner as hyaline cartilage.

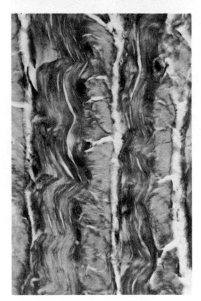

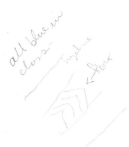

Fig. 9.4 Fibrocartilage
(H & E/Alcian blue × 320)

Fibrocartilage, which has features intermediate between cartilage and dense fibrous connective tissue, is found in the intervertebral discs, some articular cartilages, the pubic symphysis, and in association with dense connective tissue in joint capsules, ligaments and the connections of some tendons to bone. Fibrocartilage consists of alternating layers of hyaline cartilage matrix containing chondrocytes and thick layers of dense collagen fibres oriented in the direction of the functional stresses.

In this micrograph, pink-stained collagen characteristically permeates the blue-stained cartilage ground substance. Chondrocytes are usually arranged in rows between the dense collagen layers within lacunae in the glycoprotein matrix.

Fibrocartilage develops initially as dense, fibrous connective tissue, the fibroblasts of which later differentiate into chondrocytes and become surrounded by cartilaginous ground substance. Fibrocartilage can be distinguished from dense fibrous connective tissue by the absence of blood and lymphatic vessels.

Bone

Bone is a specialised form of connective tissue in which the extracellular components are mineralised, thus conferring the property of marked rigidity and strength whilst retaining some degree of elasticity. In addition to its supporting and protective function, bone constitutes a variable store of calcium and other inorganic ions, and actively participates in the maintenance of calcium homeostasis in the body as a whole. The structure of individual bones provides for the maximum resistance to mechanical stresses whilst maintaining the least bony mass. To accommodate changing mechanical stresses and the demands of calcium homeostasis, all bones in the body are in a dynamic state of growth and resorption throughout life. Like other connective tissues, bone is composed of cells and an organic extracellular matrix containing glycoprotein ground substance and collagen fibres. Inorganic salts, predominantly *calcium hydroxyapatite* crystals, form the mineral component of bone matrix.

The cells found in bone are of three types: *osteoblasts*, *osteocytes* and *osteoclasts*. These three cell types are derived from, and may revert to, mesenchymal-type cells called *osteoprogenitor cells*. Osteoblasts are immature forms of bone cells and are responsible for the synthesis and secretion of the organic component of the extracellular matrix of bone, a substance known as *osteoid*; osteoid then rapidly undergoes mineralisation to form bone. Osteoblasts become trapped within bone as osteocytes and are then responsible for maintenance of the bone matrix. Osteoclasts are multinucleate cells formed by the fusion of numerous osteoprogenitor cells, and are actively involved in resorptive processes associated with continuous remodelling of bone.

Ground substance constitutes only a small proportion of the organic extracellular matrix of bone and contains glycoproteins similar to those found in cartilage. The proportion of sulphated glycoproteins is much less than in cartilage. The fibrous component of the extracellular material is mainly collagen which exhibits a similar banding pattern to that of common collagenous connective tissues (see Fig. 3.4).

Bone exists in two main forms: *woven bone* and *lamellar bone*. Woven bone is an immature form and is characterised by a random (woven) organisation of its fibrous elements. During bone development, woven bone is the first form of bone to be produced; it is then remodelled to form lamellar bone, the form which constitutes most of the mature skeleton. Lamellar bone is composed of successive layers each of which has a highly organised infrastructure. Lamellar bone may be formed as a solid mass, when it is described as *compact bone*, or may be formed as a spongy mass, described as *cancellous bone*.

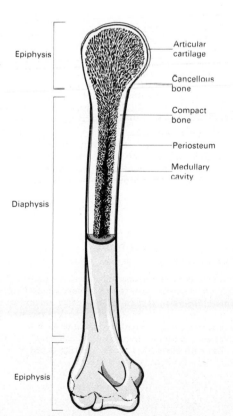

Epiphysis

Diaphysis

Epiphysis

Articular cartilage

Cancellous bone

Compact bone

Periosteum

Medullary cavity

Fig. 9.5 Long bone

This diagram illustrates the general structure of long bones and the gross morphological appearance of the two types of lamellar bone found in the mature skeleton: compact bone and (cancellous) spongy bone.

Compact bone forms the dense walls of the shaft or *diaphysis* while spongy bone occupies part of the large central *medullary cavity*. Spongy bone consists of a network of fine, irregular plates called *trabeculae* separated by intercommunicating spaces. In immature animals, the medullary cavities of most bones contain active (red) marrow which is responsible for the production of the cellular elements of blood. In the adult, active marrow is restricted to a few sites (see Chapter 2); the medullary cavities of other bones are filled with inactive (yellow) marrow which is largely composed of adipose tissue.

The articular (joint) surfaces of the expanded ends, or *epiphyses*, of long bones are protected by a layer of specialised hyaline cartilage called *articular cartilage*. The external surface of the bone is invested in a dense fibrous connective tissue layer called the *periosteum* into which are inserted muscles, tendons and ligaments. The inner surface of the bone, including the trabeculae of spongy bone, is invested by a delicate connective tissue layer called the *endosteum*. The endosteum and periosteum contain cells of the osteogenic series which are responsible for growth, continuous remodelling and repair of bone fractures.

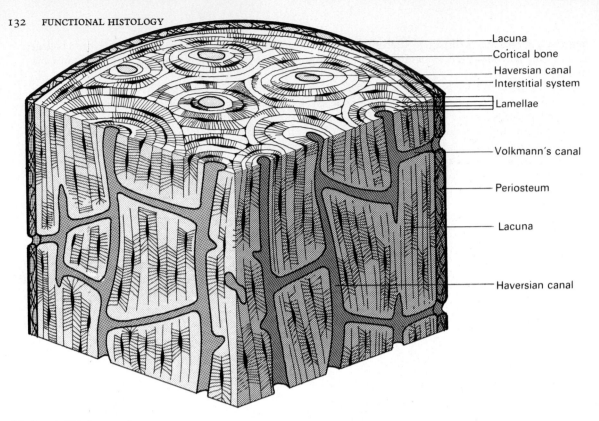

- Lacuna
- Cortical bone
- Haversian canal
- Interstitial system
- Lamellae
- Volkmann's canal
- Periosteum
- Lacuna
- Haversian canal

Fig. 9.6 Compact bone

Compact bone is basically composed of parallel columns made up of concentric bony layers or *lamellae* disposed around channels containing blood and lymphatic vessels, and nerves. The columns are arranged parallel to the long axes of long bones. The neurovascular channels are known as *canals of Havers* or *Haversian canals*, and with their concentric lamellae form *Haversian systems*. The neurovascular bundles interconnect with one another, and with the endosteum and periosteum, via *Volkmann's canals* which pierce the columns at right angles, or obliquely, to the Haversian canals.

Each Haversian system begins as a broad channel, at the periphery of which osteoblasts lay down lamellae of bone. With the deposition of successive lamellae, the diameter of the Haversian canal decreases and osteoblasts are trapped as osteocytes in spaces called *lacunae* in the matrix. The osteocytes are thus arranged in concentric rings within the lamellae. Between adjacent lacunae and the central canal are numerous minute interconnecting canals called *canaliculi* which contain fine cytoplasmic extensions of the osteocytes.

As a result of continuous resorption and redeposition of bone, complete, newly formed Haversian systems are disposed between partly resorbed systems formed earlier. The remnants of lamellae no longer surrounding Haversian canals form irregular *interstitial systems* between intact Haversian systems.

At the outermost aspect of compact bone, Haversian systems give way to concentric lamellae of dense *cortical bone* laid down at the bone surface by osteoblasts of the periosteum. At the medullary aspect, similar but irregular circumferential lamellae merge with trabeculae of spongy bone.

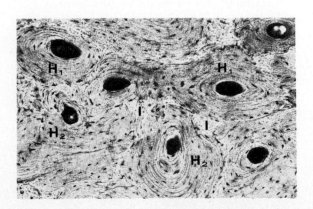

Fig. 9.7 Compact bone

(TS: Ground section: unstained ×80)

With this method, the morphology of the matrix of compact bone may be visualised. In this transverse section, newly formed Haversian systems **H₁** and older Haversian systems **H₂** are seen amongst irregular interstitial systems **I**.

Concentric rings of flattened lacunae surround the Haversian canals and numerous fine canaliculi interconnect lacunae with Haversian canals. Cellular detail of osteocytes cannot be seen with this technique.

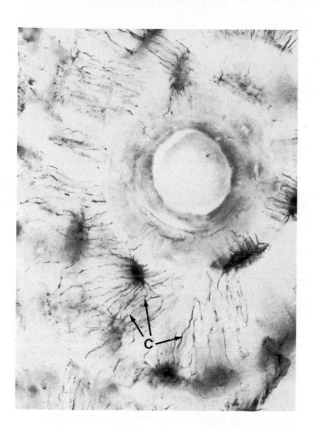

Fig. 9.8 Compact bone

(TS: Ground section: unstained × 480)

In this micrograph of a single Haversian system, canaliculi **C** can be seen to radiate from lacunae and anastomose with those of adjacent lacunae. The canaliculi provide passages for the circulation of tissue fluid and diffusion of metabolites between the lacunae and vessels of the Haversian canals. The canaliculi are partially occupied by the fine cytoplasmic extensions of osteocytes. Osteocytes are believed to maintain the dynamic state of the mineralised matrix and to mediate short-term release or deposition of calcium for the process of calcium homeostasis. The activity of osteocytes in calcium regulation is controlled directly by plasma calcium concentration and indirectly by the hormones, parathyroid hormone and calcitonin, secreted by the parathyroid and thyroid glands respectively (see Chapter 14).

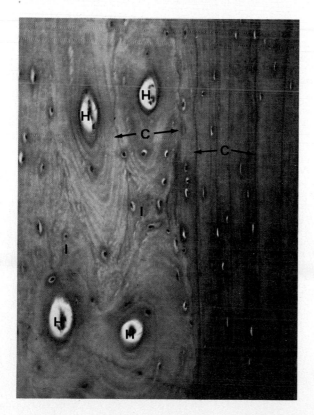

Fig. 9.9 Compact bone

(TS: H & E × 198)

The morphology of the cells and organic components of bone may be studied in standard decalcified preparations, as in this micrograph which illustrates several Haversian systems **H** in transverse section separated by irregular interstitial systems **I**. The matrix of decalcified mature bone is strongly eosinophilic because of its high content of collagen. The collagen of the lamellae is disposed in a helical manner around the long axes of the Haversian systems. At its outer aspect, the Haversian bone gives way to lamellae of cortical bone which provides a more dense, protective outer surface to most bones. Where the Haversian systems and cortical lamellae abut one-another, fine basophilic lines called *cement lines* **C**, rich in glycoprotein ground substance, are seen.

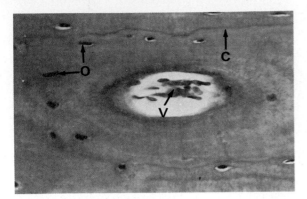

Fig. 9.10 Compact bone
(H & E × 320)

In this specimen of decalcified bone, a single Haversian system can be seen. Osteocytes **O** have densely stained, irregular nuclei and pale, basophilic cytoplasm which undergoes considerable shrinkage in routine preparations such as this. Unlike the chondrocytes of cartilage (see Fig. 9.3) osteocytes do not usually completely occupy their lacunae in bone matrix. Canaliculi, containing the fine cytoplasmic processes of osteocytes, are better demonstrated in ground sections of compact bone. Note a collapsed blood vessel **V** within the Haversian canal and the basophilic cement lines **C** between adjacent Haversian systems.

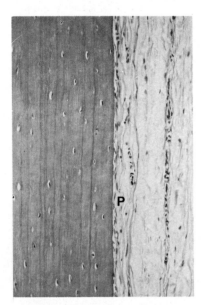

Fig. 9.11 Cortical bone and mature periosteum
(LS: H & E × 128)

In most mature long bones, the outermost compact bone, known as cortical bone, is not arranged in Haversian systems but in concentric lamellae which extend around the whole circumference of the bone shaft (see Fig. 9.6). The lamellae are characteristically separated by basophilic cement lines. As in Haversian-type compact bone, the lacunae of cortical bone are interconnected via numerous canaliculi which are not well seen in this type of preparation.

The outer surface of most bone is invested by a layer of condensed fibrous tissue, the periosteum **P**. The periosteum contains numerous osteoprogenitor cells which are practically indistinguishable from fibroblasts. During bone growth or repair the osteoprogenitor cells differentiate into osteoblasts which are responsible for the deposition of concentric lamellae of cortical bone by appositional growth. The periosteum is bound to the underlying bone by bundles of collagen fibres called *Sharpey's fibres* which may penetrate the whole thickness of the cortical bone. The periosteum is richly supplied with blood vessels from adjacent connective tissues.

Periosteum is not present on the articular surfaces of bone, the sites of insertion of tendons and ligaments, and at several other discrete sites such as the subcapsular area of the neck of the femur. The periosteum plays an important role in the repair of bone fractures; thus the absence of periosteum from the bone surface in certain sites has important implications.

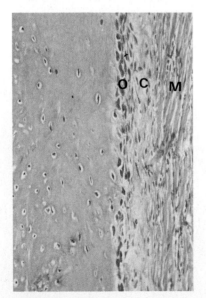

Fig. 9.12 Active periosteum
(H & E × 128)

This micrograph illustrates a highly active periosteum from a developing fetal long bone. The periosteum consists of a front of plump, basophilic osteoblasts **O** two to three cells deep on the surface of the developing bone, and a thin layer of immature, loose connective tissue **C**, into which are inserted the fibres of developing skeletal muscle **M**. The cytoplasmic basophilia of active osteoblasts is due to the large content of rough endoplasmic reticulum involved in synthesising the fibres and ground substance of bone matrix. When appositional bone growth at the periosteal surface is complete, osteoblasts revert to quiescent, osteoprogenitor cells which closely resemble fibroblasts. Note that the bone of the developing shaft is of the woven type; the process of remodelling, to form lamellar bone, occurs at a later stage (see Fig. 9.25).

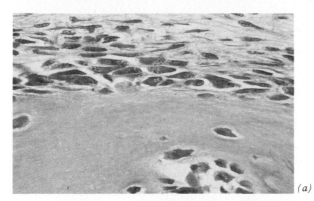

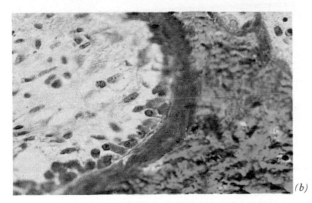

Fig. 9.13 Osteoblasts and osteoid

(a) H & E (b) undecalcified section:
Goldner's green trichrome × 320

These micrographs illustrate active osteoblasts in the process of laying down the organic components of bone matrix; before mineralisation occurs the organic matrix is known as osteoid. In comparison with mature osteocytes, osteoblasts are large cells with abundant basophilic cytoplasm, a large Golgi apparatus and a pale stained nucleus with a prominent nucleolus. These features reflect a high rate of protein and proteoglycan synthesis.

In normally developing bone, as seen in (a), osteoid becomes calcified almost immediately after deposition. Under conditions in which adequate calcium and phosphate ions are not available, for example in rickets or chronic renal failure, there is a lag in mineralisation of osteoid; under such circumstances osteoid tissue accumulates. Osteoid is readily demonstrated in undecalcified sections as shown in (b), a biopsy specimen from an individual with chronic renal failure. With this staining method, osteoid appears as an orange-stained zone between a layer of active osteoblasts and the mineralised bone (stained green).

Little is known about the process of mineralisation but it has been suggested that calcium and phosphate ions form hydroxyapatite crystals under the influence of collagen and associated ground substance; the organic components may act as nucleation centres for crystallisation.

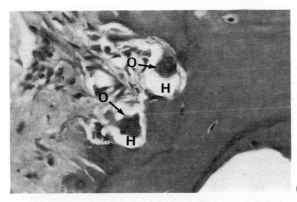

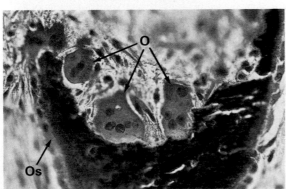

Fig. 9.14 Osteoclasts

(a) H & E (b) undecalcified section:
Goldner's blue trichrome × 320

Resorption of bone is performed by large multinucleate cells called osteoclasts **O** which are formed by the fusion of many osteoprogenitor cells. The osteoclasts are seen in depressions resorbed from the bone surface called *Howship's lacunae* **H**.

In decalcified preparations, as in (a), osteoclasts tend to shrink and become detached from the bone surface; the intimate relationship of osteoclasts with bone is seen better in (b).

Osteoclastic resorption contributes to bone remodelling in response to growth or changing mechanical stresses upon the skeleton. Osteoclasts also participate in the long-term maintenance of blood calcium homeostasis by their response to parathyroid hormone and calcitonin (see Chapter 14). Parathyroid hormone stimulates osteoclastic resorption and the release of calcium ions from bone, whereas calcitonin inhibits osteoclastic activity.

The specimen shown in (b) is from an individual with a low serum calcium level. This condition stimulates release of parathyroid hormone which promotes excessive osteoclastic resorption in an attempt to restore serum calcium levels. In addition, under these circumstances, for any newly deposited bone there is a lag in mineralisation which is manifest by the presence of osteoid **Os**.

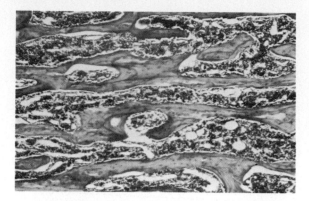

Fig. 9.15 Cancellous bone
(H & E × 50)

Cancellous (spongy) bone is composed of a network of bony trabeculae separated by a labyrinth of interconnecting spaces containing bone marrow. The trabeculae are thin and composed of irregular lamellae of bone with lacunae containing osteocytes. Spongy bone does not usually contain Haversian systems and the osteocytes exchange metabolites via canaliculi with blood sinusoids in the marrow. The trabeculae are lined by a delicate layer of connective tissue called endosteum which contains osteoprogenitor cells, osteoblasts and osteoclasts.

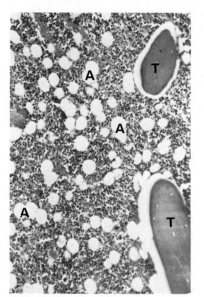

Fig. 9.16 Bone marrow
(H & E × 128)

The intertrabecular spaces of all bones are filled with bone marrow. Bone marrow contains the primitive stem cells from which all the cellular elements of blood are derived (see Chapter 2). In newborn mammals, all bone marrow participates in the process of blood cell formation. Active bone marrow is crammed with dividing stem cells and the precursors of mature blood cells. The predominance of maturing erythrocytes confers a deep red colour on active marrow and hence the name *red marrow*. With increasing age the marrow of peripheral long bones of the skeleton becomes less active and is progressively dominated by adipocytes. In mature mammals, therefore, much of the marrow is inactive and yellow in colour; *yellow marrow* may, however, be reactivated if the need arises for increased haemopoiesis.

This preparation from a seven-year-old child contains much active haemopoietic tissue and some adipocytes **A**. Note two thin trabeculae **T** of cancellous bone.

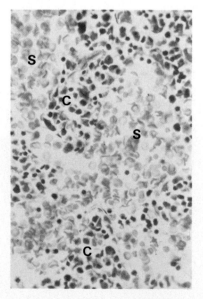

Fig. 9.17 Bone marrow
(H & E × 320)

Active bone marrow consists essentially of two components: a reticulin framework which supports developing blood cells and a system of interconnected blood sinusoids which drain towards a central vein. Haemopoiesis occurs within the reticulin framework thus forming cords of cells which contain an apparently random mixture of developing blood cell lines. When development is complete, or almost complete, blood cells pass from the cords through the delicate sinusoidal endothelium to enter the general circulation. The efflux of blood cells from the bone marrow depends on the functional demands of the body but the mechanism which controls the entry of specific blood cell types into the sinusoids is not known. This micrograph of fetal bone marrow illustrates haemopoietic cords **C** separated by broad sinusoids **S** which are filled with erythrocytes and a few leucocytes.

The functional relationship between bone and bone marrow is obscure; bone may merely provide protection and support for the delicate bone marrow tissue or there may be some specific metabolic relationship between the two tissues. In support of the latter, it has been observed that transplanted bone marrow is unable to survive in sites other than the medullary cavities of bone marrow.

Bone development and growth

The fetal development of bone occurs in two ways, both of which involve replacement of connective tissues by bone. The resulting woven bone is then extensively remodelled by resorption and appositional growth to form the mature adult skeleton which is made up of lamellar bone. Thereafter, resorption and deposition of bone occur at a much reduced rate to accommodate changing functional stresses and to effect calcium homeostasis. The bones of the vault of the skull, the maxilla and most of the mandible are formed by the deposition of bone within primitive mesenchymal tissue; this process of direct replacement of mesenchyme by bone is known as *intramembranous ossification* and the bones so formed are called *membrane bones*. In contrast, the long bones, vertebrae, pelvis and bones of the base of the skull are preceded by the formation of a continuously growing cartilage model which is progressively replaced by bone; this process is called *endochondral ossification* and the bones so formed are called *cartilage bones*. Bone development is controlled by growth hormone, thyroid hormone and the sex hormones.

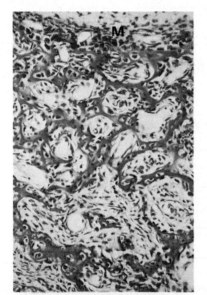

Fig. 9.18 Intramembranous ossification
(H & E × 50)

Intramembranous bone formation occurs within 'membranes' of condensed, primitive mesenchymal tissue. Mesenchymal cells differentiate into osteoblasts which begin synthesis and secretion of osteoid at so-called *centres of ossification*; mineralisation of osteoid follows closely. As osteoid is laid down, osteoblasts are trapped in lacunae to become osteocytes and their cytoplasmic extensions shrink to form the fine processes contained within canaliculi. Osteoprogenitor cells at the surface of the centres of ossification divide mitotically to produce further osteoblasts which lay down more bone. Progressive bone formation results in the fusion of adjacent bony centres to form bone which is spongy in gross appearance.

The collagen fibres of developing bone are randomly arranged in interlacing bundles giving rise to the term woven bone. The woven bone then undergoes progressive remodelling by osteoclastic resorption and osteoblastic deposition to form mature compact or spongy bone. The primitive mesenchyme remaining in the network of developing bone differentiates into bone marrow.

This preparation from the developing skull vault of a cat fetus illustrates spicules of woven bone, separated by primitive mesenchymal tissue. Note the condensed primitive mesenchyme **M** which delineates the outer margin of the developing bone.

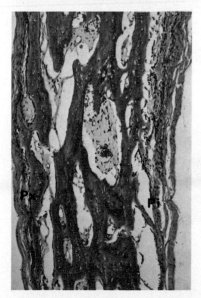

Fig. 9.19 Skull
(Cat: TS: H & E × 20)

This micrograph shows a full thickness view of the skull vault of a mature cat which, like that of the human, is formed by the process of intramembranous ossification. The skull vault consists of cancellous bone which is condensed at its internal and external aspects to form continuous, relatively smooth surfaces. The external surface of the skull is invested by periosteum **Px** which merges with the deep layers of the overlying skin. The internal surface of the skull is also lined by periosteum **Pi**; this layer also constitutes the outermost membranous covering of the brain, known as the *dura mater* (see Fig. 7.32).

During skeletal growth, the skull vault expands in response to the pressure of the growing brain within. The developing skull bones, which are bound together by sutures of loose fibrous connective tissue, are pushed outwards and new membrane bone is laid down at the sutural margins. At the same time, periosteal deposition of new bone on the outer surfaces, and corresponding osteoclastic resorption at the inner surfaces, provides for the necessary recontouring of the skull bones which become progressively flatter. At skeletal maturity the sutures between the skull bones become almost closed and filled with dense fibrous tissue which represents the periosteal layers of opposing bones. With advancing age the sutures tend to ossify.

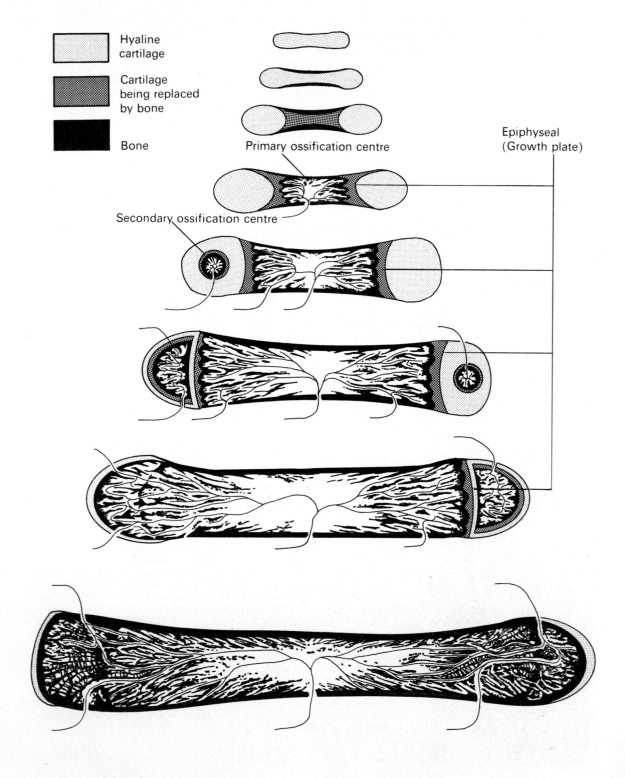

Hyaline cartilage

Cartilage being replaced by bone

Bone

Primary ossification centre

Secondary ossification centre

Epiphyseal (Growth plate)

Fig. 9.20 Endochondral ossification
(illustration opposite)

Endochondral ossification is the process by which all non-membrane bones are formed. This method of bone formation permits functional stresses to be sustained during skeletal growth and is well demonstrated in the development of the long bones.

A small model of the long bone is first formed in solid hyaline cartilage which undergoes mainly appositional growth to form an elongated, dumb-bell shaped mass of cartilage consisting of a shaft (diaphysis) and future articular portions (epiphyses) surrounded by perichondrium.

Within the shaft of the cartilage model the chondrocytes enlarge greatly, resorbing the surrounding cartilage so as to leave only slender perforated trabeculae of cartilage matrix. This cartilage matrix then calcifies and the chondrocytes degenerate leaving large, interconnecting spaces. During this period, the perichondrium of the shaft develops osteogenic potential and assumes the role of periosteum. The periosteum then lays down a thin layer of bone around the surface of the shaft. Primitive mesenchymal cells and blood vessels invade the spaces left within the shaft after degeneration of the chondrocytes. The primitive mesenchymal cells differentiate into osteoblasts and blood-forming cells of the bone marrow. Osteoblasts form a layer of cells on the surface of the calcified remnants of the cartilage matrix and commence the formation of irregular, woven bone.

The ends of the original cartilage model become separated by a large site of *primary ossification* in the shaft, the cartilaginous ends of the model, however, continue to grow in diameter. The cartilage at the ends of the shaft continues to undergo regressive changes followed by ossification so that the developing bone now consists of an elongated, diaphyseal shaft with a semilunar cartilage epiphysis at each end. The interface between the diaphysis and each epiphysis constitutes a *growth* or *epiphyseal plate* by which the shaft of the bone may elongate until inhibited by hormonal factors at physical maturity. After physical maturity, each epiphyseal plate is replaced by bone and the diaphysis and epiphyses fuse.

In the centre of the mass of cartilage of each developing epiphysis, regressive changes and bone formation similar to that in the diaphyseal cartilage occur; however, the perichondrium continues appositional growth of cartilage over the whole external surface of the epiphysis. This so-called *secondary ossification* occurs within the centre of the epiphysis always leaving a thin zone of hyaline cartilage at the surface. At physical maturity this surface cartilage remains as the articular cartilage.

Under the influence of functional stresses the calcified cartilage remnants and the surrounding irregular woven bone are completely remodelled so that the shaft of the bone consists of a compact outer layer with a medulla of cancellous bone. By maturity, the medullary bone is almost completely resorbed to leave a large medullary space filled with bone marrow.

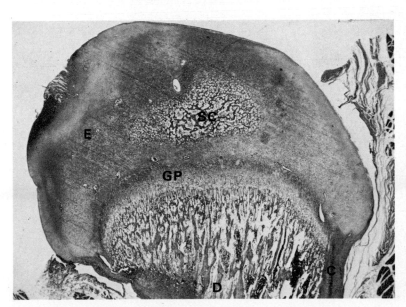

Fig. 9.21 Endochondral ossification: epiphysis
(H & E/Alcian blue × 12)

This micrograph illustrates the head of a kitten femur at an advanced stage of development.

The cartilaginous epiphysis **E** is separated from the diaphysis **D** by the epiphyseal growth plate **GP**. Note the thickening compact bone **C** at the outer aspect of the diaphysis and the trabeculae of bone in the medulla. Note also the centre of secondary ossification **SC** in the epiphyseal cartilage.

Epiphyseal growth plates provide for growth in length of long bones whilst accommodating functional stresses in the growing skeleton. The following three micrographs focus, at higher magnification, on particular regions of this field.

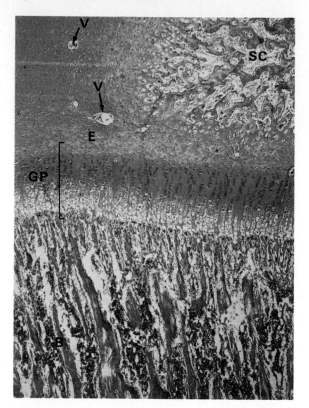

Fig. 9.22 Endochondral ossification: epiphyseal growth plate
(H & E/Alcian blue × 30)

At higher magnification, the epiphyseal growth plate **GP** shows a progression of morphological changes between the epiphyseal cartilage **E** and the newly forming bone **B** of the diaphysis. Similar, but less organised morphological changes, are seen between the epiphyseal cartilage and the centre of secondary ossification **SC** within the epiphysis although this does not represent a growth plate. Note blood vessels **V**, cut in transverse section, passing into the secondary ossification centre.

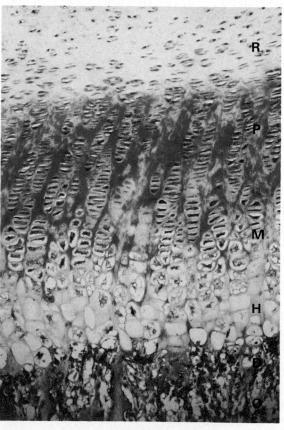

Fig. 9.23 Endochondral ossification: epiphyseal growth plate
(H & E/Alcian blue × 120)

The dynamic process of endochondral ossification is summarised in this micrograph of the epiphyseal growth plate at high magnification. The transition between epiphyseal cartilage and new bone occurs in six functional and morphological stages:

(i) Zone of reserve cartilage R: this consists of typical hyaline cartilage (see Fig. 9.1) with the chondrocytes arranged in small clusters surrounded by a large amount of moderately stained matrix.

(ii) Zone of proliferation P: the clusters of cartilage cells undergo successive mitotic divisions to form columns of chondrocytes separated by strongly stained, glycoprotein-rich matrix.

(iii) Zone of maturation M: cell division has ceased and the chondrocytes increase in size.

(iv) Zone of hypertrophy and calcification H: the chondrocytes become greatly enlarged and vacuolated and the matrix becomes calcified.

(v) Zone of cartilage degeneration D: the chondrocytes degenerate and the lacunae of the calcified matrix are invaded by osteogenic cells and capillaries from the marrow cavity of the diaphysis.

(vi) Osteogenic zone O: the osteogenic cells differentiate into osteoblasts which congregate on the surface of the spicules of calcified cartilage matrix where they commence bone formation. This transitional zone is known as the *metaphysis*.

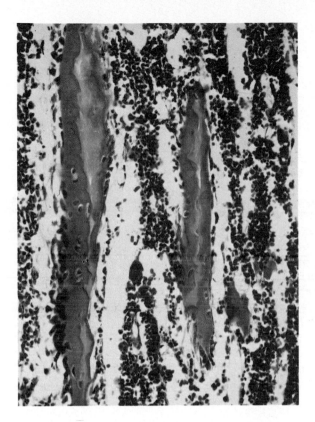

Fig. 9.24 Endochondral ossification: metaphysis

(H & E/Alcian blue × 198)

In the metaphysis seen in this preparation the blue-stained spicules of calcified cartilage matrix are surrounded by osteoblasts and newly formed woven bone which is stained pink. Further growth of metaphysial woven bone is followed by extensive remodelling to produce mature compact and spongy bone.

At physical maturity the process of endochondral ossification ceases. This stage is recognised by the fusion of the diaphysis with the epiphysis, resulting in the obliteration of the growth plates. From this point onwards no further endochondral ossification is possible. Although endochondral ossification is the means of growth in length of a long bone, growth in diameter of the shaft occurs by appositional growth at the periosteal surface and complementary osteoclastic resorption at the endosteal surface.

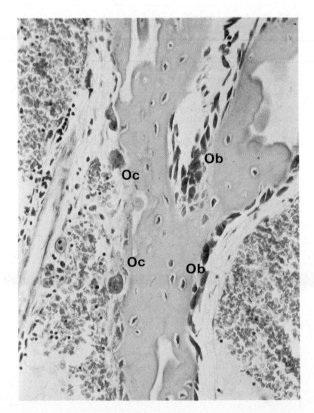

Fig. 9.25 Woven bone: remodelling and repair

(H & E × 480)

This micrograph illustrates an irregular spicule of woven bone in the process of being remodelled to form mature, lamellar bone. Some of the faces of the spicule exhibit osteoblastic deposition **Ob** whereas other faces are in the process of being resorbed by osteoclasts **Oc**.

Woven bone is not only the first type of bone to be formed during development but is also the first bone to be laid down during the repair of a fracture. Initially, a blood clot forms at the site of injury; this is replaced by highly vascular connective tissue which becomes progressively more dense and infiltrated by cartilage. This firm but still flexible bridge is known as the *provisional callus*. The provisional callus is then strengthened by deposition of calcium salts within the cartilage matrix. Meanwhile, osteoprogenitor cells in the endosteum and periosteum are activated and lay down a meshwork of woven bone within and around the provisional callus; the provisional callus thus becomes transformed into the so-called *bony callus*. *Bony union* is achieved when the fracture site is completely bridged by woven bone. Under the influence of functional stresses, the bony callus is then slowly remodelled to form mature lamellar bone.

Joints

Joints may be classified into two main functional groups both of which have wide morphological variations:

(i) synovial joints: in this type of joint there is extensive movement of bones upon one another at articular surfaces. The articular surfaces are maintained in apposition by a fibrous capsule and ligaments, and the surfaces are lubricated by *synovial fluid*. Synovial joints are known as *diarthroses*. In some diarthroses such as the temporomandibular and knee joints, plates of fibrocartilage may be completely or partially interposed between the articular surfaces but remain unattached to the articular surfaces.

(ii) non-synovial joints: these joints have limited movement; the articulating bones have no free articular surfaces but are joined by dense connective tissue which may be of three types:

(a) *dense fibrous connective tissue:* this forms the sutures between the bones of the skull, and permits moulding of the fetal skull during its passage through the birth canal. The sutures are progressively replaced by bone with advancing age. Such fibrous connective tissue joints are called *syndesmoses*, and when replaced by bone are called *synostoses*.

(b) *hyaline cartilage:* this type of joint, called a *synchondrosis* or *primary cartilaginous joint*, unites the first rib with the sternum and is the only synchondrosis found in the human adult.

(c) *fibrocartilage:* the opposing surfaces of some bones are covered by hyaline cartilage but are directly connected to each other by a plate of fibrocartilage. Such fibrocartilaginous joints are called *symphyses* or *secondary cartilaginous joints* and occur in the pubic symphysis and as the intervertebral discs. The fibrocartilage disc of the pubic symphysis develops a hollow central cavity and the intervertebral discs have a fluid-filled central cavity.

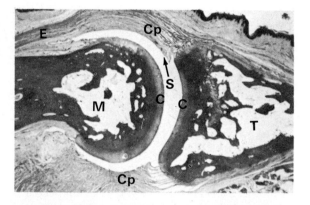

Fig. 9.26 Synovial joint: distal interphalangeal joint of finger
(Monkey: H & E × 12)

This micrograph illustrates a typical synovial joint. The articular surface of the terminal phalanx **T** and the middle phalanx **M** are covered by hyaline cartilage **C**. The joint cavity is artefactually enlarged. *In vivo* the articular surfaces are maintained in close contact by a fibrous capsule **Cp** which is inserted into the articulating bones at some distance from the articular cartilages. The *synovium* **S** is a specialised connective tissue layer on the inner aspect of the capsule. Note the extensor tendon **E** which inserts into the terminal phalanx.

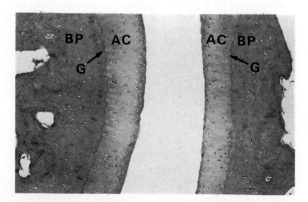

Fig. 9.27 Articular cartilage
(H & E × 20)

This micrograph focuses on the opposing articular cartilages **AC** of the synovial joint shown in Fig. 9.26.

Each articular cartilage is bonded to its long bone at a region called the *bony end plate* **BP**; this region is composed of an unusual type of bone which lacks Haversian systems, is said to lack canaliculi and in which osteocytes occupy particularly large lacunae. The articular cartilage is sharply demarcated from the underlying bony end plate by a thick layer of glycoprotein-rich substance **G** which resembles the cement lines of Haversian bone.

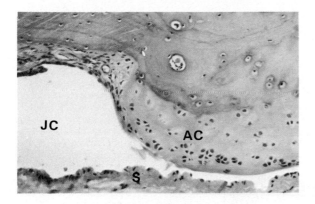

Fig. 9.28 Articular cartilage
(H & E × 128)

Articular cartilage **AC** differs from other hyaline cartilage in two respects. Firstly, the articular surface is not covered by perichondrium. Secondly, the collagen fibres of the cartilage matrix exhibit the characteristic cross-banding of the collagen fibres of loose connective tissue and bone whereas the collagen fibres of other hyaline cartilage are not cross-banded (see Fig. 3.4).

Articular cartilage, like other hyaline cartilage, is avascular; it is nourished by diffusion from the synovial fluid of the joint cavity **JC**. Note part of the synovial layer **S** of the joint capsule.

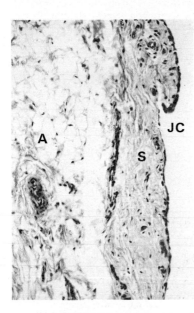

Fig. 9.29 Synovium
(H & E × 128)

The inner surface of the capsule of synovial joints is lined by a specialised connective tissue layer of variable thickness and density called the synovium **S**. The surface of the synovium is thrown up into folds which may extend for some distance into the joint cavity **JC**. The synovial connective tissue contains numerous blood and lymphatic vessels, nerves, and variable numbers of adipocytes **A**.

The free surface of the synovium is lined by a discontinuous layer of cells which are of two morphological types: fibroblast-like cells and macrophage-like cells. These cells are not connected by junctional complexes and do not rest on a basement membrane; the synovial surface, therefore, does not constitute an epithelium.

The synthesis of synovial fluid is poorly understood but it is thought to be formed by a transudate from synovial capillaries into which hyaluronic acid is secreted by the surface cells.

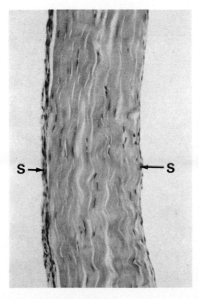

Fig. 9.30 Tendon
(H & E × 128)

Tendon is the densest form of fibrous connective tissue, consisting of parallel bundles of coarse collagen fibres. Tendons are almost inextensible but retain great flexibility. Parallel rows of fibroblasts, with extremely elongated nuclei, are the only cell type found in tendon. Each tendon is composed of small bundles bound together by a small amount of looser connective tissue. Some tendons, as shown in this micrograph, are invested in a connective tissue sheath lined by synovium **S**; movement of the tendon within this sheath is lubricated by synovial fluid.

Ligaments are dense bands of fibrous connective tissue which reinforce joint capsules and maintain bones in the correct anatomical arrangement. Ligaments are histologically similar to tendons, but have a less ordered arrangement of collagen fibres and a variable amount of elastic fibres.

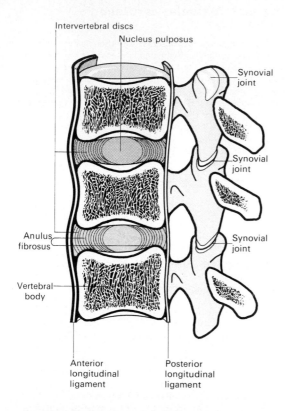

Fig. 9.31 The intervertebral joints

The vertebrae articulate by means of two different types of joints:

(i) The vertebral bodies are united by symphyseal joints, the *intervertebral discs*, which permit movement between the vertebral bodies whilst maintaining a union of great strength. The fibrocartilage of each intervertebral disc is arranged in concentric rings forming the *anulus fibrosus*. Within the disc, there is a cavity containing a viscous fluid, called the *nucleus pulposus*, which acts as a shock absorber. The anulus fibrosus is reinforced peripherally by circumferential ligaments. A thick ligament extending down the anterior aspect of the spinal column further reinforces the anulus fibrosus and a similar, but thinner, ligament reinforces the posterior aspect.

(ii) The vertebral arches articulate with each other by pairs of synovial joints. Strong elastic ligaments connecting the bony processes of the vertebral arches contribute to the stability of the spinal column.

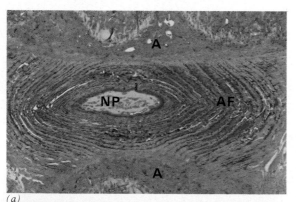

(a)

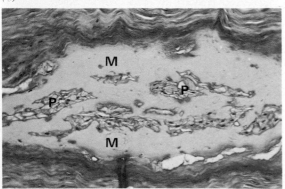

(b)

Fig. 9.32 Intervertebral disc
(Rat: H & E/Alcian blue (a) ×20 (b) ×128)

An intervertebral disc is shown in these micrographs of the tail of an immature rat. The intervertebral disc lies between the articular surfaces **A** of adjacent vertebral bodies. The disc consists of concentric layers of fibrocartilage, constituting the anulus fibrosus **AF**, which surrounds the central nucleus pulposus **NP**. This staining method distinguishes the collagen component of the fibrocartilage, which is stained pink, from the ground substance component, which is stained blue.

At high magnification, the nucleus pulposus is seen to consist of an unusual fluid form of connective tissue; this is the only remnant of the embryonic notochord persisting in adult mammals. The cells of the nucleus pulposus, called *physaliphorous cells* **P**, are scattered in irregular clumps throughout an extracellular matrix **M** which consists of ground substance only.

The intervertebral disc functions in the manner of a hydraulic shock absorber, the nucleus pulposus acting as hydraulic fluid. With advancing age, the fibrocartilage of the anulus fibrosus becomes thinned and weakened and the nucleus pulposus tends to be extruded, particularly at the posterior aspect where the disc is least reinforced by surrounding ligaments. This gives rise to the inappropriately named condition, 'slipped disc'.

10. Immune system

Introduction

All living tissues are subject to the constant threat of invasion by disease-producing organisms, or *pathogens*, such as bacteria, viruses, fungi and multicellular parasites. Mammals have three main lines of defence against invading pathogens: protective surface phenomena, non-specific cellular responses and specific immune responses.

(i) Protective surface phenomena: in man, these provide a first line of defence. The skin constitutes a relatively impenetrable surface to most micro-organisms, unless breached by injury such as abrasion or burning. The sero-mucous surfaces of the body, such as the conjunctiva and oral cavity, are protected by a variety of anti-bacterial substances including the enzyme lysozyme, secreted in tears and saliva. The respiratory tract is protected by a layer of surface mucus which is continuously disposed of by ciliary action and replaced by goblet cell activity. The maintenance of an acidic environment in the stomach, vagina and to a lesser extent the skin, inhibits the growth of bacteria in these sites. When such defences fail to prevent access of pathogens to the tissues, the two other main types of defence mechanisms are activated.

(ii) Non-specific cellular responses: many types of pathogenic bacteria are spontaneously destroyed by the phagocytic cells of loose connective tissue after breaching an epithelial surface. Macrophages and neutrophils are the principal cells which carry out this function. Viral infections induce many cell types in the body to secrete an anti-viral substance called *interferon*, which disrupts viral multiplication within cells. Many pathogens evoke a multifactorial tissue response called *acute inflammation*; this process involves local changes in blood flow and attraction of blood-borne phagocytes to the site of pathogenic insult. When both protective surface phenomena and non-specific responses fail to check the invasion of pathogenic organisms, specific responses are activated, collectively known as the *immune response*.

(iii) Specific immune responses: many pathogens activate immune responses at the time of initial invasion, these specific responses are not, however, effective until a later stage. The non-specific responses are active in the interim period. The primary function of the *immune system* is the production of specific responses directed against specific pathogens. Thus, activation of the immune system involves recognition of characteristics peculiar to a particular pathogen; such characteristics are termed *antigens* since they generate responses directed at their own destruction which at the same time also destroy the pathogenic organism as a whole.

Lymphocytes are the functional units of the immune system and express their specific activity in two main ways. Firstly, some types of lymphocyte produce *antibodies* in response to the recognition of a particular antigen. Antibodies bind to antigens to promote destruction of antigen by a variety of mechanisms to be discussed below; the defence mechanism mediated by antibody is called the *humoral immune response*. Secondly, some lymphocytes are stimulated by antigens to produce a response in which circulating antibodies are not formed but in which lymphocytes and macrophages co-operate in the destruction of pathogenic organisms. This defence mechanism is called the *cellular immune response*. Although the humoral and cellular immune responses may occur separately, a single type of antigen often evokes both responses concurrently.

The cells of the immune system, principally lymphocytes, are disseminated throughout the body either as isolated cells, diffuse aggregations, or within the *lymphoid organs*. The principal *lymphoid organs* are the *thymus, lymph nodes* and the *spleen*.

Many of the mechanisms constituting the immune response are still widely disputed; however, most of the histological features of lymphoid tissue can be interpreted in terms of known immunological defence phenomena.

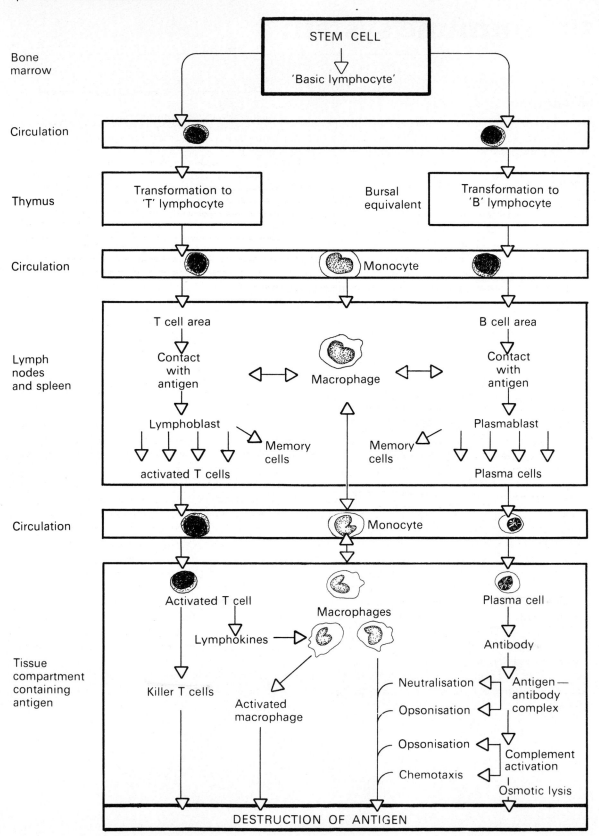

Fig. 10.1 The immune system
(illustration opposite)

This diagram summarises the principal mechanisms of the immune system. Lymphocytes are a heterogeneous population of cells all with a similar histological appearance. In functional terms, lymphocytes can be divided into a number of subpopulations, each with a different role in immunological defence.

Lymphocytes, like all other blood cells, are derived from a common stem cell in bone marrow (see Chapter 2). At some unknown point during lymphocyte development within bone marrow, each lymphocyte acquires the potential to recognise one specific antigen. These 'basic lymphocytes' are then released from bone marrow into the circulation and undergo further development in the lymphoid tissues to become mature, *immunocompetent* cells. Although basic lymphocytes have the potential to recognise specific antigens they must undergo either of two main maturation processes which determines the manner in which they will express their activity, that is via the cellular or humoral mechanism.

(i) The cellular immune response: basic lymphocytes destined to be involved in this type of response enter the thymus and undergo a series of changes before being released into the circulation; lymphocytes which mature in the thymus are called *thymus dependent* or *T lymphocytes*. From the circulation, T lymphocytes localise in the lymphoid tissues throughout the body, from which they then recirculate continuously via the blood and lymph circulations. The continuous recirculation of T lymphocytes has been interpreted as a 'quest for antigens'.

When a specific antigen is encountered in the tissues, the T lymphocytes which are programmed to recognise that particular antigen return to local lymphoid tissues and transform into *lymphoblasts*. Lymphoblasts then divide by mitosis to produce activated T lymphocytes which enter the circulation and migrate to the site of antigenic stimulation. Here they exert their destructive action in two main ways:

(a) Activated T lymphocytes produce a variety of substances, collectively called *lymphokines*, which attract and activate local and blood-borne macrophages. *Activated macrophages* possess greatly increased phagocytic activity which is directed towards destruction of antigen.

(b) Other activated T lymphocytes, called *killer T lymphocytes*, promote direct destruction of invading cells by a process termed *cytotoxic* destruction.

A small proportion of activated T lymphocytes remain in lymphoid tissues where they act as 'memory cells'; these are capable of mounting a more effective response on subsequent exposure to that particular antigen.

(ii) The humoral immune response: in mammals, those basic lymphocytes which will ultimately respond to antigens by producing antibodies, develop immunological competence in some as yet unknown organ. In birds, however, such lymphocytes mature in the *Bursa of Fabricius*, a lymphoid organ associated with the gastro-intestinal tract. Thus, these lymphocytes are called *Bursa dependent* or *B lymphocytes*. Several 'bursal equivalents'

have been suggested in mammals, including the tonsils, Peyer's patches and appendix, but recent evidence suggests that the bone marrow itself may function as the mammalian bursal equivalent. By convention, the mammalian lymphocytes involved in the humoral response are called B lymphocytes.

Immunocompetent B lymphocytes, each programmed to recognise one particular antigen only, are released into the general circulation from which they seed the lymphoid tissues, mainly lymph nodes and spleen. In contrast to T lymphocytes, it is thought that most B lymphocytes do not continuously recirculate throughout the body but rather make contact with antigens taken up and processed by macrophages. When stimulated by antigen, B lymphocytes transform into *plasmablasts* which then divide to form antibody-producing cells called *plasma cells*. A proportion of plasma cells is thought to revert to B lymphocytes and remain in lymphoid tissue as 'memory cells'.

The secretion of antibody molecules by plasma cells takes place either within lymphoid tissue or at the site of antigenic stimulation. In the first case, antibodies are carried to the appropriate site by both the lymph and blood vascular systems.

The combination of antibody and antigen produces a complex which induces antigen destruction in three main ways:

(a) Simple neutralisation of soluble antigen: the complex is destroyed by phagocytosis.

(b) opsonisation: some antigens are made more amenable to phagocytosis by combination with antibody. Antibodies which enhance phagocytosis are called *opsonins* (see also Fig. 3.20).

(c) Complement activation: the combination of antibody and antigen may activate a system of plasma factors comprising the *complement system*. Activation of complement has three main effects. Firstly, some components of complement may act as opsonins; secondly, other components of complement attract neutrophils, thus acting as *chemotaxins*; thirdly, all nine components of complement act together to create holes in the plasma membranes of pathogenic cells resulting in cell death by osmotic lysis.

Antigens often initiate co-operative responses of both the cellular and humoral type. Furthermore, the co-operation of non-specific phagocytes is often necessary to produce the final destruction of antigen. Thus the response of lymphoid tissue to any particular antigen often shows histological features of cellular, humoral and non-specific responses.

This diagram summarises the main components of the immune response and the main tissue compartments in which they occur. Lymphocyte formation (lymphopoiesis) is described in Chapter 2 and the structure of bone marrow in Chapter 9. Macrophages, which are also involved in non-specific defence mechanisms, are discussed as the macrophage-monocyte system in Chapters 2 and 3.

Thymus

The thymus is a lymphoid organ located in the anterior aspect of the thoracic cavity and lower part of the neck. During embryological development the thymus is the first lymphoid organ to appear; the major activity of the thymus takes place during childhood after which it gradually involutes such that, in human adults, the thymus is often impossible to differentiate from surrounding connective tissue. The thymus is derived from epithelial outgrowths of the primitive pharynx during embryological development; later, the primitive thymus becomes infiltrated by lymphocytes derived from haemopoietic tissue elsewhere in the developing embryo (see Chapter 2). The principal function of the thymus is the production of immunocompetent T lymphocytes by modification and proliferation of 'basic lymphocytes' produced by lymphopoiesis. It has been postulated that the thymus also controls the development of lymph nodes and spleen during infancy by the production of a hormone called *thymosine*.

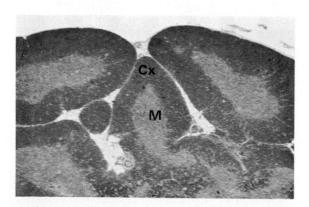

Fig. 10.2 Thymus
(H & E × 20)

The thymus is a lobulated organ invested by a loose connective tissue capsule which conducts the thymic blood supply. Fibrous septa containing blood vessels radiate into the substance of the organ from the capsule. The cells of the thymus are arranged into two distinct zones: an outer, dense *cortex* **Cx** and an inner, paler-stained *medulla* **M**.

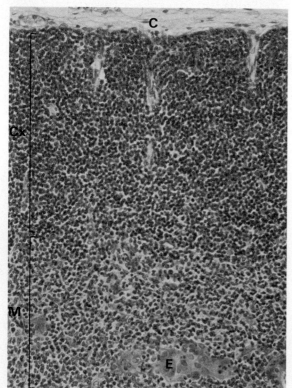

Fig. 10.3 Thymus
(H & E × 80)

At higher magnification the cortex **Cx** can be seen to contain densely packed lymphocytes whereas the medulla **M** is more loosely packed and contains fewer lymphocytes. A sponge-like framework of epithelial cells radiates in irregular, interconnected sheets from the medulla into the cortex and acts as a support for the thymic lymphocytes. The epithelial cells form a continuous sheet beneath the capsule **C** which also ensheaths the blood vessels penetrating the thymus from the outer capsule. The postulated endocrine function has been ascribed to aggregations of epithelial cells **E** seen in the medulla.

↳ Hassall's Corpuscles

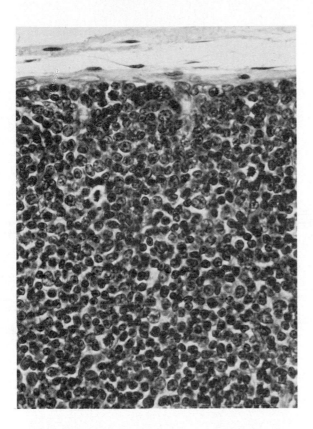

Fig. 10.4 Thymic cortex
(H & E × 480)

Developing T lymphocytes formed in the bone marrow enter the thymus from the circulation and localise in the outer part of the thymic cortex. The lymphocytes in this zone are relatively large and undergo mitosis to produce cells which become progressively smaller as they are pushed towards the medulla by subsequent cell divisions. During this period, by some unknown mechanism, developing T lymphocytes acquire immunocompetence. Mature T lymphocytes then enter the general circulation via the venules of the thymic medulla. A proportion of these cells is destroyed by macrophages in the thymic cortex; the functional significance of this process is unknown. This micrograph demonstrates large lymphocytes in the outer cortex, some of which are in mitosis. Note the generally smaller lymphocytes in the deep cortex. Epithelial support cells are distinguished by their large, pale stained nuclei. Macrophages are not readily seen in this preparation.

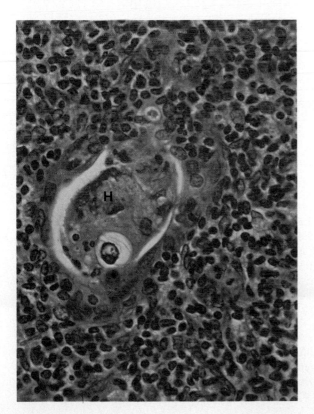

Fig. 10.5 Thymic medulla
(H & E × 480)

The thymic medulla has a prominent meshwork of epithelial cells which have an extensive eosinophilic (pink stained) cytoplasm and large, pale-stained nuclei. A characteristic feature of the medulla is the presence of bizarre, cyst-like epithelial structures called *Hassal's corpuscles* **H**, which may represent degenerated epithelial cells.

The lymphocytes of the medulla are less closely packed and smaller than those of the cortex. Mature T lymphocytes migrate through medullary post-capillary venules into the general circulation, from which they seed lymphoid tissue throughout the body.

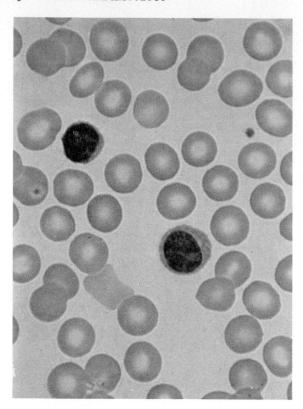

Fig. 10.6 Lymphocytes in peripheral blood

(Giemsa × 1200)

Lymphocytes in circulating blood are a mixed population of cells in various states of immunological activity. In routine tissue sections and peripheral blood smears it is usually impossible to differentiate between the various functional states. The lymphocytes seen in this micrograph are of different size but are otherwise morphologically identical. The larger lymphocytes probably represent less mature forms.

In adult humans, the principal lymphocyte found in peripheral blood is the recirculating T lymphocyte. B and T lymphocytes can be differentiated by the use of specialised techniques. The plasma membrane of each B lymphocyte contains a high density of antibody molecules of the same type as that which the B lymphocyte is programmed to produce when stimulated. B lymphocyte surface antibodies can be demonstrated by combination with fluorescent tracer molecules which are then visible in the fluorescent microscope as a bright fluorescent ring around each B lymphocyte. T lymphocytes on the other hand, contain little, if any, antibody which is amenable to demonstration by this method; T lymphocytes thus remain non-fluorescent in such preparations. T and B lymphocytes may also be differentiated by scanning electron microscopy; B lymphocytes have numerous surface projections whereas the surface of T lymphocytes is relatively smooth.

Lymph nodes

Lymphocytes are distributed throughout the body where they are arranged in aggregations which exhibit various degrees of structural organisation. Isolated lymphocytes are found in most loose connective tissues and amongst epithelial cells, particularly the epithelium of the gastro-intestinal and respiratory tracts; in addition, large diffuse aggregations of lymphocytes are found in the walls of these tracts. The vast majority of lymphocytes are, however, located in encapsulated, highly organised structures called lymph nodes, which are interposed along the larger regional vessels of the lymph vascular system (see Chapter 6).

Three principal, interrelated functions occur within lymph nodes:
(i) non-specific 'filtration' of lymph by the phagocytic activity of macrophages;
(ii) storage and proliferation of B lymphocytes;
(iii) storage and proliferation of T lymphocytes.

T and B lymphocytes occupy different areas within lymph nodes; each area undergoes characteristic histological changes when appropriately stimulated by the presence of antigens. Even in the absence of overt disease, individuals are exposed to a wide range of antigenic stimulation from both within and without. Thus the histological appearance of a lymph node at any particular time will reflect not only the response to local antigenic stimulation but also the immunological status of the individual as a whole.

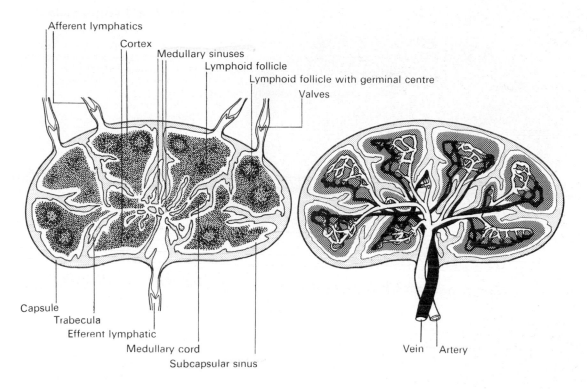

Afferent lymphatics
Cortex
Medullary sinuses
Lymphoid follicle
Lymphoid follicle with germinal centre
Valves

Capsule
Trabecula
Efferent lymphatic
Medullary cord
Subcapsular sinus

Vein Artery

Fig. 10.7 Lymph node: structural and vascular organisation

Lymph nodes are kidney-shaped organs of variable size and are found along the course of the larger lymphatic vessels. Lymph nodes tend to occur in groups, particularly in areas where the lymphatics converge to form larger trunks as in the axilla, groin and hilum of the lung.

The lymph node is encapsulated by dense connective tissue from which *trabeculae* extend for variable distances into the substance of the node. *Afferent lymphatic vessels* divide into several branches outside the lymph node, then pierce the capsule to drain into a narrow space called the subcapsular sinus. Lymph from the subcapsular sinus drains via a series of interconnected channels, *the medullary sinuses*, into the hilum of the node from which arises one or more *efferent lymphatic vessels*.

The body of the lymph node consists of an open

meshwork of fine reticular fibres which provides a loose support for the ever changing populations of lymphocytes. The *cortex* contains densely packed lymphocytes and forms extensions called *medullary cords* which project into an inner *medullary space*.

Within the cortex, lymphocytes form into a variable number of densely packed *lymphoid follicles*, many of which show less dense *germinal centres*.

The blood supply of the lymph node is derived from arteries which enter at the hilum and branch in the medulla, giving rise to capillary networks in the cortex and medullary cords. Lymphocytes enter lymph nodes mainly via the arterial system, gaining access by migrating across the walls of post-capillary venules, which have an unusual structure well adapted for this purpose.

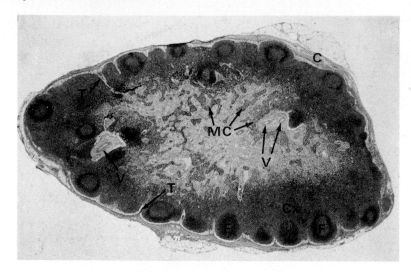

Fig. 10.8 Lymph node
(H & E × 12)

This micrograph illustrates the main geographical features of a lymph node; note that the plane of section does not pass through the hilum in this example.

Several trabeculae **T** extend from the capsule **C** into the substance of the node. The densely packed cellular mass of the cortex **Cx** contains several lymphoid follicles **F**, many of which have pale-stained germinal centres. The irregular medullary cords **MC** are continuous with the corticul cell mass. The narrow subcapsular sinus becomes continuous with the broad interconnected medullary sinuses. Blood vessels **V** are seen in trabeculae within the medulla.

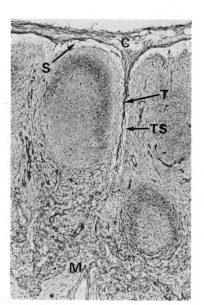

Fig. 10.9 Lymph node
(Reticulin method × 20)

This technique shows the fine reticular architecture of the lymph node; reticulin fibres are stained black and lymphocyte nuclei appear brown.

The main structural support of the lymph node is derived from the collagenous capsule **C** and trabecular extensions **T** into the body of the node. A fine meshwork of reticulin fibres extends throughout the node and provides a loose framework for aggregations of lymphocytes within the cortex and medullary cords. The subcapsular sinus **S**, trabecular sinus **TS** and medullary sinuses **M** are also kept patent by this fine skeleton of reticulin fibres. All the lymph channels of the node are continuous, allowing afferent lymph to flow throughout the node; this arrangement reduces the rate of lymph flow and increases the contact of afferent lymph with the macrophages of the node.

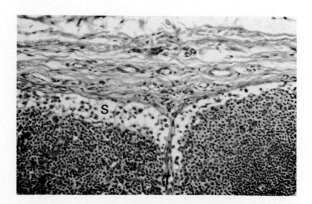

Fig. 10.10 Capsule and subcapsular sinus
(H & E × 128)

The dense fibrous capsule of the lymph node is pierced by numerous branches of afferent lymphatic vessels. The subcapsular sinus **S** extends into trabecular sinuses which pass on either side of the trabeculae **T**. The lymph node sinuses are largely involved in filtration of particulate matter from afferent lymph by the phagocytic action of macrophages.

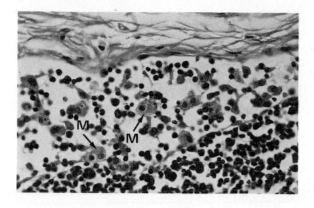

Fig. 10.11 Subcapsular sinus: macrophages

(H & E × 320)

Numerous macrophages are found on the reticulin framework and within the lymph channels of the node; their main function is to clear particles, soluble antigens and other debris from afferent lymph. Macrophages are thought to be necessary for biochemical processing of many antigens before contact with the lymphocytes of the cortex. Antigens may also be sampled in peripheral tissues by macrophages and returned to regional lymph nodes via afferent lymph where activation of appropriate immune responses follows. Cortical lymphocytes may also sample antigen directly as it percolates through the node.

Note the large, irregularly shaped macrophages **M** in this micrograph, many of which contain ingested debris.

Some macrophages, called *dendritic macrophages*, extend fine cytoplasmic processes into the follicles of the cortex; the cytoplasmic extensions are thought to be involved in transferring processed antigen to lymphocytes within the follicles.

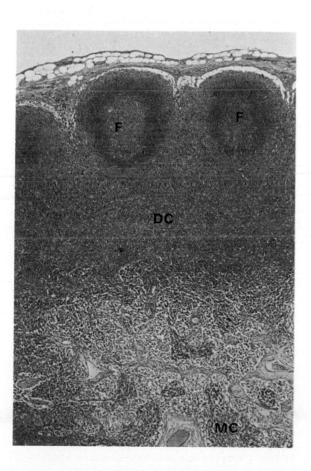

Fig. 10.12 B and T lymphocyte domains of the cortex

(H & E × 30)

The lymphocytes of the outer cortex are mainly arranged in spheroidal lymphoid follicles **F**; these are the major sites where B lymphocytes localise and proliferate. Traditionally, lymphoid follicles have been classified as 'primary follicles' if a central pale area is absent and 'secondary follicles' if such an area is present. However, the exact relationship between 'primary' and 'secondary' follicles is unclear. The pale central areas are sites of B lymphocyte proliferation and are termed germinal centres; 'primary' follicles may represent quiescent 'secondary' follicles.

The deep cortical zone **DC**, or *paracortex*, consists mainly of T lymphocytes which are never arranged as follicles; discrete B lymphocyte follicles, however, are often seen in the deep cortical zone, particularly within immunologically active lymph nodes. The medullary cords **MC** mainly contain B lymphocytes and their derivatives.

The number of cortical lymphoid follicles and the depth of the paracortex vary greatly according to the immunological state of the particular lymph node and the individual as a whole. A purely cellular response to antigen is associated with paracortical thickening whereas a humoral response to antigen is evidenced by the appearance of many cortical follicles with pale germinal centres.

Fig. 10.13 Lymphoid follicle and germinal centre
(H & E ×64)

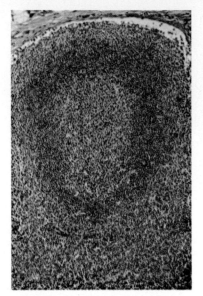

Lymphoid follicles are the principal sites of storage and proliferation of B lymphocytes; these lymphocytes include both memory cells and cells which have had no previous contact with the antigen for which they were programmed to recognise. Both types of B lymphocyte proliferate within germinal centres when appropriately stimulated by antigen; B lymphocytes transform into large cells called *plasmablasts* which then undergo mitosis to produce plasma cell precursors called *proplasmacytes*. Proplasmacytes pass to the follicle periphery and thence into the medullary cords where they mature into plasma cells and secrete antibodies into efferent lymph. Some plasma cells leave the lymph node in efferent lymph and migrate to sites of antigenic stimulation via the general circulation. At some unknown stage during the process of B lymphocyte activation, an expanded population of memory cells is formed which is capable of mounting a more rapid and intense humoral response on subsequent contact with the same antigen.

Fig. 10.14 Germinal centre
(H & E ×320)

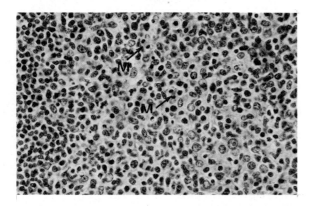

This micrograph focuses on the cells of a germinal centre; these cells are a mixed population of B lymphocytes and the plasma cell precursors, plasmablasts and proplasmacytes. The latter cells have a more extensive cytoplasm than the surrounding lymphocytes; this results in a lower density of nuclei which accounts for the paler staining characteristics of germinal centres when viewed at lower magnification. Plasma cell precursors may be seen in mitosis **M**.

Fig. 10.15 Paracortical zone
(H & E ×320)

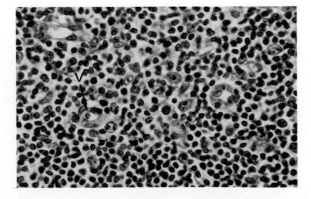

T lymphocytes are the main cell type in the deep cortical area, also called the paracortex or paracortical zone. Recirculating T lymphocytes enter the lymph node in arterial blood then migrate through the walls of post-capillary venules **V** into the paracortical zone; T lymphocytes leave the lymph node in efferent lymph. When a cell-mediated immune response is stimulated, T lymphocytes in the paracortex transform into large cells called *lymphoblasts* which divide by mitosis to produce activated T lymphocytes. In contrast to plasma cells, T lymphocytes must migrate to the site of antigenic stimulation in order to exert their locally destructive effects. When an intense cellular response is evoked within a lymph node, the paracortex expands greatly, often obliterating the entire medulla; this process is called the *paracortical reaction*.

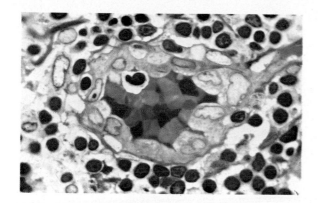

Fig. 10.16 Post-capillary venule

(Resin embedded, one micron section: toluidine blue × 800)

Post-capillary venules of the paracortex have an unusual structure which facilitates the passage of T lymphocytes from the blood circulation into the lymph node. The endothelial lining is tall cuboidal rather than the usual squamous arrangement; this may allow lymphocytes to pass through the wall, between the endothelial cells, without causing leakage of blood into the lymph node. There is evidence that the endothelial cells have surface properties which enable T lymphocytes to recognise post-capillary venules as sites of exit into lymph nodes. Note in this micrograph, three lymphocytes in various stages of progress through the wall of a post-capillary venule.

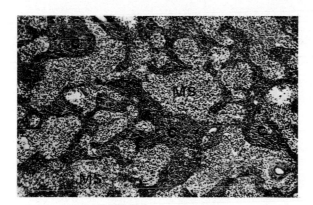

Fig. 10.17 Medullary cords and sinuses

(H & E × 20)

This micrograph illustrates medullary cords **C** with intervening wide, irregular medullary sinuses **MS**. Medullary cords largely contain B lymphocytes, proplasmacytes and plasma cells although a few macrophages and T lymphocytes may be present.

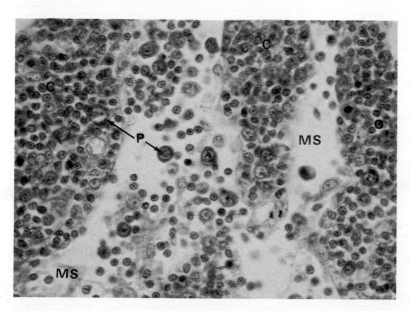

Fig. 10.18 Medullary cords and sinuses

(Methyl green/pyronin × 480)

This preparation, taken from a lymph node undergoing an intense humoral response, has been stained by a technique to demonstrate plasma cells; plasma cells **P** appear as large cells with an extensive, red-stained cytoplasm and a pale-stained nucleus with a prominent nucleolus. The red dye pyronin has a strong affinity for ribosomal RNA and hence stains the plasma cell cytoplasm strongly since it is packed with ribosomes involved in antibody synthesis. Note the presence of numerous plasma cells in both the medullary cords **C** and sinuses **MS**.

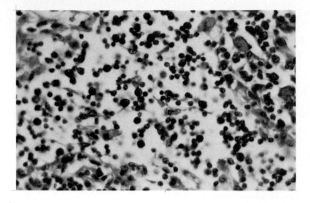

Fig. 10.19 Efferent lymph
(H & E × 320)

Efferent lymph, seen in a medullary sinus in this micrograph, differs from afferent lymph in several important respects. Afferent lymph contains particulate matter often including micro-organisms, soluble antigens and relatively few lymphocytes and macrophages. In contrast, efferent lymph contains little particulate matter or soluble antigens but contains large numbers of recirculating T lymphocytes and a variable number of B lymphocytes and plasma cells depending on the degree and type of immunological activity. Variable quantities of antibody are also carried in efferent lymph to the general circulation and thence to the site of antigenic stimulation.

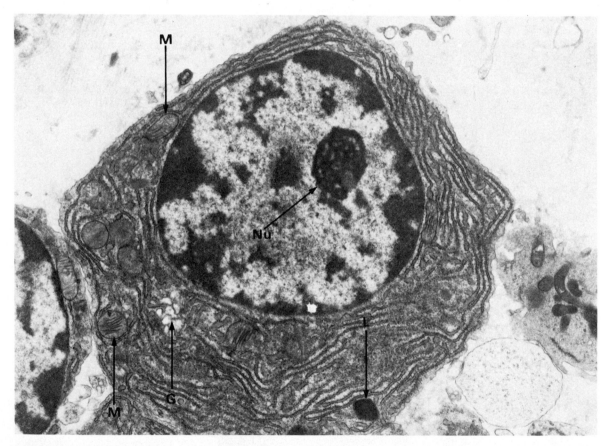

Fig. 10.20 Plasma cell
(EM × 13860)

The mature plasma cell is a large, amoeboid cell with an eccentrically placed spherical or oval nucleus. Reflecting its intense activity in protein (antibody) synthesis, the nucleus contains much dispersed chromatin; the remaining heterochromatin tends to be distributed around the nuclear envelope. A large nucleolus **Nu** is a highly characteristic feature. The cytoplasm is packed with lamellae of rough endoplasmic reticulum; during periods of active protein synthesis the lamellae become dilated and filled with amorphous material. The Golgi apparatus **G** is usually well developed. Paradoxically, antibodies do not appear to be secreted by exocytosis of Golgi-derived vesicles; the mode of antibody secretion is not known.

The cytoplasm also contains a few rounded mitochondria **M** and occasional lysosomes **L**. The plasma membrane is usually regular in outline and exhibits few microvilli or pseudopodia.

Fig. 10.21 Palatine tonsil
(H & E ×6)

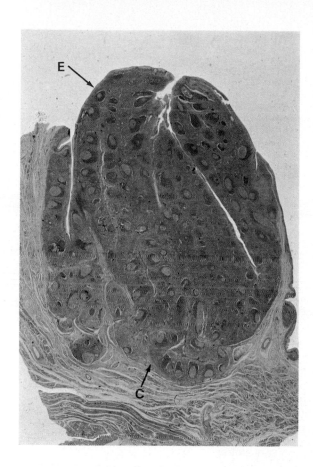

Other lymphoid tissues of the body such as the tonsils, Peyer's patches, appendix and many unnamed lymphoid aggregations in other tracts perform similar immunological functions to those performed by lymph nodes. The key difference, however, is that these lymphoid tissues are not directly disposed along the course of the lymph vascular system and are therefore not involved in filtration of lymph. The tonsils, Peyer's patches, appendix and other lymphoid aggregations are not encapsulated and often contain active lymphoid follicles which increase in number and are more prominent during an intense humoral immune response. Discrete T lymphocyte zones are not recognisable in these tissues.

The tonsils form a discontinuous ring of lymphoid tissue around the oro-pharynx. The palatine tonsil seen in this micrograph is covered on its outer surface by the stratified, squamous epithelial lining **E** of the oro-pharynx; this epithelium deeply invaginates the tonsil, almost to its base, to form blind-ended structures called *crypts*. Note that the tonsil is separated at its base from underlying muscle by a dense hemi-capsule **C**.

Lymphocytes from the tonsils pass through the crypt epithelium and thence into the oral cavity but the functional significance of the tonsils is largely unknown.

Spleen

The spleen is a large lymphoid organ situated in the left, upper part of the abdomen; it receives a rich blood supply via a single artery, the *splenic artery*, and is drained by the *splenic vein* into the hepatic portal system.

In man, the spleen has three main functions:

  (i) removal of particulate matter from circulating blood;
  (ii) production of immunological responses against blood-borne antigens;
  (iii) removal of aged or defective blood cells from the circulation.

In dogs and horses, the spleen also acts as a large reservoir of blood which can be mobilised if necessary. Despite its large size and important functions, removal of the spleen appears to have few deleterious effects on the body as a whole; its functions are assumed to be taken over by the liver and bone marrow.

The manner in which the spleen performs its functions, and many ultrastructural details, are still widely disputed; in many respects, however, the spleen may be considered analogous to a lymph node in which the lymphatic circulation is replaced by a blood circulation. The structure of the spleen provides for intimate contact to be made between blood and immunologically active cells just as the structure of lymph nodes facilitates the interaction of afferent lymph and lymphoid cells. Although it is well established that the spleen is involved in removal of aged or defective blood cells from the circulation, it is still not clear whether this is a purely mechanical process or whether immunological recognition plays an important role.

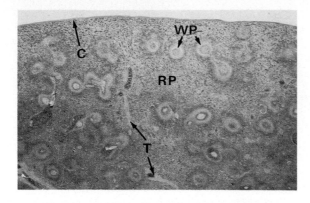

Fig. 10.22 Spleen
(H & E ×8)

Like lymph nodes, the spleen has a dense, fibrous, outer capsule **C** which is thickened at the hilum and which gives rise to supporting connective tissue trabeculae **T**. Trabeculae conduct larger arteries and veins throughout the spleen and provide major structural support for the fine reticulin network which extends throughout the organ.

Macroscopically the spleen appears to consist of discrete white nodules, the so-called *white pulp*, embedded in a red matrix called the *red pulp*. Microscopically the white pulp **WP** is seen to consist of lymphoid aggregations surrounded by a highly vascularised matrix, the red pulp **RP**.

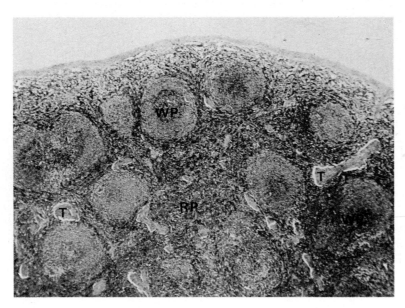

Fig. 10.23 Spleen
(H & E × 30)

The major branches of the splenic artery penetrate the spleen within connective tissue trabeculae **T**; from the trabecular arteries, arterioles branch and pass into the substance of the spleen where they are surrounded by sheaths of lymphoid tissue, the *peri-arteriolar lymphoid sheaths (PALS)* which correspond to the white pulp nodules.

In this micrograph, peri-arteriolar lymphoid sheaths **WP** are seen in various planes of section. When seen in transverse section, the lymphoid tissue bears a superficial resemblance to the follicles of lymph nodes; they are readily distinguished, however, by the presence of *central arterioles*. Little detail of the red pulp **RP** is apparent at this magnification.

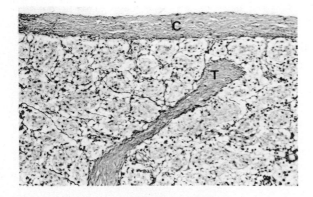

Fig. 10.24 Spleen
(Reticulin method/neutral red × 50)

This staining technique is used to demonstrate the reticular architecture of the spleen. The capsule **C** and the trabeculae **T** provide a robust framework which supports a fine, reticulin meshwork ramifying throughout the organ.

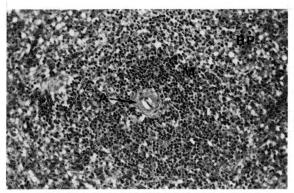

Fig. 10.25 Peri-arteriolar lymphoid sheath

(H & E ×80)

The white pulp, or peri-arteriolar lymphoid sheaths, contain populations of both T and B lymphocytes; the central region around the central arteriole **A** contains predominantly B lymphocytes which may form germinal centres if a humoral response is stimulated in the spleen by blood-borne antigen. The outer *marginal zone* **M** consists mainly of closely packed T lymphocytes. The central arterioles branch to form a capillary network in the marginal zones; thus the marginal zone is the first point of contact in the spleen between blood and immunologically active cells. Blood drains from the marginal zone capillaries into the red pulp **RP**.

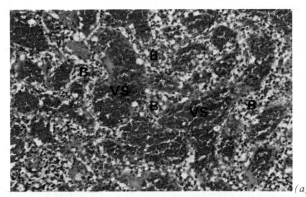

Fig. 10.26 Peri-arteriolar lymphoid sheath with germinal centre

(H & E ×80)

When blood-borne antigens evoke an active humoral response in the spleen, many of the peri-arteriolar lymphoid sheaths exhibit prominent germinal centres similar in histological structure to those seen in lymph node follicles. As in lymph nodes, germinal centre formation in the spleen is indicative of B lymphocyte proliferation and transformation into plasma cells. When this occurs, the central arteriole **A** is deflected towards the marginal zone.

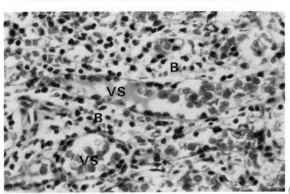

Fig. 10.27 Red pulp

(H & E (a) ×128 (b) ×320)

Red pulp consists of anastomosing cords of cells, the *cords of Bilroth* **B**, separated by broad, interconnected, venous sinuses **VS**. The pulp cords are based on a reticulin skeleton which supports a large population of highly phagocytic cells. The spaces between the meshes of the pulp cords contain variable numbers of both erythrocytes and leucocytes. The phagocytic cells of the cords are known to effect the final destruction of aged or damaged blood cells, the mechanics of this process is, however, the subject of much controversy. Similarly, the nature of the circulatory connections between the capillaries of the marginal zone and the red pulp, and the venous drainage of the red pulp are still widely disputed (see Fig. 10.28).

The venous sinuses are lined by unusual, spindle-shaped endothelial cells which lie parallel to the long axes of the sinuses. Small open spaces or pores occur between the endothelial cells; the endothelial basement membrane is discontinuous over the spaces or pores. Blood cells, particularly erythrocytes, are able to squeeze through the endothelial pores from the pulp cords into the venous sinuses.

(a) The respiratory epithelium undergoes progressive transition from a tall, pseudostratified columnar, ciliated form in the larynx and trachea to a simple, cuboidal, non-ciliated form in the smallest airways. Goblet cells are numerous in the trachea but decrease in number and are absent in the terminal bronchioles.

(b) The lamina propria consists of fibro-elastic connective tissue which contains lymphoid aggregations of variable size and density; these form part of the immune defence system (see Chapter 10).

(c) A layer of smooth muscle lies deep to the mucosa (except in the trachea) and becomes increasingly prominent as the airway diameter decreases; it reaches its greatest prominence in the terminal bronchioles. Smooth muscle tone controls the diameter of the conducting passages and thus controls resistance to air flow within the respiratory tree. Smooth muscle tone is modulated by the autonomic nervous system, adrenal medullary hormones and local factors.

(d) Submucosal connective tissue underlies the smooth muscle layer and contains serous and mucous glands which become progressively less numerous in the narrower airways and are not present beyond the tertiary bronchi.

(e) Cartilage provides a supporting skeleton for the larynx, trachea and bronchi and prevents the collapse of these airways during ventilation. This layer lies outside the submucosa and diminishes in prominence as the calibre of the airway decreases.

(f) The outermost layer of cartilage or smooth muscle is surrounded by fibro-elastic connective tissue called the *adventitia* which merges with surrounding tissues.

The lungs have a dual blood supply, the *pulmonary system* and the *bronchial system*. The pulmonary supply is the predominant system and conducts deoxygenated blood from the right side of the heart via a large pulmonary artery to each lung. The pulmonary arteries enter the roots or *hila* of the lungs with the main bronchi and then divide and course in parallel with the branching airways to supply the pulmonary capillaries surrounding the alveoli. The pulmonary arterial system is structurally unusual in two respects. Firstly, the pulmonary arterial vessels are relatively thin-walled and of large calibre, their diameter approximating that of the accompanying airway. Secondly, the pulmonary arteries have the histological characteristics of elastic arteries rather than of muscular arteries. Elastic expansion and recoil of the vessels maintains the pulmonary arterial pressure at a relatively constant level throughout the cardiac cycle. The bronchial arterial system constitutes the systemic circulation of the lower respiratory tract. It arises as small branches of the aorta and supplies oxygenated blood to the tissues of the airway walls and to the *pleura*, the layer which invests the outer surface of each lung. The bronchial vessels are of the usual type found in the rest of the systemic circulation.

A common venous system returns most of the blood to the left side of the heart via the pulmonary veins which are extremely thin-walled vessels. A small proportion of blood from the bronchial system drains to the right side of the heart via the azygos venous system.

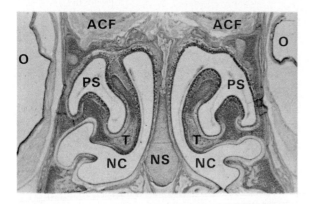

Fig. 11.1 Nasal cavity

(Kitten: coronal section: H & E/Alcian blue × 8)

The first part of the upper respiratory tract, the nose, is subdivided into two nasal cavities **NC** by the cartilaginous nasal septum **NS**; cartilage is stained blue in this preparation. The nasal cavities and paranasal sinuses **PS** are lined by respiratory mucosa, the major function of which is to filter particulate matter and to adjust the temperature and humidity of inspired air. These functions are enhanced by a large surface area provided by the turbinate system of bones **T** which project into the nasal cavities. Part of the nasal mucosa, the *olfactory mucosa*, contains receptors for the sense of smell (see Fig. 7.37). Although the olfactory mucosa is extensive in lower mammals, in man it is confined to a relatively small area in the roof of the nasal cavities. Note the close proximity of the nasal cavities to the orbital cavities **O** and the anterior cranial fossa **ACF**.

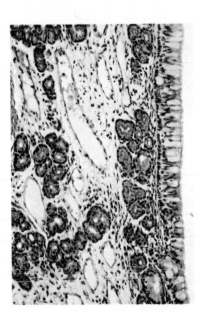

Fig. 11.2 Nasal mucosa

(H & E × 128)

The nasal mucosa consists of a pseudostratified, columnar, ciliated epithelium with numerous goblet cells supported by a richly vascular lamina propria containing serous and mucous glands. These features reflect the protective functions of the nasal mucosa, processes which begin in the nasal cavities and continue throughout the respiratory tract.

Particulate matter in inspired air is trapped in a thin layer of surface mucus secreted by the goblet cells of the surface epithelium and the mucous glands of the lamina propria. Co-ordinated, wavelike beating of cilia propels mucus with trapped particles towards the pharynx where it is swallowed and inactivated in the gastro-intestinal system. The entrance to each nasal cavity, the *nasal vestibule*, is lined by skin which has short, coarse hairs called *vibrissae* which may trap the largest particles before they reach the nasal mucosa.

The temperature of inspired air is adjusted to that of the body by heat exchange between the air and blood flowing in a rich plexus of thin-walled venules in the lamina propria. Inspired air is humidified by the watery secretions of serous glands also located in the lamina propria. A mucosa similar to that of the nasal cavities also lines the nasopharynx, paranasal sinuses and auditory tubes.

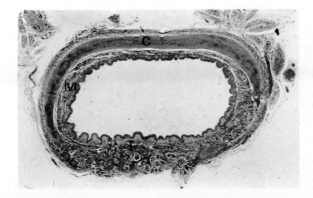

Fig. 11.3 Trachea

(TS: H & E/Alcian blue × 6)

This specimen from a newborn child shows the general structure of the trachea. The trachea is a flexible tube of fibro-elastic connective tissue and cartilage which permits expansion in diameter and extension in length during inspiration, and passive recoil during expiration. A series of C-shaped rings of hyaline cartilage **C**, stained blue in this preparation, support the tracheal mucosa **M** and prevent its collapse during inspiration. Bands of smooth muscle, called the *trachealis muscle* **T**, join the free ends of the rings posteriorly; contraction of the trachealis reduces tracheal diameter and thereby assists in raising intrathoracic pressure during coughing. A few strands of longitudinal muscle are disposed behind the trachealis muscle.

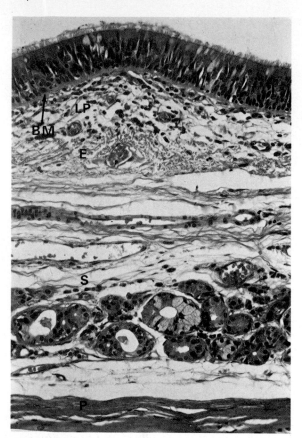

Fig. 11.4 Trachea

(LS: H & E × 198)

The layers of the tracheal wall are shown in this specimen from a young man. The respiratory epithelium of the trachea is tall, pseudostratified and ciliated and contains numerous goblet cells. In response to the irritation of tobacco smoke, the epithelium commonly undergoes morphological change (metaplasia) to a stratified squamous form with consequent loss of ciliary action; ciliary activity is essential for continuous movement of glandular secretions towards the pharynx. The tracheal epithelium is supported by a thick basement membrane **BM**, usually readily visible with light microscopy. Beneath the basement membrane, the lamina propria **LP** consists of loose, highly vascular, connective tissue which becomes condensed at its deeper aspect to form a prominent band of fibro-elastic tissue **E**. Underlying the lamina propria is the loose submucosa **S** containing numerous mixed sero-mucous glands which decrease in number in the lower parts of the trachea; the serous cells stain strongly with H & E whilst the mucous cells remain poorly stained. The submucosa merges with the perichondrium **P** of the underlying hyaline cartilage rings or with the external adventitial layer between the rings.

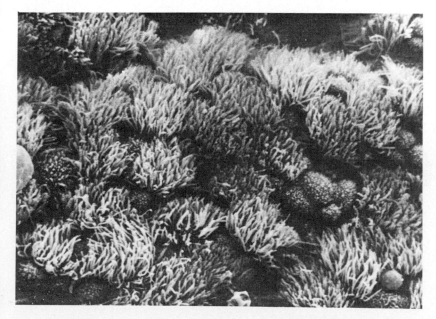

Fig. 11.5 Tracheal epithelium

(Scanning EM × 2000)

This micrograph illustrates, at high magnification, the tracheal surface; the film of surface mucus has been removed before fixation and processing. The cilia of each epithelial cell form discrete clumps on the surface. Non-ciliated goblet cells are scattered amongst the ciliated cells: note that the goblet cell surfaces exhibit a few small microvilli.

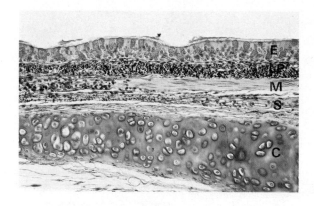

Fig. 11.6 Primary bronchus
(TS: Elastic van Gieson/Alcian blue × 80)

The basic structure of the primary bronchi is similar to that of the trachea, but it differs in several details. Firstly, the respiratory epithelium **E** is less tall and contains fewer goblet cells. Secondly, the lamina propria **LP** is denser and more elastic; elastic fibres are stained black in this preparation. Thirdly, the lamina propria is separated from the submucosa **S** by a discontinuous layer of smooth muscle **M** which becomes progressively more prominent further down the tract. Fourthly, the submucosal layer contains fewer sero-mucous glands; none are seen in this micrograph. Finally the cartilage framework **C** is arranged into flattened, interconnected plates rather than discrete C-shaped rings.

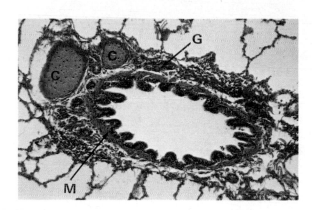

Fig. 11.7 Tertiary bronchus
(TS: Elastic van Gieson × 50)

As the bronchi diminish in diameter the structure progressively changes to more closely resemble that of large bronchioles. The respiratory epithelium, which cannot be seen at this magnification, is now tall columnar but not pseudostratified, and goblet cells have diminished in number. The lamina propria is thin, elastic and completely encircled by smooth muscle **M** which is disposed in a spiral manner. This arrangement of smooth muscle permits contraction of the bronchi in both length and diameter during expiration. Sero-mucous glands **G** are sparse in the submucosa and are rarely found in smaller airways. The cartilage framework **C** is reduced to a few irregular plates; cartilage also does not usually extend beyond the tertiary bronchi. Note that the submucosa merges with the surrounding adventitia and thence with the lung parenchyma. A small lymphoid aggregation is seen in the adventitia.

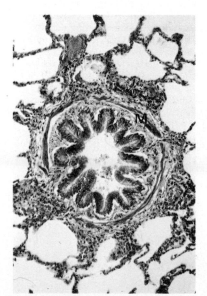

Fig. 11.8 Bronchiole
(TS: H & E × 80)

Bronchioles are airways of less than one millimetre in diameter and have no cartilaginous support. The respiratory epithelium is simple, columnar, ciliated and contains few goblet cells. Goblet cells are completely absent beyond the terminal bronchioles. The smooth muscle layer **M** is the most prominent feature of the bronchiole and is disposed in a spiral manner like that of the bronchi. The total cross-sectional area of all bronchioles combined is far greater than that of the rest of the conducting passages combined, thus the tonus of bronchiolar smooth muscle effectively controls resistance to air flow within the lungs.

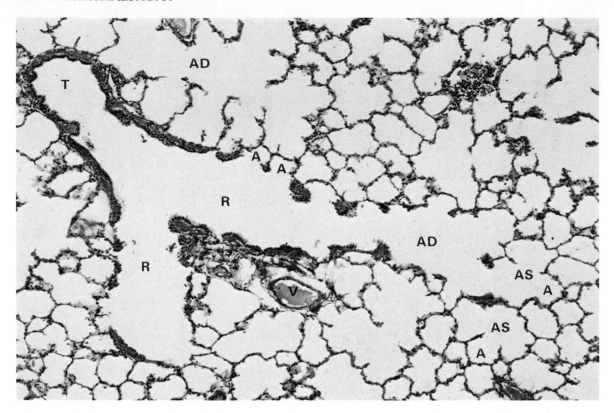

Fig. 11.9 Terminal portion of the respiratory tree

(Elastic van Gieson × 40)

Terminal bronchioles **T** are the smallest diameter passages of the purely conducting portion of the respiratory tree; further branches become increasingly involved in gaseous exchange.

Each terminal bronchiole divides to form short, thinner-walled branches called respiratory bronchioles **R**, so named because their walls contain a small number of single alveoli **A**. The epithelium of the respiratory bronchioles is devoid of goblet cells and largely consists of ciliated, cuboidal cells and smaller numbers of non-ciliated cells called *Clara cells*. The epithelium of respiratory bronchioles represents a further transition from that of the terminal bronchioles, and Clara cells become the predominant cell type in the most distal part of the respiratory bronchioles. Clara cells have the ultrastructural features of secretory cells, but the nature and function of their secretory product, if any, is poorly understood.

Each respiratory bronchiole divides further into several long, winding passages called alveolar ducts **AD** which open along their length into numerous alveolar sacs **AS** and alveoli **A**. In histological sections, all that can be seen of the walls of the alveolar ducts are minute aggregations of smooth muscle cells and associated collagen and elastic fibres which form rings surrounding the alveolar ducts and the openings of the alveolar sacs and alveoli. The smooth muscle of the respiratory bronchioles and alveolar ducts regulates alveolar air movements.

The alveolar ducts lead into alveolar sacs, distended spaces each of which gives rise to several alveoli. Each alveolus consists of a pocket, open at one side and lined by extremely flattened epithelial cells. Surrounding each alveolus is a rich network of pulmonary capillaries supplied by pulmonary vessels **V** which follow the general course of the airways. Between adjacent alveoli, the wall or *alveolar septum* consists of the flattened epithelial lining cells of each alveolus separated by capillaries and extremely delicate reticular and elastic supporting elements. Fibres condense around the opening of each alveolus and merge with those around the openings of adjacent alveoli to form a fine, supporting system for the whole lung parenchyma. The alveolar septa contain small openings called *alveolar pores* which are thought to enable equalisation of pressure between alveoli, and to provide a collateral air circulation when a bronchiole is obstructed.

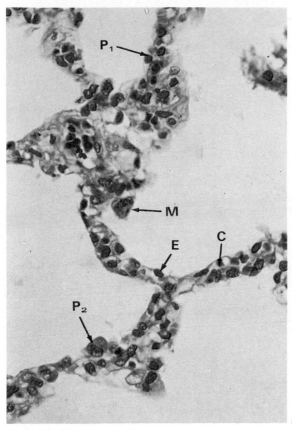

(a)

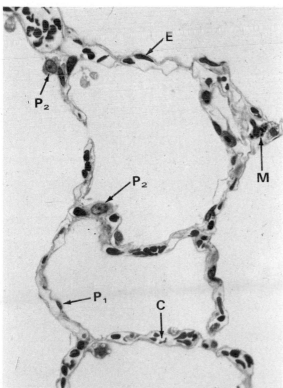

(b)

Fig. 11.10 Alveoli

(a) H & E × 480   (b) resin embedded, one micron section: toluidine blue × 480

The conventional method of studying the structure of the alveolar wall in light microscopy has been to use relatively thick (5 to 8 μm) wax-embedded tissues, stained by routine methods as in (a); the resolution obtained by such methods is limited. In contrast, thin resin sections reveal much greater structural detail since they permit better resolution. Both techniques can be compared in these preparations of lung.

In general terms, the alveolar wall consists of three tissue components: surface epithelium, connective tissue and blood vessels.

(i) Epithelium forms a continuous alveolar lining and consists of cells of two types. Most of the alveolar surface area is covered by large, extremely flattened cells called *Type I pneumocytes*; since the cytoplasm of these cells covers such an extensive area the characteristic, densely stained nuclei of Type I pneumocytes P_1 are relatively infrequently seen in histological section. A second epithelial cell type, known as the *Type II pneumocyte*, is present in larger numbers in the lining epithelium; these cells are rounded in shape and thus occupy a much smaller proportion (about three per cent) of the alveolar surface area. Type II pneumocytes P_2 have large, rounded nuclei with a prominent nucleolus and extensive, vacuolated cytoplasm. Type I pneumocytes constitute part of the extremely thin gaseous diffusion barrier, whereas Type II pneumocytes are thought to secrete a surface-active material called *surfactant* which reduces surface tension within the alveoli.

(ii) Connective tissue forms an attenuated, supporting layer beneath the epithelium and surrounding the blood vessels of the alveolar wall. This layer primarily consists of fine reticular, collagenous and elastic fibres with few fibroblasts.

(iii) Blood vessels, mainly capillaries **C** (7 to 10 μm in diameter) form an extremely rich plexus around each alveolus. In most of the alveolar wall, the basement membrane which supports the capillary endothelium is directly applied to the basement membrane supporting the surface epithelium; in such sites the two basement membranes are fused and the connective tissue layer is absent. This arrangement provides an interface of minimal thickness between alveolar air and blood. Note in these micrographs the nuclei of capillary endothelial cells **E** and the close proximity of erythrocytes to the alveolar air spaces.

Although the defence mechanisms of the conducting passages filter most particulate matter from inspired air, small particles such as carbon reach the alveoli and are engulfed by phagocytic cells found in the alveolar wall or free in the alveolar space. These phagocytes **M**, known as *alveolar macrophages* or *dust cells*, are derived from circulating blood monocytes and are usually recognisable by their content of engulfed, particulate material.

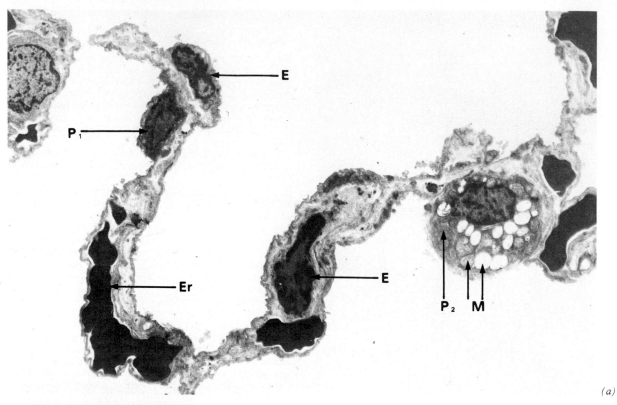

(a)

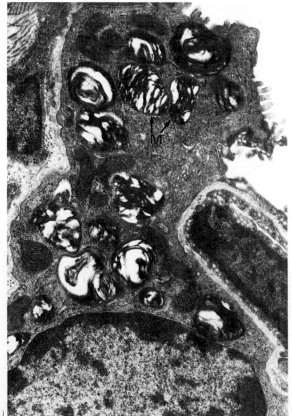

(b)

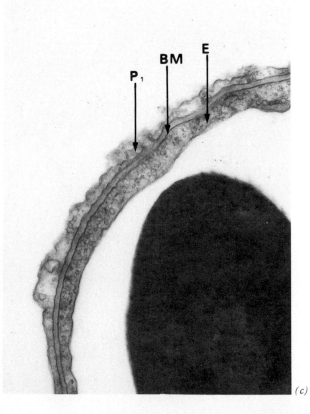

(c)

Fig. 11.11 Alveoli *(illustrations opposite)*

(EM: (a) alveolar wall × 3230
       (b) Type II pneumocyte × 17400
       (c) gaseous diffusion barrier × 30000)

These micrographs illustrate some of the ultrastructural features of the alveolar wall. At low magnification, the nuclei of two endothelial cells **E** can be seen; the capillary lumina are packed with erythrocytes **Er** in various states of deformation. A single Type I pneumocyte **P₁** is recognised by its location outside the basement membrane. A Type II pneumocyte **P₂** is seen typically located at a branching point of the inter-alveolar septum; the cytoplasm is filled with vesicles containing phospholipid in the form of multilamellate bodies **M** seen at higher magnification in (b). It is believed that these bodies are discharged into the alveolar air space where they contribute to a surfactant layer on the epithelium-air interface; Clara cells of the respiratory bronchioles (see Fig. 11.9) may synthesise other components of surfactant. Recent evidence strongly suggests that Type II pneumocytes may differentiate into Type I pneumocytes in response to damage to the alveolar lining.

At high magnification in (c), the components of the gaseous diffusion barrier between blood and alveolar air are seen to consist of the extremely attenuated cytoplasm of a Type I pneumocyte **P₁**, a common basement membrane **BM** and the thin cytoplasm of a capillary endothelial cell **E**. Note the erythrocyte in the capillary lumen.

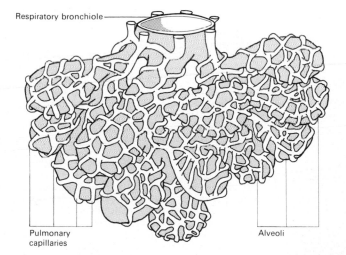

Respiratory bronchiole

Pulmonary capillaries

Alveoli

Fig. 11.12 Pulmonary capillaries

The pulmonary arterial system terminates at the alveolar ducts where arterioles ramify to form a widely interconnected capillary basket surrounding each alveolus; the capillaries are of relatively large diameter (7 to 10 μm). Control of blood flow in the pulmonary capillary bed is predominantly effected by the partial pressure of gases within the alveoli. In poorly ventilated alveoli, the partial pressure of oxygen is low and that of carbon dioxide high; this causes local vasoconstriction, thus directing blood away from poorly ventilated alveoli.

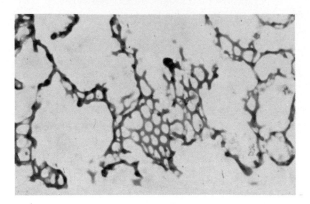

Fig. 11.13 Pulmonary capillary bed

(Dye perfused preparation × 420)

The lung tissue illustrated in this micrograph was prepared by perfusion of the pulmonary vasculature with a blue dye. This procedure outlines the pulmonary capillary bed; no other histological detail can be seen. In the centre of the field the richly anastomosing capillary network of part of an alveolar wall is demonstrated. This type of technique, in combination with the study of very thick histological sections, provided early microscopists with valuable information about the structure, function and vascular system of the lungs.

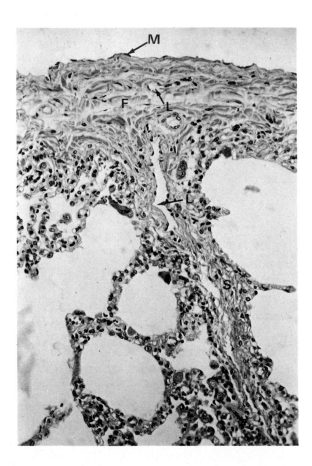

Fig. 11.14 Visceral pleura

(H & E × 198)

The cavities containing the lungs, the *pleural cavities*, are lined by a thin, flattened epithelium (mesothelium) called the *pleura* which is analogous in structure to the pericardium surrounding the heart, and the peritoneum lining the abdominal cavity. The pleura lining the thoracic wall, called the *parietal pleura*, is reflected at the hilum over the surface of the lungs to form a continuous layer called the *visceral pleura*. The visceral and parietal pleura are directly applied to one another but separated by a potential space containing a minute amount of serous fluid. The two pleural layers adhere to one another such that movements of the thoracic wall during ventilation result in corresponding expansion and contraction of the lungs. Pleural fluid is rarely present in discernable amounts in the absence of inflammation or other disease processes.

This micrograph illustrates visceral pleura. The outer surface is lined by a layer of flattened mesothelium **M** which is supported by a thin basement membrane. The underlying fibrous connective tissue **F** is particularly prominent in the human lung and consists primarily of collagen and elastic fibres; smooth muscle cells are occasionally seen. The fibrous layer of visceral pleura extends into the lung as fibrous septa **S** which are continuous with the collagenous framework of the lung.

The visceral pleura contains a superficial plexus of lymph vessels which drain via the connective tissue septa into a deep plexus surrounding the pulmonary blood vessels and airways. Lymph from the deep plexuses drains into the thoracic duct via several prominent lymph nodes in the hilar region. Lymph capillaries are not found in alveolar walls. Several lymph vessels **L** can be seen in the pleura in this micrograph. The visceral pleura also contains numerous small blood vessels and capillaries. Nerves are seen infrequently and are believed to originate from the parasympathetic and sympathetic systems supplying the airways and pulmonary vessels, and from pulmonary stretch receptors.

12. Gastro-intestinal system

Introduction

The gastro-intestinal system is primarily involved in reducing food for absorption into the body. This process occurs in five main phases within defined regions of the gastro-intestinal system: ingestion, fragmentation, digestion, absorption and elimination of waste products. The gastro-intestinal system is essentially a muscular tract lined by a mucous membrane which exhibits regional variations in structure reflecting the progressive functions of the system from the *oral cavity* to the *anus*.

Ingestion and initial fragmentation of food occur in the oral cavity, resulting in the formation of a *bolus* of food which is then conveyed to the *oesophagus* by the action of the tongue and pharyngeal muscles during swallowing (*deglutition*). Fragmentation and swallowing are facilitated by the secretion of *saliva* from three pairs of major *salivary glands* and numerous small accessory glands within the oral cavity. The oesophagus conducts food from the oral cavity to the *stomach* where fragmentation is completed and digestion initiated. Digestion is the process by which food is progressively broken down by enzymes into molecules which are small enough to be absorbed into the circulation; for example, ingested proteins are first broken down into polypeptides then further degraded to small peptides and amino-acids which can then be absorbed. Initial digestion, accompanied by intense muscular action of the stomach wall, reduces the stomach contents to a semi-digested liquid called *chyme*. Chyme is squirted through a muscular sphincter, the *pylorus*, into the *duodenum*, the short, first part of the *small intestine*, where it is neutralised partly by an alkaline secretion from the duodenal mucosa. Digestive enzymes from a large exocrine gland, the *pancreas*, enter the duodenum together with *bile* from the *liver* via the *common bile duct*; bile contains excretory products of liver metabolism, some of which act as emulsifying agents necessary for fat digestion. The duodenal contents pass onwards along the small intestine where the process of digestion is completed and the main absorptive phase occurs. After the duodenum, the next segment of the small intestine, where the major part of absorption occurs, is called the *jejunum*; the rest of the small intestine is called the *ileum*, but there is no distinct junction between these parts of the tract.

The unabsorbed liquid residue from the small intestine passes through a valve, the *ileo-caecal valve*, into the *large intestine*. In the large intestine, water is absorbed from the liquid residue which becomes progressively more solid as it passes towards the anus. The first part of the large intestine is called the *caecum*, from which projects a blind-ended sac, the *appendix*. The next part of the large intestine, the *colon*, is divided anatomically into *ascending*, *transverse*, *descending* and *sigmoid* segments although histologically the segments are similar. The terminal portion of the large intestine, the *rectum*, is a holding chamber for faeces prior to defaecation via the *anal canal*.

Food is propelled along the gastro-intestinal tract by two main mechanisms: voluntary muscular action in the oral cavity, pharynx and upper third of the oesophagus is succeeded by involuntary waves of smooth muscle contraction called *peristalsis*. Peristalsis and the secretory activity of the entire gastro-intestinal system are modulated by the autonomic nervous system and variety of hormones, some of which are secreted by endocrine cells located within the gastro-intestinal tract itself. These cells constitute a diffuse endocrine organ, called the *gastro-intestinal endocrine system*, which not only regulates gastro-intestinal functions but also has a wide range of metabolic influences; this system is discussed in Chapter 14.

Because of its continuity with the external environment, the gastro-intestinal system is a potential portal of entry for pathogenic organisms. Thus the system incorporates a number of defence mechanisms which include prominent aggregations of lymphoid tissue distributed throughout the tract.

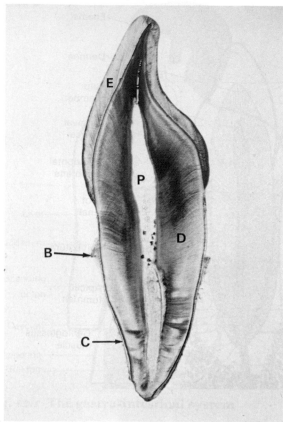

(a)

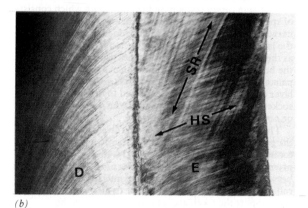

(b)

Fig. 12.3 Incisor tooth

(Undecalcified section: unstained (a) × 5 (b) × 50)

These undecalcified sections cut with a diamond wheel demonstrate the arrangement of the calcified tissues of an upper central incisor tooth.

The dentine **D** which forms the bulk of the crown and root is composed of a calcified organic matrix similar to that of bone. The inorganic component constitutes a somewhat larger proportion of the matrix of dentine than that of bone and exists mainly in the form of hydroxyapatite crystals. From the pulp cavity **P**, minute parallel tubules, called *dentine tubules*, radiate to the periphery of the dentine; in longitudinal sections of teeth, the tubules appear to follow an S-shaped course.

The crown of the tooth is covered by enamel **E**, an extremely hard, translucent substance composed of parallel rods or prisms of extremely calcified material cemented together by an almost equally highly calcified interprismatic material. The enamel prisms have a highly ordered arrangement generally perpendicular to the enamel surface; this arrangement is represented by an optical effect of alternating dark and light bands almost perpendicular to the surface (*Hunter-Schreger bands* **HS**), seen only at higher magnification. Oblique lines representing rest periods between developmental phases can also be seen in the enamel (*striae of Retzius* **SR**).

The root is invested by a thin layer of cementum **C** which is generally thicker towards the apex of the root. The cementum is an amorphous calcified tissue into which the fibres of the periodontal membrane are anchored. Fragments of alveolar bone **B** have remained attached to the root after extraction of this specimen.

The morphological form of the tooth crown and roots varies considerably in different parts of the mouth, nevertheless the basic arrangement of the dental tissues is the same in all teeth.

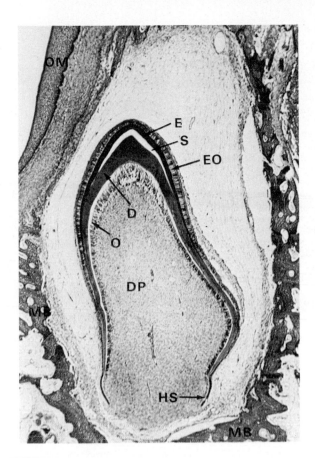

Fig. 12.4 Unerupted tooth

(Kitten: Decalcified section/H & E × 30)

This micrograph of a tooth at an intermediate stage of formation illustrates some important features of developing teeth.

The tissues of the teeth are derived from two embryological sources. An epithelial downgrowth of the fetal oral mucosa forms the so-called *enamel organ*, the *ameloblasts* of which are responsible for the formation of enamel. The enamel organ forms a cap over a papilla of mesenchymal tissue called the *dental papilla* which is responsible for the formation of dentine. As enamel and dentine are laid down in apposition, the enamel organ becomes progressively separated from the dental papilla which shrinks in size and, in the mature tooth, remains as the dental pulp. The dentine-forming cells of the dental pulp are known as *odontoblasts*.

In this micrograph, a densely stained, thin layer of poorly mineralised enamel **E** can be seen covered at its external surface by the enamel organ **EO**. At the tip of the tooth, an unstained space **S** represents fully mineralised enamel laid down at an earlier stage but which has been dissolved away during tissue preparation. Underlying the enamel is a layer of progressively thickening dentine **D** which encloses the highly cellular dental papilla **DP**. Note the layer of odontoblasts **O** immediately underlying the forming dentine. The tip of the tooth crown is formed first, followed by the root which is not fully formed until after tooth eruption. Once the shape of the crown has been established, the shape of the root is determined by an extension of the enamel organ called *Hertwig's sheath* **HS** which, however, does not lay down enamel on the surface of the root. Note the membranous bone **MB** surrounding the developing tooth and the close proximity of the oral mucosa **OM**.

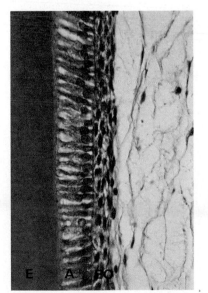

Fig. 12.5 Ameloblasts

(Decalcified section/H & E × 320)

This micrograph, taken from the same specimen of unerupted tooth shown in Fig. 12.4, illustrates the characteristic appearance of ameloblasts, the cells responsible for enamel formation. Active ameloblasts **A** are tall, columnar, epithelial cells which form a single layer apposed to the forming surface of the enamel **E**. Each ameloblast elaborates a column of organic enamel matrix which undergoes progressive mineralisation by the deposition of calcium phosphate mainly in the form of hydroxyapatite crystals. Fully formed enamel contains less than one per cent organic material and is the hardest and most dense tissue in the body.

The structure of mature enamel is not fully understood, but it appears that the process of mineralisation of the enamel matrix is not uniform and, as a result, mature enamel consists of highly calcified prisms separated by so-called *interprismatic material* which may differ only in the orientation of its crystals. Each prism extends from the dentino-enamel junction to the enamel surface and may represent the enamel laid down by a single ameloblast.

Underlying the ameloblast layer are several layers of cells, also of epithelial origin, which constitute the remainder of the enamel organ **EO**. As enamel formation progresses, the enamel organ becomes much reduced in thickness compared with earlier stages of its development. At tooth eruption, the enamel organ, including the ameloblasts, degenerates leaving the enamel exposed to the hostile oral environment, completely incapable of regeneration.

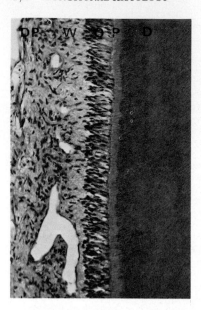

Fig. 12.6 Odontoblasts and dentine
(Decalcified section/H & E × 128)

Dentine, the dense calcified tissue which forms the bulk of the tooth, is broadly similar to bone in composition but is more highly mineralised and thus much harder than bone. The cells responsible for dentine formation, the odontoblasts, differentiate as a single layer of tall, columnar cells on the surface of the dental papilla, apposed to the ameloblast layer of the enamel organ. The odontoblasts initiate tooth formation by deposition of organic dentine matrix between the odontoblastic and ameloblastic layers; calcification of this dentine matrix then induces enamel formation by ameloblasts (see Fig. 12.5). Dentine formation proceeds by continuing odontoblastic deposition of dentine matrix and its subsequent calcification; unlike ameloblasts, each odontoblast leaves behind a slender cytoplasmic process, within a fine dentinal tubule. When dentine formation is complete, the dentine is thus pervaded by parallel odontoblastic processes radiating from the odontoblast layer on the dentinal surface of the reduced dental papilla which now constitutes the dental pulp. After tooth formation is complete, a small amount of less organised *secondary dentine* continues to be laid down resulting in the progressive obliteration of the pulp cavity with advancing age.

This micrograph illustrates active odontoblasts **O** forming a pseudostratified layer of columnar cells at the dentine surface. Parallel dentine tubules containing odontoblastic processes extend through a narrow, pale-stained zone of uncalcified dentine matrix called *predentine* **P** into the mature dentine **D**. Underlying the odontoblastic layer, a relatively acellular layer, called the *cell free zone of Weil* **W**, gives way to the highly cellular dental pulp **DP**.

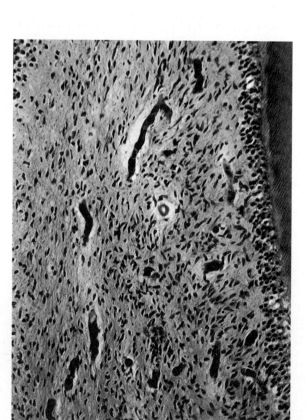

Fig. 12.7 Dental pulp
(Decalcified section/H & E × 198)

The dental pulp consists of a delicate connective tissue resembling primitive mesenchyme (see Fig. 3.1); it contains numerous stellate fibroblasts, reticulin fibres, fine poorly organised collagen fibres and much ground substance. The pulp contains a rich network of thin-walled capillaries supplied by arterioles which enter the pulp canal from the periodontal membrane, usually via one foramen at each root apex. The pulp is also richly innervated by a plexus of myelinated nerve fibres from which fine, unmyelinated branches extend into the odontoblastic layer. Despite the acute sensitivity of dentine, nerve fibres are rarely demonstrable in dentine and the mechanism of sensory reception is unknown; it has been suggested that the odontoblastic processes may act as sensory receptors.

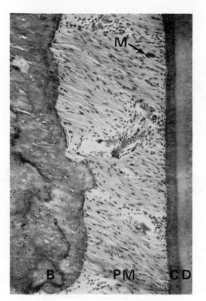

Fig. 12.8 Periodontal membrane and cementum
(Decalcified section/H & E × 128)

The periodontal membrane **PM** forms a thin fibrous attachment between the tooth root and the alveolar bone. The dentine **D**, comprising the root, is covered by a thin layer of cementum **C** which is elaborated by cells called *cementocytes* lying on the surface of the cementum. Cementum consists of a dense, calcified organic material similar to the matrix of bone, and is generally acellular. Towards the root apex, the cementum layer becomes progressively thicker and cementocytes are often entrapped in lacunae within the cementum.

The periodontal membrane consists of dense, fibrous connective tissue. The collagen fibres, known as *Sharpey's fibres*, run obliquely downwards from their attachment in the alveolar bone **B** to their anchorage in the cementum at a more apical position on the root surface. The periodontal membrane thus acts as a sling for the tooth within its socket, permitting slight movements which cushion the impact of masticatory forces. The points of attachment of the collagen fibres in both cementum and bone are in a constant state of reorganisation to accommodate changing functional stresses upon the teeth. Osteoclastic resorption (see Fig. 9.14) is often seen at one aspect of a tooth socket and complementary osteoblastic deposition (see Fig. 9.13) at the opposite side, thus indicating bodily movement of the tooth through the bone; this is the mechanism which permits tooth movement during orthodontic treatment.

The periodontal membrane is richly supplied by blood vessels and nerves from the surrounding alveolar bone, the apical region and the gingiva. Small clumps of epithelial cells are often found scattered throughout the periodontal membrane; these cells are remnants of Hertwig's sheath (see Fig. 12.4) and are known as *epithelial rests of Malassez* **M**.

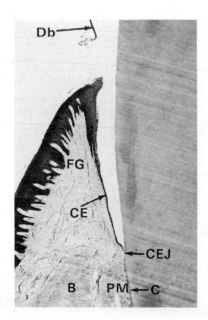

Fig. 12.9 Gingival attachment
(Decalcified section/H & E × 20)

This micrograph shows the relationship of the gingiva or gum to the neck of the tooth. During tissue preparation the enamel has been completely dissolved from the surface of the crown, but the extent of the outer surface of the enamel can be visualised by shreds of remaining organic debris **Db** which had been adherent to the tooth surface.

The gingiva may be divided into the *attached gingiva* which provides a protective covering to the alveolar bone **B**, and the *free gingiva* **FG** which forms a cuff around the enamel at the neck of the tooth. Between the enamel and the free gingiva is a potential space, the gingival crevice, which extends from the tip of the free gingiva to the cemento-enamel junction **CEJ**.

The thick, stratified squamous epithelium, which constitutes the oral aspect of the gingiva, undergoes abrupt transition at the tip of the free gingiva to form a thin layer of epithelial cells tapering to only two or three cells thick at the base of the gingival crevice. This crevicular epithelium **CE** is easily breached by pathogenic organisms and the underlying connective tissue is thus frequently infiltrated by lymphoid cells.

Collagen fibres of the periodontal membrane **PM** radiate from the cementum **C** near the cemento-enamel junction into the dense connective tissue of the free gingiva; these fibres, together with circular fibres surrounding the neck of the tooth, maintain the role of the gingiva as a protective cuff.

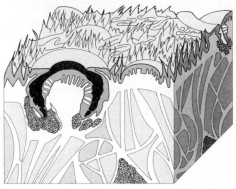

Fig. 12.10 Tongue

The tongue is a muscular organ covered by oral mucosa which is specialised for manipulating food, general sensory reception and the special sensory function of taste (see Fig. 7.39). Four types of papillae crowd the tongue surface: *filiform, fungiform, circumvallate* and *foliate papillae*. In man, the taste buds containing taste receptors are found mainly on the circumvallate papillae, twelve to twenty of which form a V-shaped row which divides the anterior two-thirds of the tongue from the posterior third. The other papillae have mainly general sensory and mechanical functions.

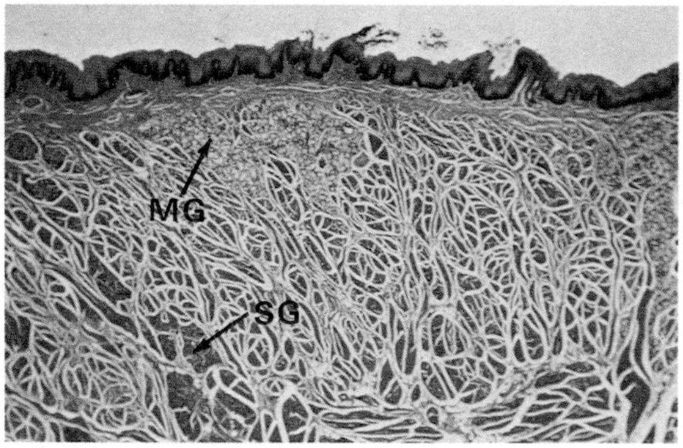

Fig. 12.11 Tongue

(H & E × 8)

The body of the tongue consists of a mass of interlacing bundles of skeletal muscle fibres which permit an extensive range of tongue movements. The mucous membrane covering the tongue is firmly bound to the underlying muscle by a dense, collagenous, lamina propria which is continuous with the epimysium of the tongue muscle. Note the papillary nature of the surface epithelium.

Numerous small serous and mucous accessory salivary glands are scattered throughout the muscle and lamina propria of the tongue. In this preparation the serous glands **SG** are stained strongly whereas the mucous glands **MG** are poorly stained.

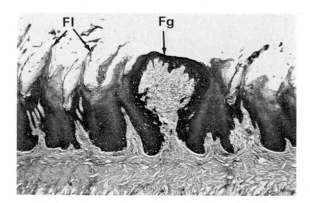

Fig. 12.12 Filiform and fungiform papillae

(H & E × 20)

This micrograph illustrates several filiform papillae **Fl** and a fungiform papilla **Fg**. Filiform papillae are the most numerous type and consist of a dense, connective tissue core and a heavily keratinised surface projection. Fungiform papillae have a thin, non-keratinised epithelium and a richly vascularised connective tissue core giving them a red appearance macroscopically amongst the much more numerous, whitish, filiform papillae.

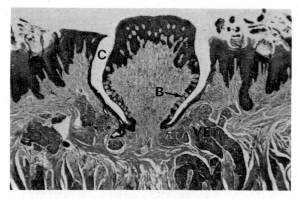

Fig. 12.13 Circumvallate papilla

(H & E × 20)

Circumvallate papillae are the largest and least common type of papilla on the tongue. They are set into the tongue surface and encircled by a deep cleft **C**. The papillary epithelium of the cleft contains numerous taste buds **B**, the detail of which is shown in Fig. 7.39. Aggregations of serous glands, called Von Ebner's glands **VE**, secrete a watery fluid into the cleft; this secretion dissolves food components thus facilitating taste reception.

Salivary glands

Saliva is produced by three pairs of major salivary glands, the *parotid, submandibular* and *sublingual glands*, and numerous minor accessory glands scattered throughout the oral mucosa. The minor salivary glands secrete continuously and are, in general, under local control, whereas the major glands mainly secrete in response to parasympathetic activity which is produced by physical, chemical and psychological stimuli.

Saliva is a hypotonic, watery secretion containing variable amounts of mucus, enzymes (principally *amylase* and the antibacterial enzyme *lysozyme*), antibodies and inorganic ions. Two types of secretory cells are found in the major salivary glands: serous cells and mucous cells. The parotid glands consist mainly of serous cells and produce a thin, watery secretion rich in enzymes and antibodies. The sublingual glands have predominantly mucous secretory cells and produce a viscid secretion. The submandibular glands contain both serous and mucous secretory cells and produce a secretion of intermediate consistency. The overall composition of saliva varies according to the degree of activity of each of the major gland types.

Traditionally, the role of salivary amylase has been considered to be the initiation of starch digestion in the oral cavity; its primary role, however, is more likely to be as a cleansing agent for starch debris retained around the teeth. The protective role of salivary antibodies is poorly understood; they may be associated functionally with leucocytes also found in saliva.

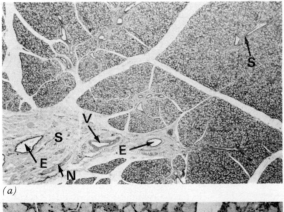

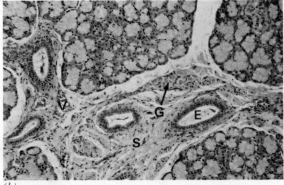

(a)

(b)

Fig. 12.14 Salivary gland: submandibular gland

(H & E (a) ×8 (b) ×80)

The general architecture of the major salivary glands follows the pattern shown in these preparations. The glands are divided into numerous lobules, each containing many secretory units. In H & E preparations, serous secretory cells are stained strongly whereas mucous cells are poorly stained. Connective tissue septa **S** radiate between the lobules from an outer capsule and convey blood vessels **V**, nerves **N** and large excretory ducts **E**. Note that the large excretory ducts have a stratified cuboidal epithelial lining seen at higher magnification in (b). Small parasympathetic ganglia **G** may be seen in the connective tissue septa.

Fig. 12.15 Salivary gland secretory unit

The salivary secretory unit consists of a terminal, branched, tubulo-acinar structure composed exclusively of either serous or mucous secretory cells or a mixture of both types. In mixed secretory units where mucous cells predominate, serous cells often form semilunar caps called *serous demilunes* surrounding the terminal part of the mucous acini. The terminal secretory units merge to form larger, so-called *intercalated ducts* which are also lined by secretory cells. The intercalated ducts drain into larger ducts called *striated ducts* which are named for their striated appearance in light microscopy. The striations result from the presence of numerous, deep infoldings of the basal plasma membranes of the large cuboidal cells which line these ducts.

In addition to the salivary proteins, the serous cells are involved in active secretion of a watery fluid containing a variety of inorganic ions; this basic secretion is isotonic with plasma. In the striated ducts, the ionic content of the basic secretion is modified by active reabsorption and further secretion of ions to produce saliva which is hypotonic with respect to plasma. The ionic composition of saliva varies at different flow rates, but in general, the concentrations of sodium and chloride ions are below that of plasma, and the concentrations of potassium and bicarbonate ions are above that of plasma. The transport processes in the striated ducts are facilitated by the large surface area offered by the basal infoldings of the lining cells and fuelled by their numerous associated mitochondria.

The secretory acini are enveloped by the processes of cells of epithelial origin which are packed with contractile filaments similar to those of smooth muscle; contraction of these so-called myoepithelial cells mediates salivary secretion by forcing the contents of secretory acini into the duct system and thence into the oral cavity.

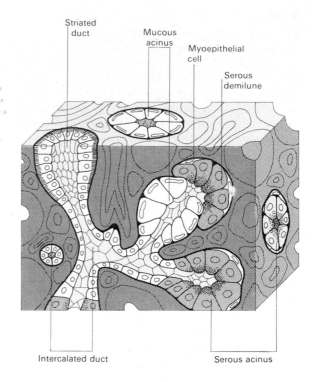

Striated duct

Mucous acinus

Myoepithelial cell

Serous demilune

Intercalated duct

Serous acinus

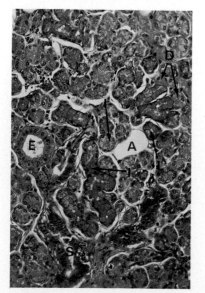

Fig. 12.16 Submandibular salivary gland

(H & E/Alcian blue × 128)

This preparation of a mixed sero-mucous salivary gland has been counterstained with alcian blue to highlight mucous secretory cells. This field is mostly occupied by pure serous secretory units; most of the mucous secretory units are capped by serous demilunes **D**. Serous secretory cells have a round nucleus which is located near to the centre of the cell; in contrast, the mucous cells have a flattened nucleus which is pressed against the base of the cell by densely packed mucigen granules in the cytoplasm. Serous and mucous intercalated ducts **I** can be seen in both transverse and longitudinal section. Striated ducts **S** are more intensely stained due to their numerous mitochondria. A small excretory duct **E** is characterised by its larger diameter and the relatively pale stained cytoplasm of its lining cells. No modification of saliva occurs in the excretory ducts. All salivary glands contain a variable number of adipocytes which increase in number with advancing age; a single large adipocyte **A** is seen in this micrograph.

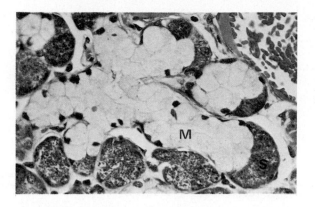

Fig. 12.17 Salivary gland: mixed secretory unit

(H & E × 320)

This micrograph of a mixed sero-mucous secretory unit shows several mucous acini **M** with serous demilunes **S**. In H & E stained preparations, mucigen granules within mucous acini are poorly stained whereas the enzyme-containing (zymogen) granules of serous acini are strongly stained. The nuclei of mucous cells are characteristically condensed and flattened against the basement membrane. The nuclei of serous cells are rounded, with dispersed chromatin, and usually occupy a more central position within the cell.

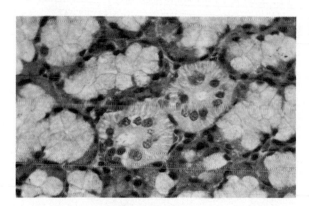

Fig. 12.18 Striated ducts

(H & E × 320)

The striated ducts are lined by large cuboidal cells with large nuclei located between the centre and luminal surface of the cell. The basal cytoplasm appears striated, reflecting the presence of deep basal infoldings of the plasma membrane and associated columns of mitochondria; the apical cytoplasm is uniformly stained and not striated. In predominantly serous salivary glands, the striated ducts are larger than in predominantly mucous glands, a feature associated with the role of the striated duct in modifying isotonic basic saliva to produce hypotonic saliva.

Note in this micrograph that the two striated ducts are surrounded by predominantly mucous secretory units some of which have small serous demilunes. Note also the rich capillary network in the sparse supporting tissue between the secretory acini.

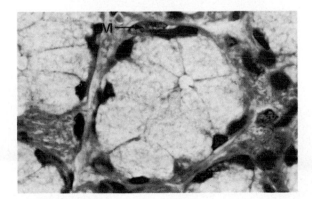

Fig. 12.19 Mucous acinus

(H & E × 800)

Both serous and mucous acini are embraced by the processes of contractile cells called myoepithelial cells which, on contraction, force secretion from the acinar lumen into the duct system. Myoepithelial cells are located between the basal plasma membranes of secretory cells and the epithelial basement membrane. These cells are flattened and have long processes which extend around the secretory acinus but in sections they can only be recognised by their large, flattened nuclei lying within the basement membrane surrounding the acinus. This micrograph shows the typical appearance of a myoepithelial cell **M** embracing a mucous acinus.

General structure of the gastro-intestinal tract

The structure of the gastro-intestinal tract conforms to a general plan which is clearly evident from the oesophagus to the anus and is illustrated in Fig. 12.20. The oral cavity and pharynx also conform to this general pattern, but this is less evident due to the extreme specialisation of these regions.

The tract is essentially a muscular tube lined by a mucous membrane. The arrangement of the major muscular component remains relatively constant throughout the tract whereas the mucosa shows marked variations in the different regions of the tract. At several points along the tract the mucosa undergoes abrupt transition from one form to another: these points are the *oesophageo-gastric junction*, the *gastro-duodenal junction*, the *ileo-caecal junction* and the *recto-anal junction*. Between these epithelial junctions the mucosa generally undergoes only a gradual transition in structure along the length of the tract.

Fig. 12.20 General structure of the gastro-intestinal tract

The gastro-intestinal tract has four distinct functional layers: *mucosa*, *submucosa*, *muscularis* and *adventitia*.

(i) The mucosa: the mucosa is divided, histologically, into three layers: an epithelial lining, a supporting connective tissue lamina propria and a thin smooth muscle layer, the *muscularis mucosae*, which produces local movements and folding of the mucosa.

(ii) The submucosa: this layer of loose connective tissue supports the mucosa and contains the larger blood vessels, lymphatics and nerves.

(iii) The muscularis: this functional layer consists of smooth muscle which is subdivided usually into two histological layers: an inner circular layer and an outer longitudinal layer. The action of these smooth muscle layers, opposed at right angles to one another, is the basis of peristaltic contraction.

(iv) The adventitia: this outer layer of connective tissue conducts the major vessels and nerves. In the abdominal cavity it is continuous with the connective tissue of the mesenteries and in other sites it is continuous with the surrounding connective tissues. Where the adventitia is exposed to the abdominal cavity it is referred to as the *serosa* and is lined by a simple squamous epithelium called mesothelium.

Parasympathetic ganglia are concentrated in so-called plexuses in the wall of the tract. In the submucosa, isolated or small clusters of parasympathetic ganglion cells give rise to post-ganglionic fibres which supply the mucosal glands and the smooth muscle of the muscularis muscosae; this submucosal plexus is sometimes referred to as *Meissner's plexus*. Larger clusters of parasympathetic ganglion cells are found between the two layers of the muscularis; the post-ganglionic fibres mainly supply the surrounding smooth muscle. This plexus is known as the *myenteric plexus* or *Auerbach's plexus*.

Glands are found throughout the tract at various depths in the tract wall. In some parts of the tract, the mucosal lining is arranged into glands which have a variety of secretory functions. In some regions, glands penetrate the muscularis mucosa to lie in the submucosa. The pancreas and liver are large glands draining into the gastro-intestinal lumen but lying entirely outside the tract wall.

Lymphoid tissue is distributed throughout the tract in aggregations of variable size; these are predominantly located within the mucosal layer.

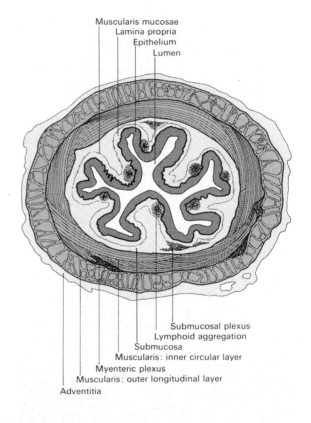

Muscularis mucosae
Lamina propria
Epithelium
Lumen

Submucosal plexus
Lymphoid aggregation
Submucosa
Muscularis: inner circular layer
Myenteric plexus
Muscularis: outer longitudinal layer
Adventitia

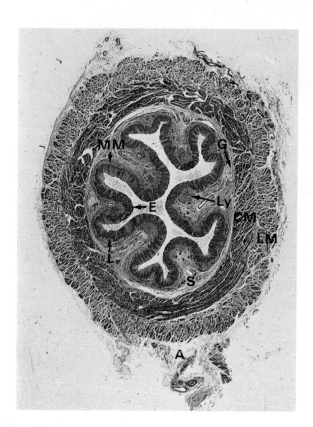

Fig. 12.21 Oesophagus

(TS: Masson's trichrome ×6)

This section from the lower third of the oesophagus demonstrates all the basic layers of the gastro-intestinal tract. The lumen of the oesophagus is lined by a thick, protective, stratified squamous epithelium **E** which in some animals with coarse diets, e.g. rodents, may be keratinised. The underlying lamina propria **L** contains lymphoid aggregations **Ly**. The muscularis mucosae **MM** is barely visible at this magnification. The submucosa **S** contains small mucous glands **G** which are mainly confined to the lower third of the oesophagus. In the muscularis, inner circular **CM** and outer longitudinal **LM** layers of smooth muscle are clearly distinguishable. Since the first part of swallowing is under voluntary control, fasciculi of skeletal muscle predominate in the muscularis of the upper third of the oesophagus. Outside the muscularis, the richly vascular adventitia **A** is continuous with the surrounding connective tissue. In the relaxed state, the oesophageal mucosa is deeply folded; this arrangement permits gross distension during the passage of a food bolus.

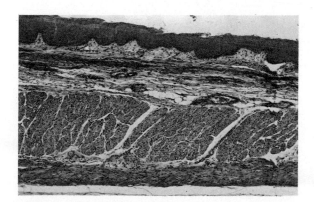

Fig. 12.22 Oesophagus

(LS: H & E ×20)

This micrograph illustrates at higher magnification similar features of the oesophageal wall as seen in Fig. 12.21 but in longitudinal section.

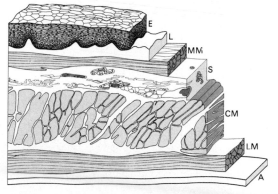

Fig. 12.23 Explanatory diagram for Fig. 12.22

E   —stratified squamous epithelium
L   —lamina propria
MM —muscularis mucosae
S   —submucosa
CM —circular layer of muscularis
LM —longitudinal layer of muscularis
A   —adventitia

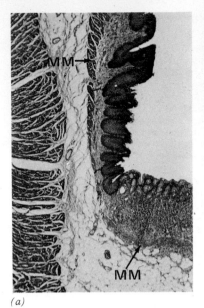

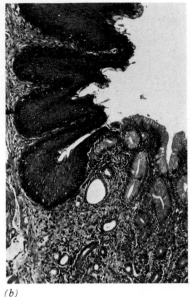

(a)　　　　　*(b)*

Fig. 12.24 Oesophageo-gastric junction

(H & E (a) ×20 (b) ×128)

At the junction of the oesophagus and stomach the mucosa of the tract undergoes an abrupt transition from a protective, stratified squamous epithelium to a highly glandular mucosa. The muscularis mucosae **MM** is continuous across the junction but becomes less clearly definable in the stomach. The underlying layers continue uninterrupted beneath the mucosal junction. The muscularis does not form a thick anatomical sphincter; increased tone in the muscularis of the terminal part of the oesophagus provides a physiological sphincter mechanism which, under normal circumstances, prevents reflux of gastric contents into the oesophagus.

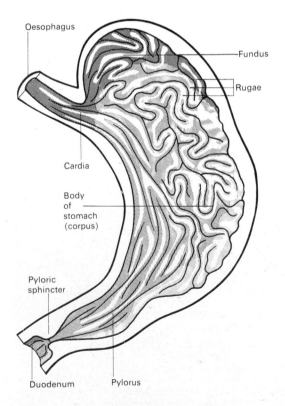

Fig. 12.25 Stomach

The stomach is a dilated part of the gastro-intestinal tract in which ingested food is retained for two hours or longer so as to undergo mechanical and chemical reduction to form chyme. Mechanical reduction is produced by a strong, muscular, churning action whilst chemical reduction is produced by gastric juices secreted by the glands of the stomach mucosa. There is little absorption of food products from the stomach, although alcohol is a notable exception. Once chyme formation is completed, the pyloric sphincter relaxes and allows the liquid chyme to be squirted into the duodenum. In the non-distended state, the stomach mucosa is thrown into prominent longitudinal folds called *rugae* which permit great distension after eating.

Anatomically the stomach is divided into four regions: the *cardia, fundus, body (corpus)* and *pylorus (pyloric antrum)*. The pylorus terminates in a strong muscular sphincter surrounding the gastro-duodenal junction.

The mucosa of the whole stomach is glandular and there are three distinctly different histological zones:

(i) The cardia is a small area of predominantly mucus-secreting glands surrounding the entrance of the oesophagus (see Fig. 12.24).

(ii) The mucosa of the fundus and body forms the major histological region and consists of glands which secrete gastric juices as well as some protective mucus.

(iii) The pylorus has a different glandular conformation; here the glands secrete mucus, and associated endocrine cells secrete the hormone *gastrin* into the blood vessels of the lamina propria.

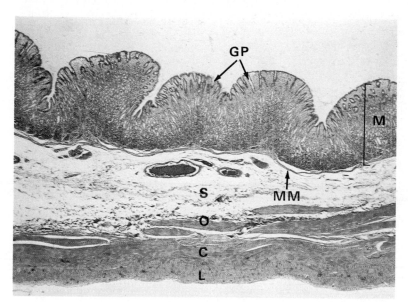

Fig. 12.26 Body of the stomach
(H & E × 12)

This micrograph of the body of the stomach in the non-distended state shows the mucosa thrown into prominent folds or rugae. The mucosa **M** consists of *gastric glands* which extend from the level of the muscularis mucosae **MM** to open into the stomach lumen via *gastric pits* **GP**. The muscularis comprises the usual inner circular **C** and outer longitudinal **L** layers but the inner circular layer is reinforced by a further inner oblique layer **O**. Note the relatively large blood vessels coursing in the submucosa **S**.

Fig. 12.27 Gastric glands
(H & E × 120)

The mucosa of the fundus and body of the stomach consists of straight, tubular glands which synthesise and secrete gastric juice. Gastric juice is a watery secretion containing hydrochloric acid (pH 0·9 to 1·5) and the digestive enzyme *pepsin* which hydrolyses proteins into polypeptide fragments. The stomach mucosa is protected from self-digestion by a thick surface covering of mucus.

The gastric glands contain a mixed population of cells of three main types:

(i) Mucus-secreting cells **M** cover the luminal surface of the stomach and line the gastric pits **GP** into which the gastric glands open; the cytoplasmic mucigen granules which pack these cells are stained poorly by H & E. Another type of mucous cell, the *neck mucous cell*, is found in the necks of the glands.

(ii) Hydrochloric acid-secreting cells, called *parietal* **Pl** or *oxyntic cells*, are distributed along the length of the glands but tend to be most numerous in the middle portion. These large, rounded cells have an extensive eosinophilic (oxyntic) cytoplasm and a centrally located nucleus.

(iii) Pepsin-secreting cells, called *peptic* **Pc**, *chief*, or *zymogenic cells*, tend to be clustered at the base of the gastric glands. Peptic cells are recognised by their strongly basophilic, granular cytoplasm and dense, basally located nuclei.

Thin strands of the muscularis mucosae extend between the gastric glands from the base; contraction of this muscle expels gastric secretions into the stomach lumen.

In addition to the exocrine cells of the gastric mucosa, endocrine secretory cells are found scattered throughout the gastric mucosa as in the mucosa of the rest of the gastro-intestinal tract (see Chapter 14).

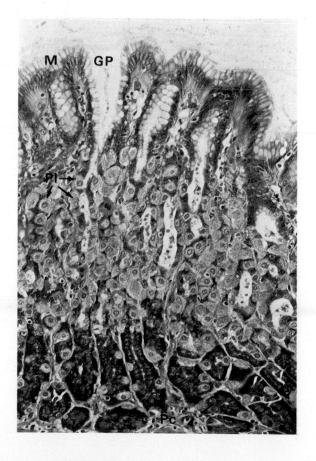

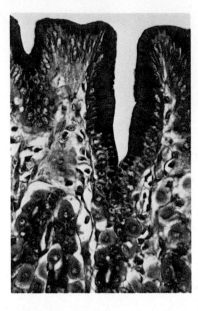
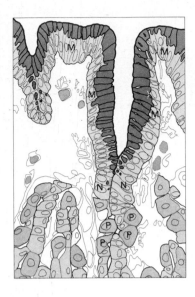

Fig. 12.28 Gastric pit

LS: (a) PAS/Haematoxylin/ Orange G × 320
(b) explanatory diagram for (a)

The PAS method has been used in this preparation to highlight the mucous cells of the gastric mucosa. The stomach surface is lined by a single layer of tall columnar, mucus-secreting cells **M** which are shed continuously and replaced by cells which migrate from the gastric pits. Other mucus-secreting cells in the necks of the gastric glands, called neck mucous cells **N**, secrete a less viscous mucus which may protect the gland duct from autodigestion.

Parietal (acid-secreting) cells **P** are recognised by their characteristic 'fried egg' appearance; in this preparation their acidophilic cytoplasm is stained strongly with Orange G.

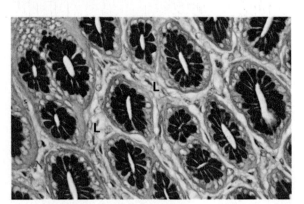

Fig. 12.29 Gastric pits

(TS: PAS/Haematoxylin/Orange G × 128)

In transverse section, the tubular nature of the gastric pits is clearly evident. Note the richly vascularised, loose connective tissue of the supporting lamina propria **L**.

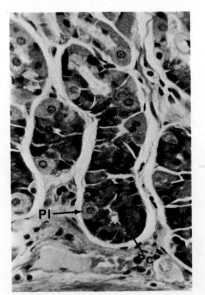

Fig. 12.30 Base of gastric gland

(H & E × 320)

Peptic **Pc** (chief) cells, which synthesise and secrete the proteolytic enzyme pepsin, are the principal cell type in the basal third of the gastric glands, although parietal cells **Pl** are also found at this level. Peptic cells have a basally located nucleus and extensive, granular cytoplasm packed with the inactive pepsin precursor, *pepsinogen*. Pepsinogen remains inactive until it reaches the lumen of the stomach where it is activated by the gastric juices; this mechanism prevents destruction of the gastric glands by autodigestion.

In contrast to the peptic cells, the parietal cells are rounded with large, centrally-located nuclei and strongly eosinophilic (pink stained) cytoplasm. Whereas peptic cells tend to occur in clusters at the base of the gastric glands, parietal cells are scattered throughout the gland from neck to base.

The secretory activity of both parietal and peptic cells is controlled by the autonomic nervous system and the gastro-intestinal hormone gastrin secreted by endocrine cells mainly located in the pylorus.

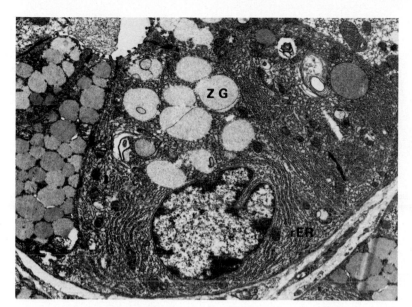

Fig. 12.31 Peptic cells
(Rat: EM × 7900)

This electron micrograph illustrates a peptic cell at the base of a gastric gland. The ultrastructural features of peptic cells are those of protein secreting (zymogenic) cells in general; these features include an extensive rough endoplasmic reticulum **rER** and membrane bound secretory vesicles **ZG** (zymogen granules) crowded in the apical cytoplasm, thus restricting the nucleus to the base of the cell. The extensive rough endoplasmic reticulum accounts for the intense basophilia of peptic cells seen with light microscopy.

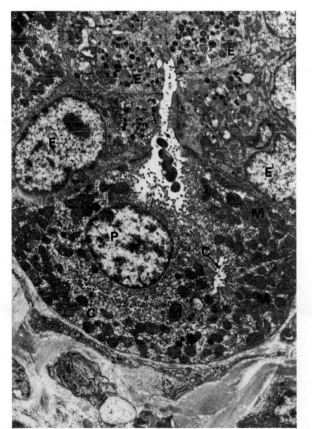

Fig. 12.32 Parietal cell
(Rat: EM × 4800)

This micrograph shows a parietal cell **P** within a gastric gland. The luminal plasma membrane of the parietal cell forms deep, branching canaliculi **C** which extend throughout the cytoplasm. Numerous short microvilli project into the lumina of the intracellular canaliculi. The cytoplasm is crowded with mitochondria **M** which have closely packed cristae; an extensive labyrinth of smooth endoplasmic reticulum pervades the cytoplasm. The mechanism by which parietal cells produce hydrochloric acid is poorly understood. The concentration of hydrogen ions, by the order of one million times compared with plasma, and the equivalent concentration of chloride ions, is a highly energy-dependent process; this energy is provided by the extremely numerous mitochondria. Parietal cells are also thought to secrete the substance called *intrinsic factor* which is essential for the absorption of vitamin B12 in the ileum.

Also seen in this micrograph are several endocrine cells **E** of the gastro-intestinal endocrine series (see Chapter 14); these cells contain small electron-dense secretory granules. Special histochemical techniques must be used to identify the precise nature of their secretory product.

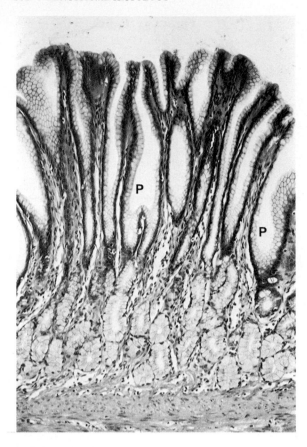

Fig. 12.33 Pyloric stomach
(H & E × 120)

In contrast to the simple tubular glands of the fundus and body, the pyloric glands are branched, and are composed of mucus-secreting cells only. The glands open into deep, irregularly shaped pits **P**. The function of the mucus secreted by the pyloric glands is to lubricate and protect the entrance to the duodenum.

Scattered amongst the pyloric mucous cells are endocrine cells which secrete the peptide hormone gastrin and are thus called 'G' cells. Demonstration of G cells requires special histochemical methods. The presence of food in the stomach stimulates secretion of gastrin into the bloodstream; gastrin then stimulates secretion of pepsin and acid by the gastric glands of the fundus and body, and also stimulates gastric motility. Gastrin-secreting cells are also found in smaller numbers in other sites along the gastro-intestinal tract (see Chapter 14).

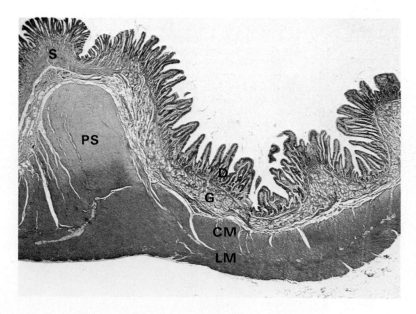

Fig. 12.34 Gastro-duodenal junction
(Monkey: H & E × 12)

The pyloric sphincter **PS** marks a dramatic transition in the gastro-intestinal mucosa from the glandular arrangement of the stomach **S** to a villous arrangement which characterises the whole of the small intestine from the duodenum to the ileo-caecal junction. The duodenal mucosa **D** is arranged into villi and crypts, the detailed structure of which is described in later sections. The duodenum is characterised by the presence of numerous mucus-secreting glands **G** in the submucosa. The submucosal glands are called *Brunner's glands* and are not found elsewhere in the small intestine.

The pyloric sphincter consists of an extreme thickening of the circular layer of the muscularis at the gastro-duodenal junction. Note the continuity of both the circular **CM** and longitudinal **LM** layers of the muscularis between the pylorus and duodenum.

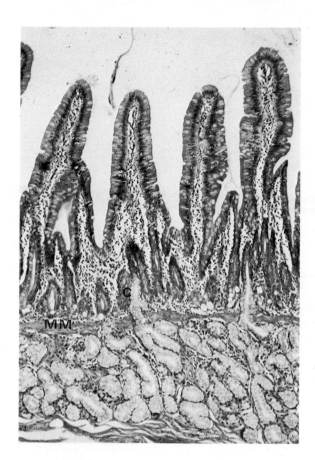

Fig. 12.35 Duodenum
(Monkey: H & E × 50)

This micrograph illustrates the extensive aggregation of Brunner's glands underlying the muscularis mucosae **MM** of the duodenum. The glands have a branched, coiled arrangement and the excretory ducts penetrate the muscularis mucosae to open into the bases of the mucosal crypts **C**.

The duodenum constitutes the first ten inches of the small intestine and undergoes gradual transition into the jejunum. The functions of the duodenum are similar to those of the rest of the small intestine, that is the completion of the digestive process and the absorption of digestive products. In addition, the duodenum has two specialised secretory functions related to the reception of acidic chyme from the stomach.

(i) The presence of chyme in the duodenum stimulates Brunner's glands to secrete a thin, alkaline mucus which helps to neutralise the acidic chyme and to protect the duodenal mucosa from autodigestion.

(ii) Chyme also stimulates the release of two peptide hormones, *secretin*, and *cholecystokinin-pancreozymin* (*CCK*) from endocrine cells scattered throughout the duodenal mucosa. Secretin and CCK promote pancreatic secretion into the pancreatic duct, and CCK also stimulates contraction of the gall bladder thus propelling bile into the common bile duct. The pancreatic and bile ducts merge to empty their contents into the duodenum via a single short duct.

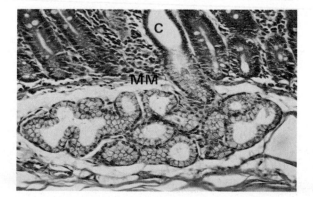

Fig. 12.36 Brunner's gland
(H & E × 128)

This micrograph shows a Brunner's gland from the distal part of the duodenum where the glands tend to be smaller and less branched than in the proximal section. The duct of a Brunner's gland is seen penetrating the muscularis mucosae **MM** to enter a mucosal crypt **C**. The tall, columnar cells of Brunner's glands have extensive, poorly stained, mucigen-filled cytoplasm and dense, basally located nuclei.

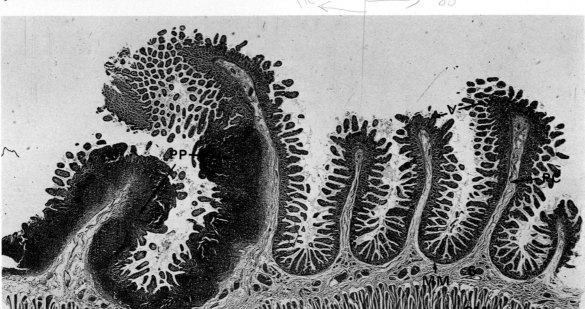

Fig. 12.37 Small intestine
(H & E × 16)

The small intestine, comprising the duodenum, jejunum and ileum, is the principal site for absorption of digestion products from the gastro-intestinal tract. Digestion begins in the stomach and is completed in the small intestine in intimate association with the absorption process. Intestinal digestion occurs in two ways: *luminal digestion* and *membrane digestion*.

(i) Luminal digestion: this involves the mixing of chyme with pancreatic enzymes with subsequent molecular breakdown occurring within the intestinal lumen. Luminal digestion is greatly facilitated by adsorption of pancreatic enzymes on to the mucosal surface.

(ii) Membrane digestion: this type of digestive process involves enzymes located within the luminal plasma membranes of the cells lining the small intestine; these digestive enzymes do not occur free in the intestinal lumen.

Digestion and absorption are enhanced by the provision of an enormous surface area in the small intestine by virtue of four main features:

(a) the great length of the small intestine (four to six metres long in man);

(b) the presence of circularly arranged folds of the mucosa and submucosa called *plica circulares* or *valves of Kerckring*; the plica are particularly numerous in the jejunum;

(c) the arrangement of the mucosa into extremely numerous finger-like projections, called *villi*, and the invagination of the mucosa between the bases of the villi into crypts, called *crypts of Lieberkuhn*;

(d) the presence of extensive microvilli on the surface of each intestinal lining cell.

This micrograph, taken at very low magnification, illustrates plica circulares **PC** covered with villi **V**. The muscularis mucosae **MM** immediately underlies the villi. The vascular submucosa **S** extends into, and forms the core of, the plica circulares. The inner circular **CM** and outer longitudinal **LM** layers of the muscularis produce continuous peristaltic activity of the small intestine. The peritoneal aspect of the muscularis is invested by the loose connective tissue serosa **Sr** which is lined on its peritoneal surface by mesothelium.

A prominent feature of the small intestine is the presence of lymphoid aggregations of various size within the lamina propria; the larger aggregations are known as *Peyer's patches* **PP**. The functional significance of the gastro-intestinal lymphoid tissues is poorly understood and is discussed in Chapter 10.

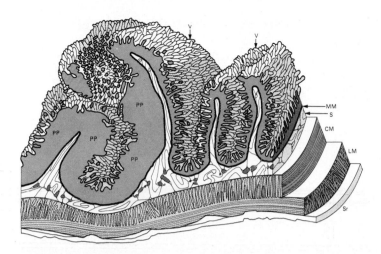

Fig. 12.38 Explanatory diagram for Fig. 12.37

V —villi
MM —muscularis mucosae
S —submucosa
CM —circular layer of smooth muscle
LM —longitudinal layer of smooth muscle
Sr —serosa
PP —Peyer's patch

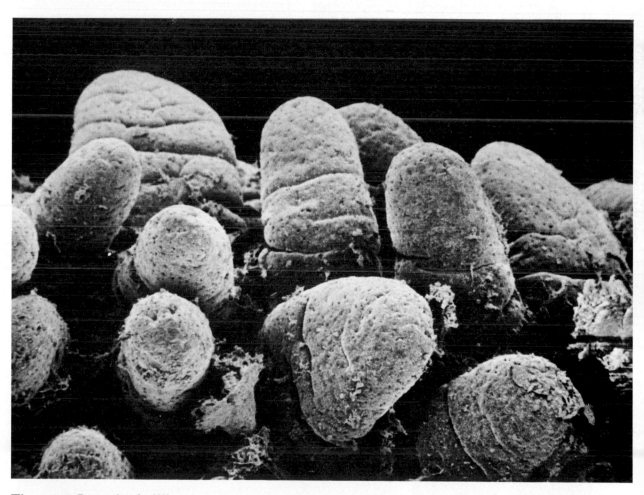

Fig. 12.39 Intestinal villi

(Scanning EM × 100)

This preparation of small intestine taken from the same biopsy specimen as Fig. 12.37 demonstrates, in three dimensions, the intestinal villi along the crest of a plica circularis. Crypts of Lieberkuhn open into the spaces between the bases of the villi but are obscured by residual mucus. Surface openings of scattered goblet cells give each villus the appearance of a pepper pot in this type of preparation.

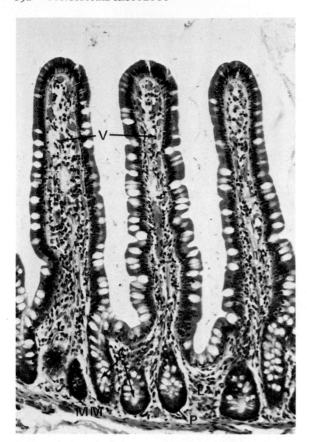

Fig. 12.40 Intestinal villi and crypts
(H & E × 120)

The intestinal villi **V** are lined by a simple, columnar epithelium which is continuous with that of the crypts **C**. The cells of this epithelium are of two main types: *enterocytes* and goblet cells. The enterocytes, which are involved in membrane digestion and absorption, are tall columnar cells with basally located nuclei; goblet cells are scattered among the enterocytes. The entire epithelial lining of the intestine is replaced every three to five days by the continual shedding of cells from the tips of the villi into the lumen. Mitotic activity in the crypts produces a continuous supply of new cells which progress up the villi where they mature before degenerating and being shed.

A third cell type, with no known digestive or absorptive function, is found in clusters at the base of the crypts. These cells, called *Paneth cells* **P**, are packed with strongly eosinophilic granules and are a prominent feature of the small intestine in man, although absent in some mammals. Paneth cells are known to be a stable population of cells and to have the ultrastructural characteristics of exocrine, protein-secreting cells yet their function remains obscure.

The lamina propria **L** extends between the crypts and into the core of each villus and contains a rich vascular and lymphatic network into which digestive products are absorbed. The muscularis mucosae **MM** lies immediately beneath the base of the crypts.

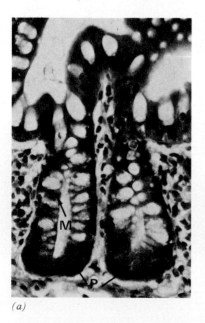

(a)

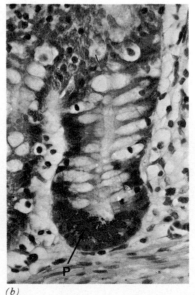

(b)

Fig. 12.41 Crypts of Lieberkuhn
(a) H & E × 320
(b) Phloxine-tartrazine × 320

At high magnification, mitotic figures **M** can be seen in the crypts. With such a high rate of cell turnover, more mitotic figures might by expected to be seen; the mitotic phase, however, occupies only a small proportion of the cell cycle (see Fig. 1.18), thus at any one point in time relatively few mitotic figures are seen.

With H & E staining, cells with intensely eosinophilic, cytoplasmic granules are seen in the base of the crypts; these cells, Paneth cells **P**, are more clearly demonstrated by the phloxine-tartrazine method which stains the granules scarlet.

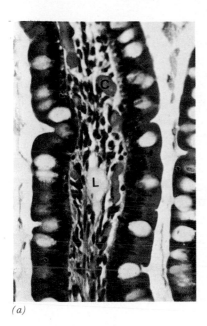
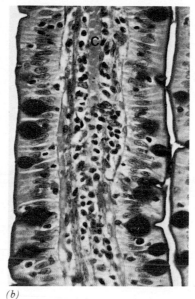

(a)   *(b)*

Fig. 12.42 Intestinal villus

(LS: (a) H & E × 320
(b) PAS/Iron haematoxylin/Orange G × 320)

In the longitudinal sections of intestinal villi seen in these micrographs the tall columnar nature of enterocytes can be seen. The luminal surface of the enterocytes seen in (b) is strongly PAS positive due to the presence of a particularly thick glycocalyx (see Fig. 1.2) and a surface layer of goblet cell derived mucus; both these surface features protect against auto-digestion. It has been suggested that the glycocalyx acts as the site for adsorption of pancreatic digestive enzymes. Lymphocytes and plasma cells are often scattered between the enterocytes; plasma cells are thought to secrete antibodies of the IgA class which pass readily into the intestinal lumen where they may provide defence against invading pathogens.

Capillaries **C** lie immediately beneath the layer of enterocytes and transport amino-acids, monosaccharides and other digestive products to the hepatic portal vein. Small lymphatic vessels drain into a single, larger vessel called a *lacteal* **L** located in the centre of the core of the villus; lacteals, which often contain lymphocytes, may be difficult to distinguish. The lacteals transport absorbed lipids into the circulatory system via the thoracic duct, thus bypassing the liver.

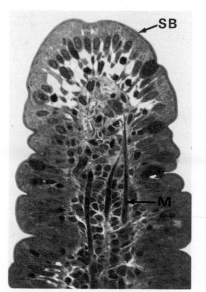

Fig. 12.43 Tip of intestinal villus

(LS: Resin embedded, one micron section: toluidine blue × 320)

This method of tissue preparation shows several features of the intestinal villus which are more difficult to demonstrate in thicker, conventional paraffin wax-embedded sections.

Firstly, degenerating enterocytes and goblet cells are seen about to be shed from the tip of the villus. Secondly, a striated or brush border **SB** can be seen on the luminal surface of the enterocytes; this represents a row of tall microvilli present on each enterocyte. Individual microvilli are too small to be resolved by light microscopy. Thirdly, occasional smooth muscle fibres **M** are seen within the connective tissue core of the villus; these muscle cells are extensions of the muscularis mucosae from beneath the base of the crypts. Contraction of the smooth muscle strands enhances drainage of lymph from the lacteals.

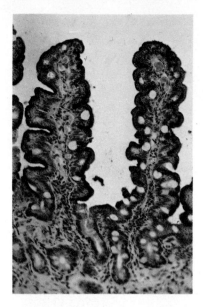

Fig. 12.44 Intestinal villi

(LS: Enzyme histochemical method for alkaline phosphatase × 128)

This frozen section from an intestinal biopsy has been stained for the enzyme alkaline phosphatase which is one of the many membrane-bound enzymes characteristic of enterocyte microvilli; alkaline phosphatase activity is represented by a red deposit. Alkaline phosphatase is thought to be involved in the transport of calcium ions from the intestinal lumen. Other membrane-bound enzymes are involved in the breakdown of peptides and disaccharides to amino-acids and monosaccharides respectively. The membrane-bound enzymes of the striated border are structurally integrated into the plasma membrane and are synthesised by enterocytes, in contrast to those enzymes adsorbed on to the surface which are synthesised by the pancreas (see Fig. 12.37). Note that the relatively immature enterocytes in the intestinal crypts show little alkaline phosphatase activity.

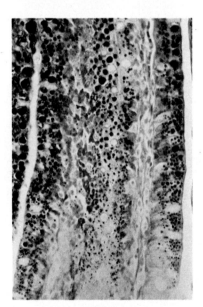

Fig. 12.45 Intestinal villus

(LS: Sudan black × 320)

This frozen section from the intestine of a rat fed with milk has been stained to demonstrate the presence of absorbed lipids within a villus. Ingested triglycerides are emulsified by bile and hydrolysed by the pancreatic enzyme, *lipase*; the degradation products, mainly free fatty acids and monoglycerides, are absorbed by enterocytes where they are resynthesised into triglycerides.

   The triglycerides, with the addition of protein and carbohydrate components, are packaged into membrane-bound vesicles called *chylomicrons* by the enterocyte Golgi apparatus, then passed towards the base of the cell where they are released by exocytosis into intercellular clefts; from here they pass into the lacteals from which they enter the general circulation. Note the high concentration of black-stained lipid in the enterocyte cytoplasm and in chylomicrons within the central lacteal.

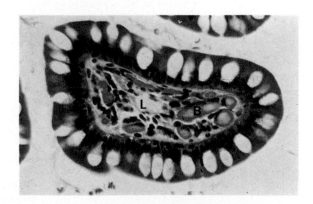

Fig. 12.46 Intestinal villus

(TS: H & E × 320)

In transverse section, the arrangement of the blood and lymphatic systems within a villus can be seen. Blood capillaries **B** tend to be disposed at the periphery, immediately beneath the enterocyte lining. Lymph drains into a single, central lacteal **L** via minute lymphatic tributaries.

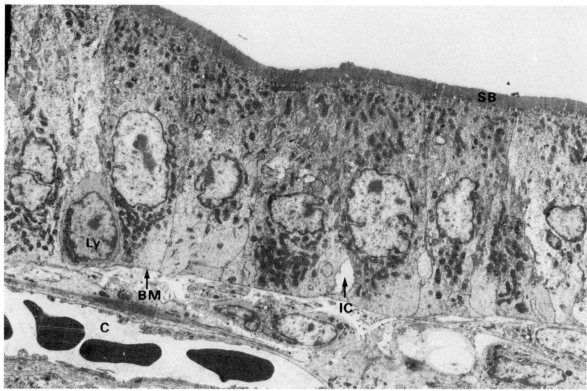

(a)

Fig. 12.47 Intestinal epithelium: enterocytes

(EM (a) ×4540 (b) ×50000)

These micrographs illustrate the main ultrastructural features of the absorptive cells of the small intestine, the enterocytes. Enormous numbers of microvilli, up to 3000 per cell, increase about thirtyfold the surface area of the plasma membrane exposed to the lumen. The microvilli are of uniform length, approximately 1 μm, and constitute the striated border **SB** of light microscopy. The glycocalyx of the enterocyte microvilli is usually prominent and is thought not only to provide protection against autodigestion but also to act as the site for adsorption of pancreatic digestive enzymes. Note in (b) the filamentous cytoskeleton of the microvilli **Mv** extending into the terminal web **TW**. Enterocytes are tightly bound near their luminal surface by junctional complexes (see Fig. 4.24) which prevent direct access of luminal contents to the intercellular spaces.

Most absorption in the small intestine is thought to occur by direct passage of low molecular weight digestion products across the luminal plasma membrane. Mitochondria are particularly abundant within enterocytes reflecting the high energy demands of active absorptive processes. In actively absorbing enterocytes, endocytotic vesicles are often seen between the bases of microvilli. The importance of this mode of absorption in the small intestine is not well understood although endocytosis may be a minor pathway of lipid absorption.

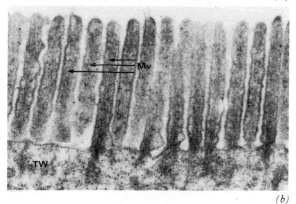

(b)

Between the bases of the enterocytes are intercellular clefts **IC** into which chylomicrons are first passed after processing by the Golgi apparatus. From the clefts, the chylomicrons pass across the thin basement membrane **BM** to be preferentially absorbed into the lacteals. Lymphocytes **Ly** and plasma cells are commonly found in the intercellular clefts between enterocytes but their precise role in the immunological defence of the tract is unclear. Note the close proximity of a blood capillary **C** to the enterocyte basement membrane.

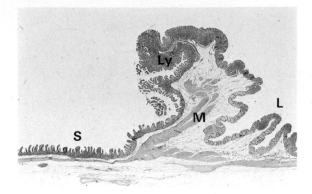

Fig. 12.48 Ileo-caecal junction
(LS: H & E × 5)

Unabsorbed and indigestible food residues from the ileum are forced, by peristalsis, into the distended first part of the large intestine, the caecum, through a simple cone-shaped valve which marks the ileo-caecal junction. There is an abrupt transition in the lining of the valve from the villiform pattern in the small intestine **S** to the glandular form in the large intestine **L**. This mucosal change reflects the different functions of the small and large intestines. Whereas the small intestine is predominantly the site of digestion and absorption, the large intestine is principally involved in the formation of faeces by the absorption of excess water from the liquid residue of the small intestine.

The ileo-caecal valve consists of a thickened extension of the muscularis **M** which provides robust support for the mucosa. Variable quantities of lymphoid tissue **Ly** are found in the mucosa.

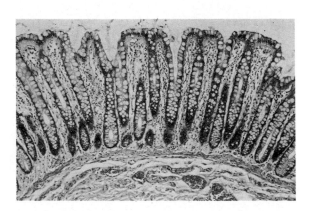

Fig. 12.49 Mucosa of the large intestine
(LS: H & E × 50)

The mucosa of the entire large intestine, which includes the appendix, caecum, colon and rectum, has a similar structure and function. The mucosa consists of closely packed, straight, tubular glands containing cells of two main types: absorptive cells and goblet cells. The glands are analogous to the crypts of Lieberkuhn of the small intestine and this term may also be applied to the glands of the large intestine. Like the stomach and small intestine, the epithelium undergoes continual turnover at the luminal surface, the cells being replaced by mitosis at the base of the glands.

As the residue passes along the large intestine and is progressively dehydrated, mucus derived from the intestinal glands becomes increasingly important as a lubricant.

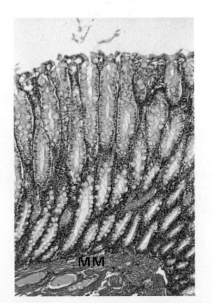

Fig. 12.50 Mucosa of the large intestine
(LS: Alcian blue/van Gieson × 80)

This staining method permits ready differentiation of the two major cell types which comprise the glands of the large intestine; goblet cell mucus is stained a greenish-blue colour whilst the absorptive cells remain poorly stained. The simple, tubular glands extend from the luminal surface to the muscularis mucosae **MM** and are separated from each other by thin plates of lamina propria, the collagen of which is stained red in this preparation. The lamina propria is rich in capillaries and diffusely infiltrated by leucocytes. Thin strands of the muscularis mucosae extend into the lamina propria between the glands; contraction of these strands facilitates the expulsion of mucus into the bowel lumen. Goblet cells predominate in the base of the glands whereas the luminal surface is almost entirely lined by columnar absorptive cells; the middle part of the glands represents a transition between these two extremes.

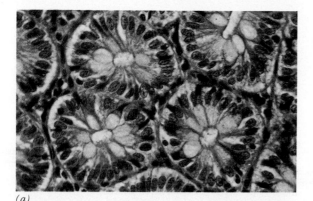

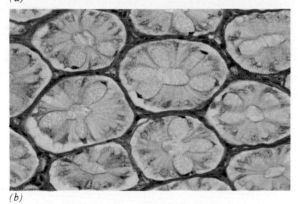

(a)

(b)

Fig. 12.51 Glands of the large intestinal mucosa

(TS: (a) H & E × 320 (b) Alcian blue/Van Gieson × 320)

These transverse sections through the upper part of the large intestinal glands highlight the closely packed arrangement of the glands in the mucosa. The absorptive cells are tall columnar with large, ovoid, basally located nuclei; in contrast, goblet cell nuclei are small and condensed. Lamina propria fills the spaces between the glands and contains numerous blood and lymphatic vessels into which water is absorbed by passive diffusion.

The large intestine is inhabited by a variety of commensal bacteria which further degrade food residues. Bacterial degradation is an important mechanism for the digestion of cellulose in ruminants, but in man this function is of little importance. Small quantities of fat-soluble vitamins derived from bacteria are absorbed in the large intestine of man.

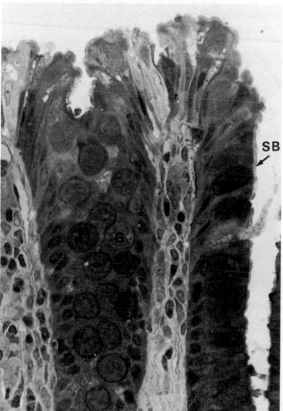

SB

Fig. 12.52 Glands of the large intestinal mucosa

(Resin embedded, one micron section: toluidine blue × 480)

This micrograph illustrates the similarity of the epithelium in the large intestine to that of the small intestine as shown in Fig. 12.43. As in the small intestine, the absorptive cells of the large intestine have a striated border **SB** formed by microvilli which increase greatly the surface area exposed to the lumen, thus enhancing passive water absorption. The epithelial lining of the large intestine is replaced every three to five days like that of the small intestine; note several degenerating cells in the process of being shed from the luminal surface. Goblet cells **G** are seen in different phases of secretory activity.

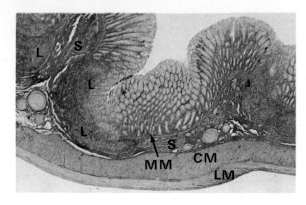

Fig. 12.53 Colon

(LS: Alcian blue/van Gieson × 12)

This micrograph demonstrates the main histological layers of the wall of the large intestine. The thick, glandular mucosa is highly folded in the non-distended state, but it does not exhibit distinct plica circulares like those of the small intestine (see Fig. 12.37). Immediately above the anal valves, the mucosa forms longitudinal folds called the *columns of Morgagni*.

The muscularis mucosae **MM** is a prominent feature of the large intestine, but in many places it is traversed by large lymphoid aggregations **L** which extend from the lamina propria into the submucosa **S**; the collagen of the submucosa is stained red in this preparation. As in the rest of the gastro-intestinal tract, the muscularis of the large intestine consists of an inner circular **CM** and outer longitudinal layer **LM**, but, except in the rectum, the longitudinal layer does not completely surround the tract but rather forms three separate longitudinal bands called *taeniae coli*.

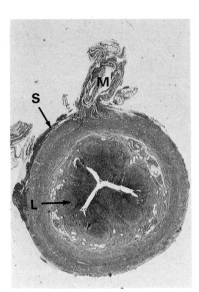

Fig. 12.54 Appendix

(TS: H & E × 5)

The appendix is a small, blind-ended sac extending from the caecum just below the ileo-caecal junction. The appendix is not known to have any digestive or absorptive function in man. The general structure of the appendix conforms to that of the rest of the digestive tract as can be seen in this specimen, taken from a young person. The specimen also illustrates the suspensory mesentery **M** which becomes continuous with the outer serosal layer and is a feature of all parts of the gastro-intestinal tract which lie free in the peritoneal cavity. In this specimen, the serosa **S** contains a moderate amount of haemorrhage resulting from surgical removal. The mesenteries conduct blood vessels, lymphatics and nerves to and from the gastro-intestinal tract.

The most characteristic feature of the appendix, particularly of a young person, is the presence of masses of lymphoid tissue **L** in the lamina propria. This lymphoid tissue often forms follicles containing germinal centres (see Chapter 10).

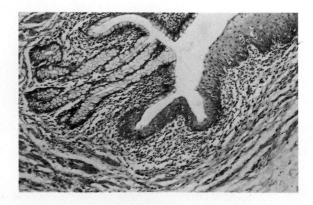

Fig. 12.55 Recto-anal junction

(H & E × 128)

The rectum is the short, dilated, terminal portion of the large intestine, the main function of which is to store semi-solid faeces immediately prior to defaecation. The mucosa of the rectum, which is similar to that of the rest of the large bowel except that it has even more numerous goblet cells, undergoes an abrupt transition at the recto-anal junction to become stratified squamous epithelium in the anal canal. The anal canal forms the last two or three centimetres of the gastro-intestinal tract and is surrounded by an external skeletal muscle mass which constitutes the anal sphincter. At the anal sphincter, the stratified squamous epithelium undergoes a gradual transition to that of skin containing sebaceous glands and large apocrine sweat glands (see Fig. 8.16).

Pancreas

The pancreas is a major gland which develops embryologically as an outgrowth of the primitive gut. The pancreas has both exocrine and endocrine functions; the endocrine pancreas is described in detail in Chapter 14. The exocrine pancreas, which forms the bulk of the gland, secretes an alkaline, enzyme-rich fluid into the duodenum via the pancreatic duct. The alkalinity of pancreatic secretion is due to a high content of bicarbonate ions and serves to neutralise the acidic chyme as it enters the small intestine from the stomach. The pancreatic enzymes degrade proteins, carbohydrates, lipids and nucleic acids by the process of luminal digestion (see Fig. 12.37). Like pepsin in the stomach, the pancreatic proteolytic enzymes *trypsin* and *chymotrypsin* are secreted in an inactive form. *Enterokinase*, an enzyme secreted by the duodenal mucosa, activates protrypsin to form trypsin; trypsin then activates prochymotrypsin to form chymotrypsin. This mechanism prevents autodigestion of the pancreas. The other pancreatic enzymes are secreted in the active form.

Pancreatic secretion occurs continuously, the rate, however, is modulated by hormonal and nervous influences. Secretin, a hormone released by endocrine cells scattered in the duodenum, promotes the secretion of copious watery fluid rich in bicarbonate. Cholecystokinin-pancreozymin (CCK), also derived from duodenal endocrine cells, stimulates the secretion of enzyme-rich pancreatic fluid. Gastrin, secreted by endocrine cells of the pyloric mucosa, has a similar action on the pancreas to that of CCK. The pancreas is richly innervated by the autonomic nervous system, but the significance of its influence on pancreatic secretion is incompletely understood.

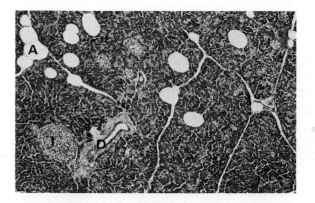

Fig. 12.56 Pancreas
(H & E × 20)

The pancreas is a highly lobulated gland invested by a loose connective tissue capsule which extends as delicate septa between the lobules. The exocrine component of the pancreas consists of closely packed, secretory acini which drain into a highly branched duct system. Most of the secretions drain into the main *pancreatic duct* which joins the common bile duct to drain into the duodenum via the *ampulla of Vater*; a small, accessory pancreatic duct drains into the duodenum at a more proximal site. Note a duct **D** of moderate size in this micrograph.

The endocrine tissues of the pancreas form islets **I** of various sizes, the *islets of Langerhans* (see Chapter 14), which are scattered throughout the exocrine tissue. In man, adipocytes **A** appear in increasing number with advancing age.

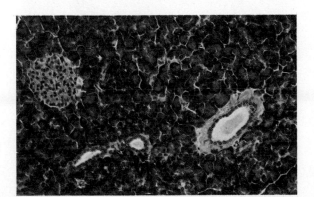

Fig. 12.57 Pancreas
(H & E × 128)

At higher magnification, more detail of the pancreatic acini and duct system can be seen. Each acinus is made up of an irregular cluster of secretory cells which drain into a minute, central duct. These minute ducts then drain into a system of ducts of progressively increasing size. The small ducts are lined by simple cuboidal epithelium which becomes stratified cuboidal in the larger ducts. With increasing size, the ducts are supported by a progressively thicker layer of dense connective tissue and the wall of the main pancreatic duct contains smooth muscle. Note in this micrograph, the structure of ducts of various sizes and the non-acinar nature of an islet of Langerhans.

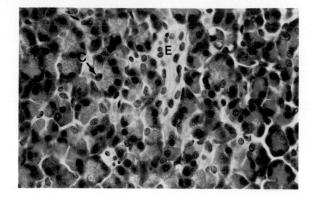

Fig. 12.58 Exocrine pancreas
(H & E × 320)

With further magnification, the pancreatic acini are seen to consist of roughly pyramidal-shaped cells with their apices projecting towards the lumen of a minute duct. The acinar cells are typical protein-secreting (zymogenic) cells. The nuclei are basally located and surrounded by basophilic cytoplasm rich in rough endoplasmic reticulum; the apices of the cells are packed with eosinophilic, zymogen secretory granules. The smallest excretory ducts merge with the lumina of acini, and duct lining cells are often seen in the centre of secretory acini; these duct lining cells are thus described as *centroacinar cells* **C** and are recognised by their pale-stained nuclei and sparse, pale-stained cytoplasm. The cells lining the small ducts are responsible for elaborating the bicarbonate component of pancreatic secretion. Note a small excretory duct **E** in longitudinal section.

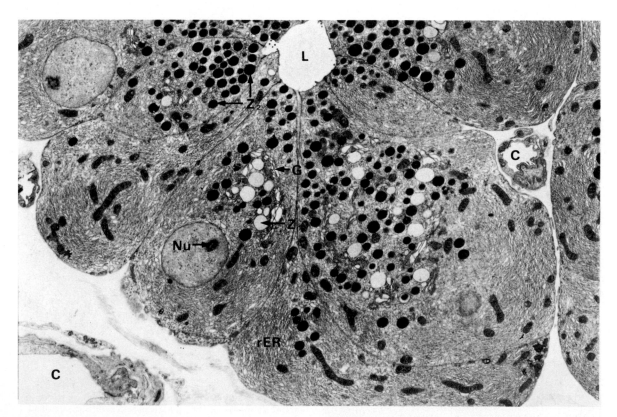

Fig. 12.59 Pancreatic acinus
(EM × 4270)

This micrograph illustrates part of a pancreatic acinus with its central lumen **L**. The pyramidal-shaped secretory cells have round, basally located nuclei with dispersed chromatin and prominent nucleoli **Nu**, both characteristic features of highly active cells. The basal cytoplasm is crammed with lamellar profiles of rough endoplasmic reticulum **rER**. The large Golgi apparatus **G** is located in a supranuclear position and is responsible for packaging enzymes synthesised on the rough endoplasmic reticulum to form zymogen granules. Newly packaged zymogen granules Z_1 are larger and much less electron-dense than the smaller, mature granules Z_2 which aggregate in the apical cytoplasm. Zymogen granules (pancreatic enzymes) are released into the acinar lumen by exocytosis; small, irregular microvilli associated with this process are seen projecting into the lumen. Note small capillaries **C** in the fine supporting connective tissue which surrounds the acini.

Liver and biliary system

The liver, like the pancreas, also develops embryologically as an outgrowth of the primitive gut. Although the liver is often described as a gland it has numerous other concurrent metabolic functions. The major functions of the liver may be summarised as follows:

(i) detoxification of metabolic waste products;

(ii) destruction of spent red cells and reclamation of their constituents (alone and in conjunction with the spleen);

(iii) synthesis and secretion of bile into the duodenum via the biliary system; bile contains many of the end products of the processes described in (i) and (ii) above, thus bile may be considered as both an excretory product and an exocrine secretion;

(iv) synthesis of the plasma proteins including the clotting factors but excluding the immunoglobulins (antibodies);

(v) synthesis of plasma lipoproteins.

Many of these biosynthetic functions directly utilise the products of digestion. With the exception of most lipids, absorbed food products pass directly in venous blood from the small intestine to the liver via the *hepatic portal system* before entering the general circulation. Thus the vascular bed of the liver is perfused by blood rich in amino-acids, simple sugars and other products of digestion but relatively poor in oxygen. Oxygen required to support the intense metabolic activity of the liver is supplied in arterial blood via the *hepatic artery*. The liver, therefore, is unusual in that it has a dual blood supply that is both arterial and venous. Venous drainage of the liver occurs via the *hepatic vein* and lymph from the liver is drained directly into the thoracic duct.

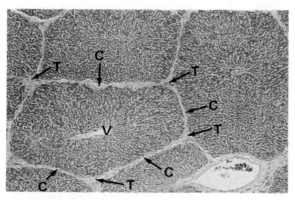

Fig. 12.60 Liver
(Pig: H & E ×20)

The principal cells of the liver, called *hepatocytes*, are arranged into structures called *lobules*. Lobules have a sub-structure which maximises contact of hepatocytes with blood flowing through the liver. In pigs, the 'classical' liver lobule is particularly well delineated by connective tissue boundaries **C**. The liver lobules are roughly hexagonal in shape when seen in any section, reflecting a compact, regular, polyhedral shape in three dimensions. Branches of the hepatic artery and hepatic portal vein ramify throughout the liver within the connective tissue bounding the liver lobules, the larger vessels tending to be concentrated at the angles of the lobule margins in the so-called *portal tracts* **T**. Blood from the portal tracts percolates towards a central vein **V** of each lobule via sinusoids which pass between plates of hepatocytes. The central vein drains into the hepatic vein.

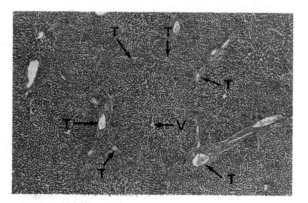

Fig. 12.61 Liver
(H & E ×20)

The human liver has a similar lobular pattern to that of the pig but the boundaries of the lobules are not defined by distinct connective tissue. Portal tracts **T** define the angles of the lobule margins and a central vein **V** defines the centre of each lobule. Note that each portal tract and its branches supplies more than one lobule whereas each central vein drains only a single lobule.

Blood flows between plates of hepatocytes which are usually only one cell thick; thus each hepatocyte is bathed by blood on at least two sides. The plates of hepatocytes branch and anastomose to form a three-dimensional structure like a honeycomb.

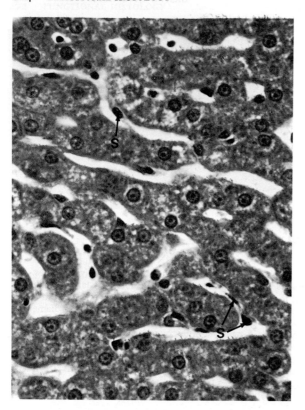

Fig. 12.67 Hepatocytes
(H & E × 480)

Hepatocytes are large, polyhedral cells which have a variable cytoplasmic appearance depending on the nutritional status of the body. In well nourished individuals, hepatocytes store significant quantities of glycogen and process large quantities of lipid; both these metabolites are partially removed during routine histological preparation thereby leaving irregular, unstained areas within the cytoplasm. The remaining cytoplasm is strongly eosinophilic due to a high content of organelles. The nuclei of hepatocytes are large with peripherally dispersed chromatin and prominent nucleoli. The nuclei, however, vary greatly in size, reflecting an unusual cellular feature; more than half the hepatocytes contain twice the normal (diploid) complement of chromosomes within a single nucleus (i.e. they are tetraploid) and some contain four or even eight times this amount (polyploid). Occasional binucleate cells are seen in section although up to twenty-five per cent of all hepatocytes are binucleate. The significance of the polyploid state exhibited by normal, mature hepatocytes is obscure.

Sinusoid lining cells **S** are readily distinguishable from hepatocytes by their flattened, condensed nuclei and attenuated, poorly stained cytoplasm.

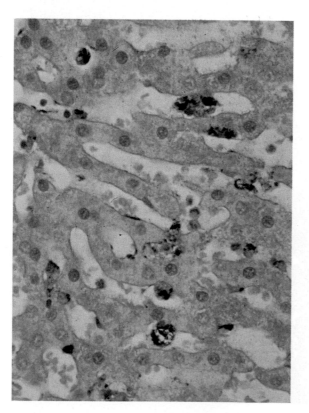

Fig. 12.68 Sinusoid lining cells
(Perls' Prussian blue × 480)

The nature and function of the sinusoid lining cells has been in dispute ever since the liver was first studied. At least a proportion of these cells can be shown to be highly phagocytic when 'fed' either artificially or under pathological conditions with appropriate particulate matter. The animal used for this preparation was injected intravenously with a particulate iron-sugar compound which, with this staining method, is demonstrated as a dark deposition appearing within sinusoid lining cells. Some authorities believe that all sinusoid lining cells are capable of intense phagocytosis when appropriately stimulated, whereas others believe that a distinct population of phagocytic cells exists amongst endothelial-like, sinusoid lining cells. In either case, the intensely phagocytic cells probably represent cells analogous to, or identical with, the cells of the monocyte-macrophage defence system (see Chapters 2 and 3). The phagocytic cells of the liver are commonly referred to as *Kupffer cells*. Kupffer cells participate, with the spleen, in the removal of spent erythrocytes and other particulate debris from the circulation.

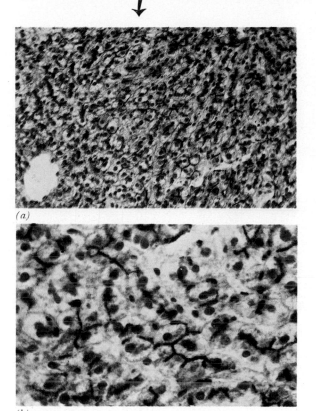

(a)

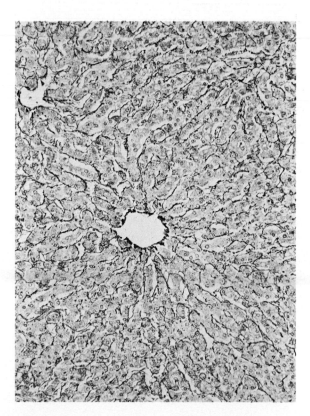

(b)

Fig. 12.69 Bile canaliculi

*(Enzyme histochemical method for ATP-ase (a) × 80
(b) × 320)*

Bile is synthesised by all hepatocytes and secreted into a
system of minute canaliculi which form an anastomosing
network between hepatocytes. The canaliculi have no
discrete structure of their own but consist merely of fine
channels running between adjacent hepatocytes, the walls of
the canaliculi being formed by the plasma membranes of
adjacent hepatocytes; the ultrastructural features are shown
in Fig. 12.71. Thus within each plate of hepatocytes, which
is one cell thick, the canaliculi form a regular, hexagonal
network in the plane of the plate, each mesh enclosing a
single hepatocyte.

From within each lobule, bile canaliculi drain towards
bile collecting vessels of the portal tracts. The hepatocyte
plasma membranes forming the walls of the canaliculi
contain the enzyme ATP-ase on the basis of which it has
been suggested that bile secretion is an energy-dependent
process. In these preparations, a histochemical method for
ATP-ase has been used to demonstrate bile canaliculi
(stained brown) which are difficult to demonstrate with
routine methods for light microscopy.

Fig. 12.70 Liver

(Reticulin method × 50)

Hepatocytes and sinusoid lining cells are supported by a
fine meshwork of reticulin fibres which radiate from around
the central vein of each lobule to merge with the reticular
and sparse connective tissue framework of the portal tracts
and lobule boundaries. Reticulin is thus almost the only
connective tissue element supporting the liver. This
framework becomes continuous with a thin but tough
connective tissue capsule, called *Glisson's capsule*, which
invests the external surface of the liver.

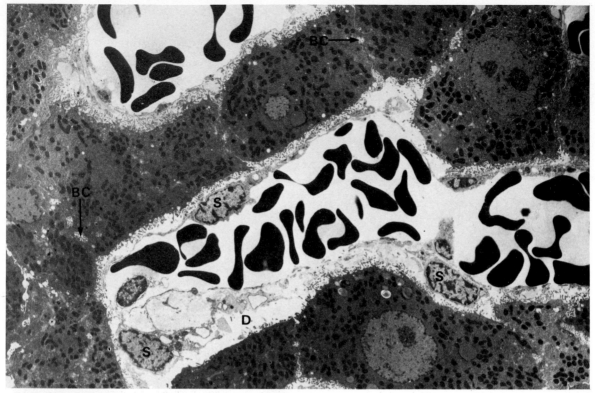

(a)

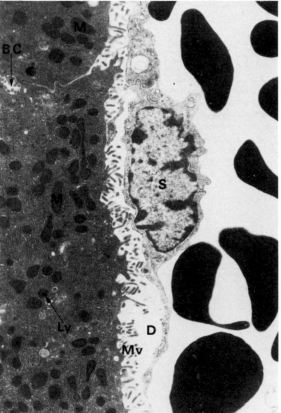

(b)

Fig. 12.71 Liver
(EM (a) × 2890 (b) × 7560)

These micrographs demonstrate the main ultrastructural features of the liver. Each hepatocyte is bathed on at least two sides by blood within the sinusoids which are lined by a discontinuous layer of sinusoid lining cells **S**. Sinusoid lining cells are supported by the fine reticular framework of the liver (see Fig. 12.70) such that a space, known as the *space of Disse* **D**, remains between the lining cells and the hepatocyte surface. Since the sinusoid lining cells form a discontinuous layer, the space of Disse is continuous with the sinusoid lumen. Numerous irregular microvilli **Mv** extend from the hepatocyte surface into the space of Disse thus greatly increasing the plasma membrane surface available for bidirectional exchange of metabolites between liver and blood.

Reflecting the extraordinary range of biosynthetic and degradative activities, the hepatocyte cytoplasm is crowded with organelles, particularly rough and smooth endoplasmic reticulum, mitochondria **M** and lysosomes **Ly**. Lipid droplets and glycogen rosettes are present in variable numbers depending on nutritional status (see Fig. 1.15).

Bile canaliculi **BC** are seen to be formed from the plasma membranes of adjacent hepatocytes, the plasma membranes being tightly bound by junctional complexes; small microvilli project into the canaliculi.

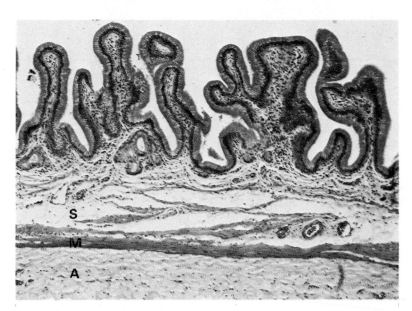

Fig. 12.72 Gall bladder

(H & E × 30)

The intrahepatic bile collecting system merges to form a single large duct, the common bile duct, which joins the pancreatic duct to form the short ampulla of Vater before entering the duodenum. The duodenal opening is guarded by the muscular *sphincter of Oddi*. Immediately after leaving the liver, the common bile duct has a major branch, the *cystic duct*, which connects the common bile duct to the *gall bladder*.

Most of the bile does not pass directly down the common bile duct but is shunted into the gall bladder where it is temporarily stored and concentrated. The walls of the common bile duct contain both longitudinal and circular smooth muscle layers which increase in thickness towards the duodenum. A well developed biliary sphincter regulates bile flow from the common bile duct into the ampulla of Vater. The tonus of this smooth muscle also controls the flow of bile into the gall bladder.

The gall bladder is a muscular sac lined by a simple columnar epithelium; it has a capacity of about 100ml in man. The presence of lipid in the duodenum promotes the secretion of the hormone cholecystokinin-pancreozymin (CCK) by endocrine cells of the duodenal wall. CCK stimulates contraction of the gall bladder smooth muscle thus forcing bile along the biliary tract into the duodenum Bile is essentially an emulsifying agent which facilitates the hydrolysis of dietary lipids by pancreatic lipases.

This micrograph shows the wall of a gall bladder in the non-distended state in which the lining mucosa is thrown up into many folds. The relatively loose submucosal connective tissue **S** is rich in elastic fibres and contains many blood and lymphatic vessels which drain water reabsorbed from bile during the concentration process. The muscle layer **M** is seen to separate the submucosa from the outer adventitial connective tissue **A**. In the neck of the gall bladder, mucous glands are often found in the submucosa; this mucus may provide a protective surface film for the biliary tract.

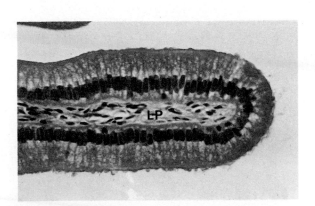

Fig. 12.73 Gall bladder epithelium

(H & E × 480)

The simple epithelial lining of the gall bladder consists of very tall columnar cells with basally located nuclei. Although not usually evident with light microscopy, the luminal surface of the cells is formed into very numerous, short irregular microvilli. The primary functions of the gall bladder are to store and concentrate bile prior to expulsion into the gastro-intestinal tract. Bile is concentrated 5 to 10 fold by an active process, mediated by the lining cells, which involves absorption of water into the vessels of the lamina propria **LP**.

13. Urinary system

Introduction

The urinary system is the principal organ system responsible for water and electrolyte homeostasis. The maintenance of homeostasis requires that any input into a system is balanced by an equivalent output; the urinary system provides the mechanism by which excess water and electrolytes are eliminated from the body. A second major function of the urinary system is the excretion of many toxic metabolic waste products, particularly the nitrogenous compounds urea and creatinine; this excretory function is intimately related to water and electrolyte elimination which provides an appropriate fluid vehicle. The end product of these processes is *urine*. Since all body fluids are maintained in dynamic equilibrium with one another via the circulatory system, any adjustment in the composition of the blood is reflected in complementary changes in the other fluid compartments of the body. Thus regulation of the osmotic concentration of blood plasma ensures the osmotic regulation of all other body fluids. The process, primarily performed by the urinary system, is called *osmoregulation*.

The functional units of the urinary system are the *nephrons*, of which there are approximately one million in each human kidney. Nephrons perform the functions of osmoregulation and excretion by the following processes:

(i) filtration of most relatively small molecules from blood plasma to form a filtrate;

(ii) selective reabsorption of most of the water and other molecules from the filtrate, leaving behind excess and waste materials to be excreted;

(iii) secretion of some excretory products directly from blood into the filtrate.

The kidney is also involved in two other homeostatic mechanisms which are mediated via hormones. The *renin-angiotensin-aldosterone mechanism* contributes to the maintenance of blood pressure, and the hormone *erythropoietin* stimulates erythrocyte production in bone marrow and hence contributes to the maintenance of the oxygen-carrying capacity of blood.

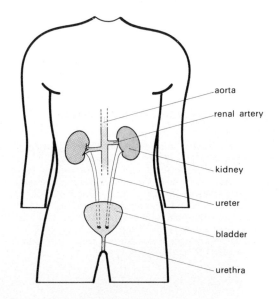

Fig. 13.1 The urinary system

The urinary system comprises two *kidneys*, two *ureters*, a *bladder* and a *urethra*. Urine is produced in the kidneys and conducted by the ureters to the bladder where it is stored until voided via the urethra.

Blood is supplied to each kidney by *renal arteries* which arise from the aorta. The total blood volume of the body is circulated through the kidneys about 300 times each day.

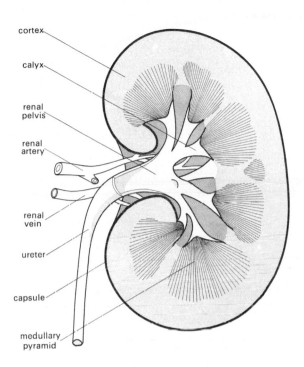

cortex

calyx

renal
pelvis

renal
artery

renal
vein

ureter

capsule

medullary
pyramid

Fig. 13.2 Kidney

The gross structure of the kidney reflects the arrangement
of nephrons within it. The substance of the kidney may be
divided into an outer *cortex* and inner *medulla*. A portion of
each nephron is located in both the cortex and the medulla,
although the major part of each nephron is found in the
cortex. The medulla is arranged into pyramid-shaped units
called *medullary pyramids* which are separated by extensions
of cortical tissue. The medullary pyramids convey ducts
which converge to discharge urine at their apices; the apices
of the pyramids are known as *renal papillae*. *Calyces* are
funnel-shaped spaces into which one or more renal papillae
project. The calyces converge to form the larger, funnel-
shaped *renal pelvis* from which urine is conducted to the
bladder by the ureter.

The kidney is invested in a capsule of tough fibrous
tissue. The renal artery and renal vein enter and leave the
kidney above the ureter at the region known as the *hilum*.

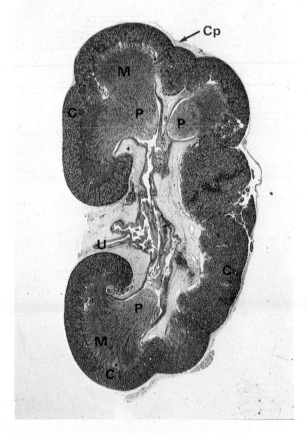

Fig. 13.3 Kidney
(LS: H & E × 3)

This micrograph of a kidney from a newborn child
illustrates the gross features of the kidney as described in
Fig. 13.2. In histological section, only a single plane
through the pelvi-calyceal system can be visualised.

The darker-stained cortex **C** can be clearly differentiated
from the paler-stained medulla **M**. Note the continuity of
the cortex throughout the outer zone of the kidney and the
cortical extensions between the medullary pyramids. Three
renal papillae **P** are seen projecting into the pelvi-calyceal
system which becomes continuous with the ureter **U** at the
hilum. Note that the fibrous capsule **Cp** of the kidney is
continuous, at the hilum, with connective tissue which
packs the spaces between the hilar structures. In later life,
the hilum often contains significant quantities of adipose
tissue. The kidney is cushioned by a thick pad of adipose
tissue, not seen in this preparation, and is protected by the
lower ribs retroperitoneally.

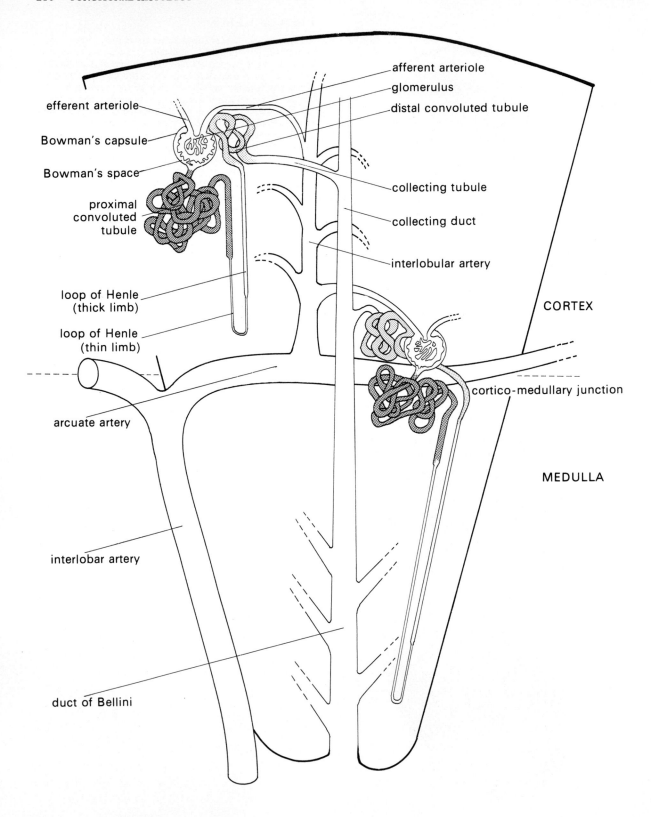

afferent arteriole

glomerulus

distal convoluted tubule

efferent arteriole

Bowman's capsule

Bowman's space

proximal
convoluted
tubule

collecting tubule

collecting duct

interlobular artery

loop of Henle
(thick limb)

loop of Henle
(thin limb)

CORTEX

cortico-medullary junction

arcuate artery

MEDULLA

interlobar artery

duct of Bellini

Fig. 13.4 The nephron *(illustration opposite)*

The nephron, the functional unit of the kidney, consists of two major components, the *renal corpuscle* and the *renal tubule*.

(i) Renal corpuscle: the renal corpuscle is that part of the nephron responsible for the filtration of plasma and is a combination of two structures, *Bowman's capsule* and the *glomerulus*.

(a) Bowman's capsule consists of a single layer of flattened cells resting on a basement membrane; it forms the distended, blind end of an epithelial tubule, the renal tubule.

(b) The glomerulus is a tightly coiled network of anastomosing capillaries which invaginates Bowman's capsule. Within the capsule, the glomerulus is invested by a layer of epithelial cells, called *podocytes*, which constitutes the *visceral layer of Bowman's capsule*; the visceral layer is reflected around the vascular stalk of the glomerulus to become continuous with the *parietal layer*, the Bowman's capsule proper. The space between the visceral and parietal layers is known as *Bowman's space* and is continuous with the lumen of the renal tubule; the parietal epithelium of Bowman's capsule is continuous with the epithelium lining the renal tubule.

In the renal corpuscle, elements of plasma are filtered from the glomerular capillaries into Bowman's space, and the *glomerular filtrate* then passes into the renal tubule. Thus the filtration barrier between the capillary lumen and Bowman's space consists of the capillary endothelium, the podocyte layer and a common basement membrane, the *glomerular basement membrane*, separating these two cellular layers.

The *afferent arteriole* which supplies the glomerulus, and the *efferent arteriole* which drains the glomerulus, enter and leave the corpuscle at the so-called *vascular pole* which is usually situated opposite the entrance to the renal tubule, the so-called *urinary pole*.

(ii) Renal tubule: the renal tubule extends from Bowman's capsule to its junction with a *collecting duct*. The renal tubule is up to 55 mm long in man and is lined by a single layer of epithelial cells. The primary function of the renal tubule is the selective reabsorption of water, inorganic ions and other molecules from the glomerular filtrate. In addition, some inorganic ions are secreted directly from blood into the lumen of the tubule. In man, glomerular filtrate is produced at a steady rate of approximately 120 ml per minute; of this, approximately 119 ml per minute are reabsorbed in the renal tubules. The highly convoluted renal tubule has four distinct histo-physiological zones, each of which has a different role in tubular function.

(a) *The proximal convoluted tubule (PCT):* this is the longest, most convoluted section of the tubule; PCTs make up the bulk of the renal cortex. Approximately seventy-five per cent of all the ions and water of the glomerular filtrate are reabsorbed from the PCT.

(b) *The loop of Henle:* this arises from the PCT as a straight, thin-walled limb (*the thin limb*) which descends from the cortex into the medulla; here it loops closely back on itself to ascend as a straight, thicker-walled limb (*the thick limb*) into the renal cortex. The limbs of the loop of Henle are closely associated with parallel, wide capillary loops, the *vasa recta* (not shown in this diagram). The vasa recta, which arise from glomerular efferent arterioles, descend into the medulla then loop back on themselves to drain into veins at the junction of the medulla and cortex. In man, only a relatively small proportion of the water in glomerular filtrate is absorbed from the loops of Henle into the vasa recta. The main function of the loops of Henle is to generate a high osmotic pressure in the extracellular fluid of the renal medulla; the mechanism by which this is achieved is known as the *counter-current multiplier system*, the details of which are beyond the scope of this discussion.

(c) *The distal convoluted tubule (DCT):* this is shorter and less convoluted than the PCT. Sodium ions are actively reabsorbed from the DCT by a process which is controlled by the adreno-cortical hormone *aldosterone* (see Chapter 14). Sodium reabsorption is in some way coupled with the secretion of hydrogen or potassium ions into the DCT.

(d) *The collecting tubule:* this is the terminal portion of the DCT and conducts urine to the *collecting ducts* which merge to form the large *ducts of Bellini* in the renal medulla. The collecting tubules and ducts are not normally permeable to water; however, in the presence of antidiuretic hormone (ADH), secreted by the posterior pituitary, the collecting tubules and ducts become permeable to water which is then drawn out by the high osmotic pressure of the medullary extracellular fluid; reabsorbed water is returned to the general circulation via the vasa recta. The activity of the loops of Henle and ADH thus provide a mechanism for the production of urine which is hypertonic with respect to plasma.

This diagram also illustrates the arterial supply of the renal cortex. In the hilum, the renal artery divides into two main branches. Each of these gives rise to several *interlobar arteries* which ascend between the pyramids to the cortico-medullary junction. Here they branch to form the *arcuate arteries* which run parallel to the capsule of the kidney. The arcuate arteries give rise to numerous *interlobular arteries* which extend towards the capsule and branch to form the glomerular afferent arterioles.

Fig. 13.5 Kidney

(Monkey: TS: Jones' methenamine silver/H & E ×8)

The basic geography of the kidney can be seen in this micrograph of a transverse section through the kidney at the level of the ureter **U**.

In the cortex, numerous renal corpuscles **RC** are just visible at this magnification. The corpuscles tend to be arranged in parallel rows at right angles to the capsule, corresponding to the course of the interlobular arteries from which they derive their blood supply. In a corresponding manner, the venous system converges upon the medulla; venous elements appear as thin-walled vessels **V**.

Most of the tissue mass surrounding the renal corpuscles in the cortex consists of proximal and distal convoluted tubules. From the cortex, pale-stained lines appear to radiate towards the medulla and thence to the tip of the renal papilla **RP**. These lines, which are called *medullary rays* **MR**, are bundles of collecting tubules and ducts derived from nephrons located high in the cortex. The collecting ducts merge to form the larger ducts of Bellini which drain urine into the pelvi-calyceal space through the renal papilla. Although not visible at this magnification, the limbs of the loops of Henle dip into the medulla between, and parallel with, the collecting tubules and ducts. The vasa recta, the long, straight vessels into which water is absorbed from the collecting tubules and ducts, also dip down into the medulla alongside the loops of Henle; these vessels are also too small to be seen at this magnification.

Note two large interlobar branches of the renal artery **Ai** in the hilar connective tissue surrounding the pelvi-calyceal space. At the cortico-medullary junction, several arcuate arteries **Aa** can be seen in transverse section.

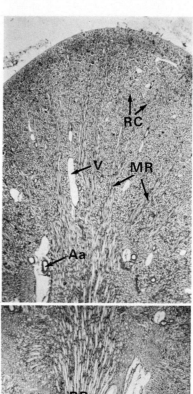

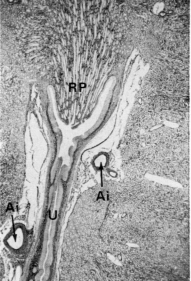

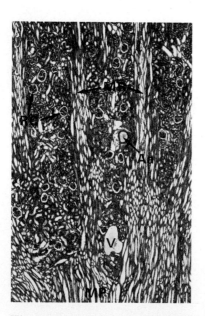

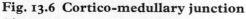

Fig. 13.6 Cortico-medullary junction

(Azan ×20)

With increased magnification, greater detail of the cortico-medullary junction can be resolved. The collecting tubules and ducts of several medullary rays **MR** are seen to enter a medullary pyramid **MP**. Towards the cortico-medullary junction, the medullary rays divide the cortical tissue into *cortical lobules* each containing renal corpuscles **RC** surrounded by an assortment of renal tubular components. Note an arcuate artery **Aa** and a corresponding tributary of the renal vein **V**.

Fig. 13.7 Renal cortex

(Azan ×80)

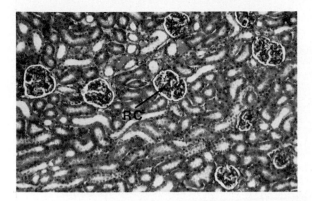

Further magnification reveals more details of the cortical tissue. Renal corpuscles **RC** appear as dense, rounded structures, the glomeruli, surrounded by narrow spaces, Bowman's spaces. Even at this magnification, it is evident that the tubules comprising the tissue between the renal corpuscles differ from one another in diameter, staining intensity and shape. The mass of cortical tubules seen in section mainly consists of proximal convoluted tubules with smaller numbers of distal convoluted tubules and a lesser number of other segments of renal tubules.

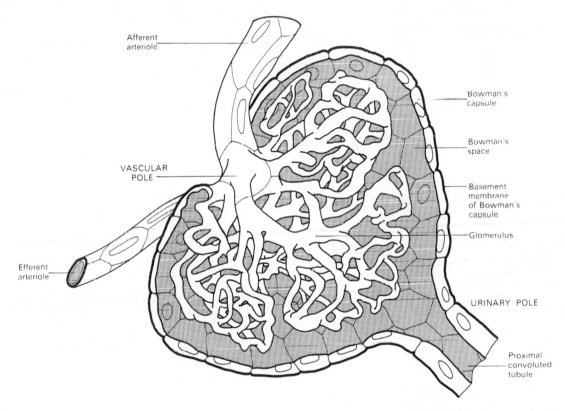

Fig. 13.8 Renal corpuscle

The main structural features of the renal corpuscle are demonstrated in this idealised diagram.

The relatively wide-diameter afferent arteriole pierces Bowman's capsule at the vascular pole of the renal corpuscle and then branches to form a tightly anastomosing network of capillaries, the glomerulus. The glomerulus is thus suspended in Bowman's space from the vascular pole. Although not shown in this diagram, the capillary loops are supported by stalks of specialised connective tissue called *mesangium* extending into the glomerulus through the vascular pole. If the capillary loops are likened to the coils of the small bowel lying in the abdominal cavity, then the mesangium forms the equivalent of the mesenteries.

The efferent vessel which drains the glomerulus is unusual in that it has the structure of an arteriole and is thus called the efferent arteriole (rather than the efferent venule). The efferent arteriole is of smaller diameter than the afferent arteriole and a pressure gradient is thus maintained which drives the filtration of plasma into Bowman's space.

The layer of podocytes which invests the glomerular capillaries is not represented in this diagram. At the vascular pole, the podocyte layer is reflected to become continuous with the epithelium of Bowman's capsule which in turn becomes continuous with the first part of the renal tubule, the proximal convoluted tubule.

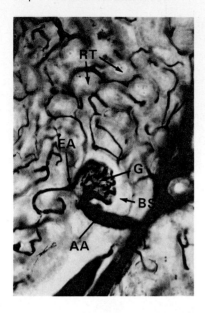

Fig. 13.9 Blood supply of the glomerulus
(Carmine-gelatine perfused × 128)

This is a section of a kidney which has been perfused with a red dye in order to demonstrate the renal blood supply. The kidney tissue remains unstained in this preparation.

An interlobular artery (see Fig. 13.4) can be seen branching to form the afferent arteriole **AA** of a glomerulus **G**. Note that the afferent arteriole has a greater diameter than the efferent arteriole **EA**. This arrangement maintains the pressure within glomerular capillaries necessary for blood plasma to be filtered into Bowman's space **BS**. Blood pressure within the glomerulus is controlled by appropriate variation of the diameter of the afferent and efferent arterioles.

The efferent arteriole gives rise to a network of capillaries which surround the renal tubules **RT**. The efferent arterioles also give rise to the vasa recta which loop into the medulla and are therefore not seen in this section of the renal cortex. Molecules reabsorbed from glomerular filtrate are returned to the general circulation via this capillary network which drains into the renal venous system.

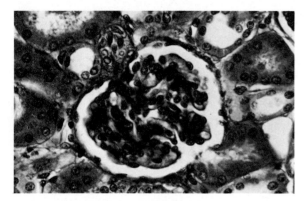

Fig. 13.10 Renal corpuscle
(Azan × 320)

The renal corpuscle in this micrograph has been sectioned through both the vascular and urinary poles. At the vascular pole, the afferent arteriole is seen entering the corpuscle to supply the glomerulus; the lumen of this vessel cannot be seen. Glomerular capillaries are cut in transverse, longitudinal and oblique section but little detail can be resolved in this type of preparation. The numerous nuclei (stained red) in the glomerulus are those of capillary endothelial cells, *mesangial cells* of the supporting mesangium, and podocytes.

Note the flattened nuclei of the squamous cells lining Bowman's capsule. In this preparation the basement membranes of the glomerulus and Bowman's capsule are stained a prominent blue. Note the continuity of Bowman's space with the lumen of the proximal convoluted tubule. Due to shrinkage of the glomerulus, inevitable in this type of tissue preparation, Bowman's space appears artefactually enlarged; *in vivo*, Bowman's space is filled with glomerular filtrate which is at much lower pressure than that of the plasma within the glomerular capillaries; this pressure gradient forces the glomerular filtrate down the renal tubular system.

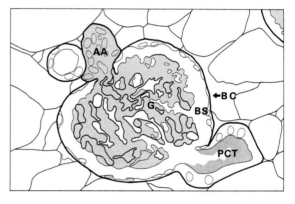

Fig. 13.11 Explanatory diagram for Fig. 13.10

AA —afferent arteriole
G —glomerulus
BC —Bowman's capsule
BS —Bowman's space
PCT —proximal convoluted tubule

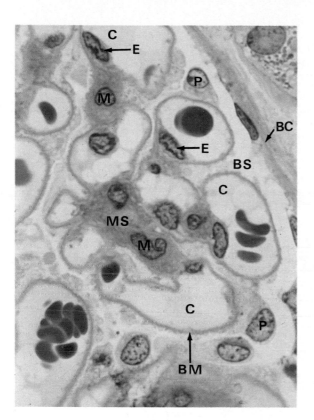

Fig. 13.12 Glomerulus

(Resin-embedded, one micron section: toluidine blue × 1200)

Using resin-embedding techniques it is possible to cut thin sections (approximately 0·5 to 1·0 μm thick) which permit much greater resolution at high magnification.

In this preparation, the glomerular capillaries **C**, some of which contain erythrocytes, are defined by their prominent basement membranes **BM**. Occasional capillary endothelial cell nuclei **E** are seen bulging into the capillary lumina. Mesangium, which consists of mesangial cells **M** and densely stained extracellular substance called *mesangial substance* **MS**, provides support for the capillary loops particularly at their branching points. Mesangium is thought to represent specialised connective tissue but its physiological role is poorly understood.

The surface of the glomerular capillary loops exposed to Bowman's space **BS** is invested by a continuous but irregular layer of podocytes. The podocytes are epithelial in origin since they represent that part of Bowman's capsule pushed inwards by the invagination of the glomerulus during embryonic development. The podocytes **P** have an extensive, branching, pale-stained cytoplasm and large rounded pale-stained nuclei. Thus, the glomerular filtrate must traverse capillary endothelium, basement membrane and the podocyte layer before reaching Bowman's space. Bowman's space is much less prominent in this type of preparation in which little glomerular shrinkage occurs. Note the nuclei of two squamous cells of Bowman's capsule **BC**, the outline of which may be traced by its prominent basement membrane.

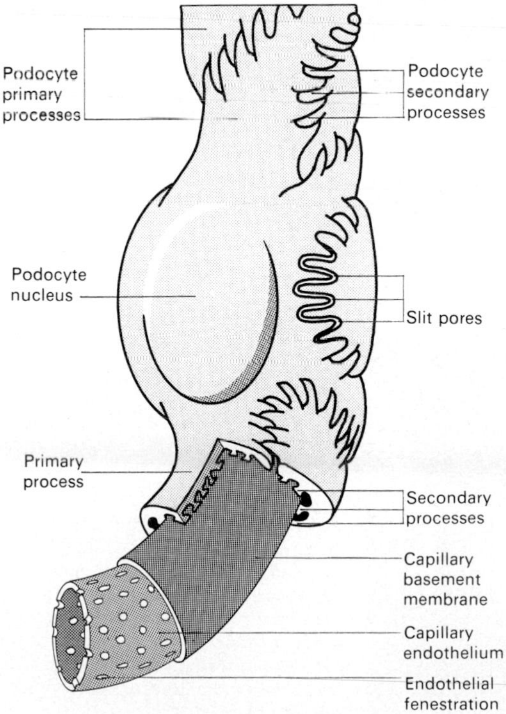

Fig. 13.13 Components of the glomerular filter

During filtration of plasma from glomerular capillaries into Bowman's space, the filtrate passes through three layers:

(i) Capillary endothelium: glomerular capillary endothelial cells contain numerous pores or fenestrations which are large enough to permit the passage of all the non-cellular elements of blood.

(ii) Capillary basement membrane: this layer is continuous and non-fenestrated. Clinical evidence has demonstrated that free haemoglobin (molecular weight 65000) and smaller molecules pass freely through the glomerular filter, whereas albumin (molecular weight 68000) and larger molecules are retained. Experimental evidence, based on the use of tracer molecules, suggests that the basement membrane acts as the glomerular *ultrafilter*.

(iii) Podocytes: these cells, which envelop the glomerular capillaries, have long cytoplasmic extensions called *primary processes*. The primary processes in turn give rise to short *secondary foot processes (pedicels)* which closely interdigitate with those of other primary processes and are directly applied to the glomerular basement membrane. The gaps between these interdigitations are of uniform width (25 nm) and are called *slit pores*. The role of slit pores in the filtration process is poorly understood. Plasma molecules, too large to be filtered, remain within the glomerular capillaries and maintain a colloidal osmotic pressure which prevents filtration of all the water from plasma.

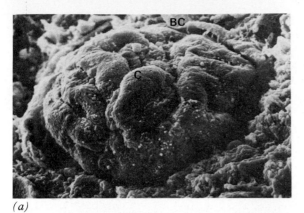

(a)

Fig. 13.14 Glomerulus
(Scanning EM (a) ×450 (b) ×1000 (c) ×4500)

Scanning electron microscopy readily demonstrates the three-dimensional relationships of podocytes and their processes which extend like octopus tentacles over the whole surface of the glomerulus.

(a) Part of Bowman's capsule **BC** has been removed to reveal a three-dimensional view of the glomerulus. Note the tightly packed capillary loops **C**.

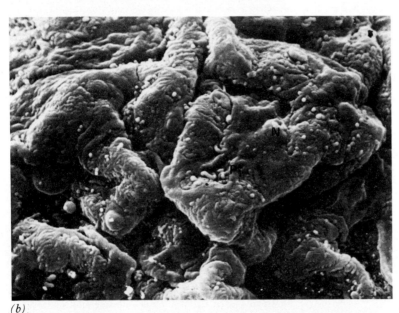

(b)

(b) At higher magnification, the capillaries can be seen to be enveloped by podocytes which have large, flattened cell bodies and bulging nuclei **N**. Each podocyte has several long primary processes P_1 which embrace one or more capillaries. Each primary process has numerous secondary foot processes.

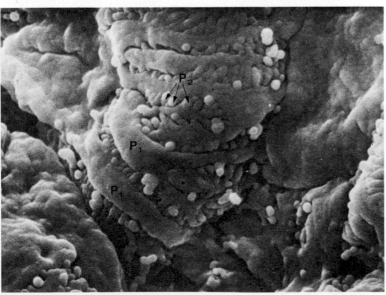

(c)

(c) With further magnification the secondary foot processes P_2 can be seen as extensions of the larger processes P_1. The secondary foot processes interdigitate with those of other primary processes. The slit pores between interdigitating secondary foot processes are of approximately uniform width (25 nm).

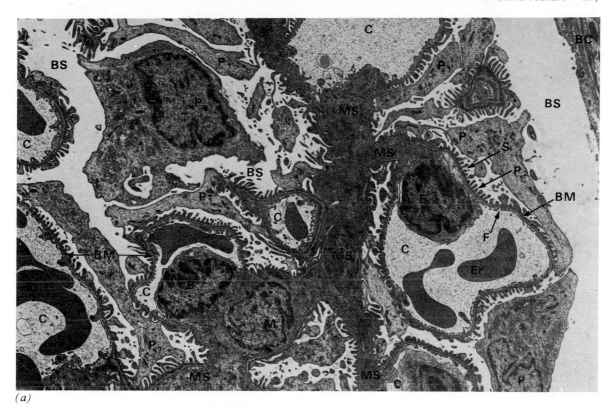

(a)

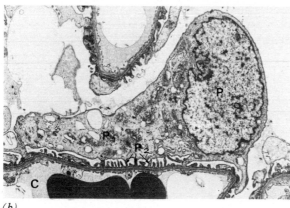

(b)

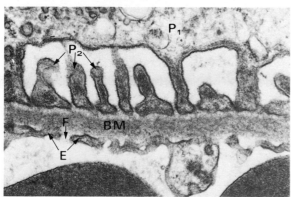

(c)

Fig. 13.15 Glomerulus

(EM (a) ×2400 (b) ×4275 (c) ×44000)

At low magnification, several capillary loops **C** are recognised by their content of erythrocytes **Er** and precipitated plasma proteins. The nuclei of two capillary endothelial cells **E** can be seen bulging into the capillary lumina. Capillary endothelial fenestrations **F** are better seen at higher magnification in (c). A branched mesangial stalk comprising a mesangial cell **M** and dense mesangial substance **MS** provides support for several capillary loops. The nuclei of two podocytes **P** can be seen. Several podocyte primary processes **P₁** give rise to numerous secondary foot processes **P₂** which rest on the glomerular basement membrane **BM**. Part of Bowman's capsule **BC** is seen at the periphery. Note the labyrinth of Bowman's space **BS** which pervades the glomerulus. At higher magnification, the intimate relationship of a podocyte **P** and its primary **P₁** and secondary **P₂** foot processes with the basement membrane of a glomerular capillary **C** is demonstrated. With further magnification, the three components of the glomerular filter are seen. The fenestrated capillary endothelium **E** is closely applied to the luminal surface of the glomerular basement membrane **BM**. The outer aspect of the basement membrane supports podocyte secondary foot processes **P₂**, separated by slit pores of approximately uniform width. Parts of two erythrocytes are seen in the capillary lumen.

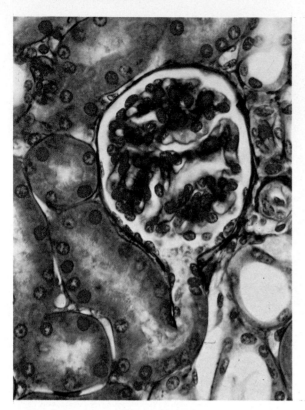

Fig. 13.16 Proximal convoluted tubule

(*Azan* × *480*)

A proximal convoluted tubule (PCT) can be seen to arise from a renal corpuscle; convolutions of this PCT are seen in longitudinal, oblique and transverse sections.

Approximately seventy-five per cent of the glomerular filtrate is reabsorbed from the PCT and this reabsorptive function is reflected in the structure of the epithelial lining. The simple, tall cuboidal epithelium has a prominent brush border which almost completely fills the lumen. The brush border greatly increases the surface area of plasma membrane through which molecules can be reabsorbed from the glomerular filtrate. The cytoplasm of PCT epithelial cells stains intensely due to a high content of organelles, principally mitochondria. The bulk of the renal cortex is composed of proximal tubules since the PCT is the longest and most convoluted part of the nephron.

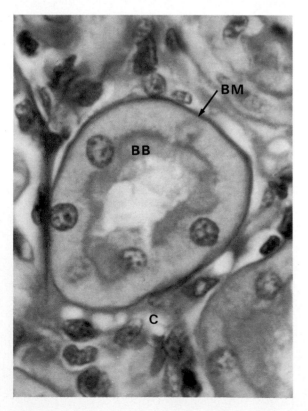

Fig. 13.17 Proximal convoluted tubule

(*PAS/Haematoxylin* × *1200*)

This staining method has been used to demonstrate the prominent brush border **BB** of microvilli projecting into the lumen of the PCT. The brush border is PAS-positive since the surfaces of the microvilli are coated with a particularly dense glycocalyx (see Fig. 1.2). The glycocalyx is thought to afford physical and chemical protection to the microvilli. Like all other basement membranes, the basement membrane **BM** supporting the tubular epithelium is strongly PAS-positive due to its condensed ground substance.

A rich capillary network **C** arising from the efferent arteriole of the glomerulus (see Fig. 13.9) surrounds the PCT and returns molecules reabsorbed from the glomerular filtrate back into the general circulation.

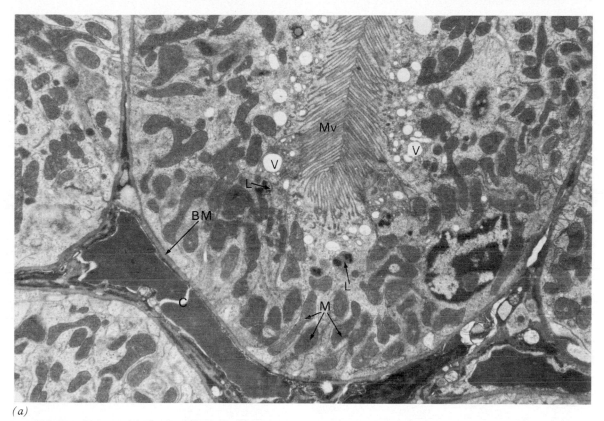

(a)

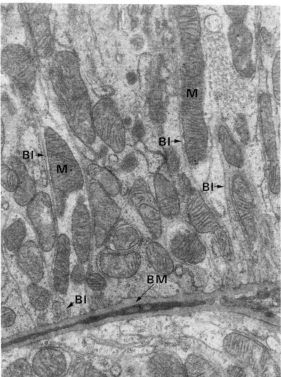

(b)

Fig. 13.18 Proximal convoluted tubule

(EM (a) ×3000   (b) ×6500)

Electron microscopy of the PCT reveals profuse, tall
microvilli **Mv** constituting the brush border seen with light
microscopy. The plasma membrane of the microvilli
contains a variety of transport proteins and enzymes
involved in selective reabsorption of solutes from the
glomerular filtrate. Some of these transport processes are
dependent on energy which is supplied in the form of ATP
by mitochondria **M** which crowd the cytoplasm of PCT
cells. The cytoplasm immediately beneath the brush border
contains many pinocytotic vesicles **V** and lysosomes **L**
which are thought to be involved in reabsorption and
degradation of small amounts of protein which have leaked
through the glomerular ultrafilter. Reabsorbed solutes are
transported through the basal plasma membrane **BM** into
surrounding capillaries **C**.

At high magnification, the basal plasma membrane
of the PCT is seen to exhibit deep basal infoldings **BI** into
the cell. These infoldings are closely related to columns of
elongated mitochondria **M**. This mitochondrial
arrangement may give rise to the appearance of basal
striations in light microscopy. The basal infoldings of the
plasma membrane increase the surface area for transport of
reabsorbed molecules from PCT cells into the extracellular
fluid and thence into capillaries. The presence of numerous
mitochondria reflects the high energy demands of this
process.

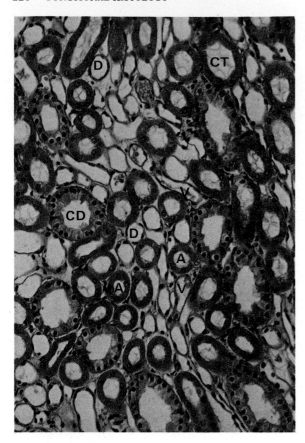

Fig. 13.19 Loop of Henle
(H & E × 198)

The loop of Henle is a continuation of the PCT and constitutes the second histo-physiological zone of the renal tubule (see Fig. 13.4). Each loop of Henle arises in the renal cortex, dips down into the medulla as the descending limb, then returns to the cortex as the ascending limb before becoming continuous with the distal convoluted tubule. Thus loops of Henle are best seen in sections of renal medulla and are most easily recognised in transverse section as in this micrograph. In addition to loops of Henle, the medulla also contains the vasa recta, collecting tubules and collecting ducts. All these structures are seen in this micrograph and may be distinguished by the following features.

The thin descending limbs **D** have a simple squamous epithelium but may be differentiated from the vasa recta **V** by their regular, rounded shape and the absence of erythrocytes. The thick ascending limbs **A** are lined by low cuboidal epithelium and are also round in cross-section. Neither limb of the loop of Henle has a brush border. Collecting tubules **CT** have a similar epithelial lining to the ascending limbs but are of wider and less regular diameter. The collecting ducts **CD** are easily recognised by their large diameter and columnar, pale-stained epithelial lining.

The function of the loop of Henle is to produce an increasing osmotic gradient from the cortex to the tip of the renal medulla. The high osmotic pressure in medullary extracellular fluid permits the removal of water, by osmosis, from fluid in the collecting tubules and ducts in the presence of ADH (see Fig. 13.24). The vasa recta take up water from the medullary extracellular fluid and return it to the general circulation.

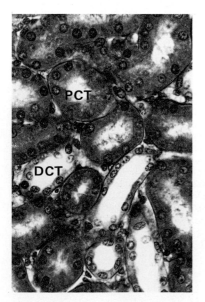

Fig. 13.20 Distal convoluted tubule
(Azan × 320)

The distal convoluted tubule (DCT) extends from the ascending limb of the loop of Henle after its return to the cortex, and forms the third histo-physiological zone of the renal tubule. Therefore, DCTs are found mainly within the cortex where they are entangled with proximal convoluted tubules.

As seen in this micrograph of the renal cortex, distal convoluted tubules **DCT** may be differentiated from surrounding proximal convoluted tubules **PCT** on the basis of the following characteristic features: absence of a brush border; a larger, more clearly defined lumen; more nuclei are seen in transverse section (since DCT cells are smaller than those of the PCT); less affinity for cytoplasmic stains (due to a smaller content of organelles). In addition, sections of the DCT are seen much less frequently than sections of the PCT since the DCT is a much shorter segment of the renal tubule than the PCT.

The DCT is mainly involved in reabsorption of sodium ions from the tubular fluid; this process is directly coupled to the secretion of hydrogen and potassium ions into the tubular fluid. One hydrogen ion or one potassium ion is secreted for every one sodium ion reabsorbed. This process is controlled by the hormone aldosterone secreted by the adrenal cortex (see Chapter 14).

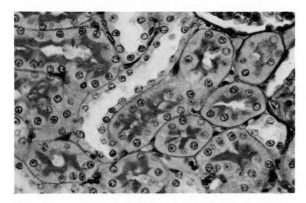

Fig. 13.21 Renal tubules

(PAS/Haematoxylin × 320)

This micrograph demonstrates a method of differentiating between proximal and distal convoluted tubules on the basis of the presence or absence of a brush border. The PCT has a profuse PAS-positive brush border (see Fig. 13.17) whereas a brush border is almost completely absent from the DCT. Note the characteristic star-shaped lumina of the PCTs.

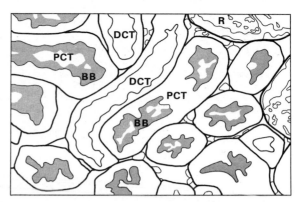

Fig. 13.22 Explanatory diagram for Fig. 13.21

DCT —distal convoluted tubule
PCT —proximal convoluted tubule
BB —brush border
R —renal corpuscle

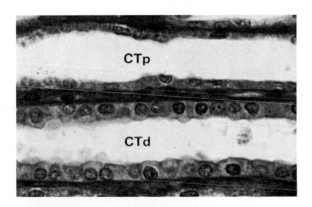

Fig. 13.23 Collecting tubules

(LS: Azan × 500)

The collecting tubule continues from the terminal part of the DCT and constitutes the fourth histo-physiological zone of the nephron. The collecting tubules converge in the renal cortex to form bundles of tubules termed medullary rays (see Fig. 13.6). As the medullary rays approach the medulla, the cuboidal epithelium lining the collecting tubules becomes progressively taller. This micrograph illustrates a proximal section of a collecting tubule **CTp** and a more distal section **CTd** of an adjacent tubule within a medullary ray. The absence of a brush border and a clear cytoplasm are consistent with the evidence that no active reabsorption takes place within collecting tubules.

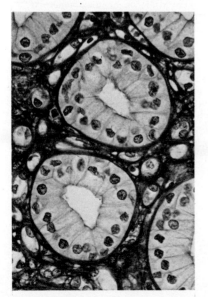

Fig. 13.24 Collecting ducts

(TS: Azan × 320)

The collecting ducts are formed by the fusion of collecting tubules and convey urine into the pelvi-calyceal space. As they converge upon the renal papilla the collecting ducts merge to form progressively larger ducts, the largest ducts being known as the ducts of Bellini.

This micrograph of the renal medulla illustrates two collecting ducts surrounded by thin limbs of the loop of Henle and vasa recta. Collecting ducts are characterised by tall columnar epithelium, well defined cellular outlines, pale-stained cytoplasm and the absence of a brush border.

No active reabsorption takes place from the collecting ducts, but in the presence of anti-diuretic hormone (ADH) secreted by the pituitary, the collecting ducts become permeable to water. Water is drawn out of collecting ducts, by osmosis, into extracellular fluid and thence into adjacent vasa recta. Release of ADH from the pituitary is stimulated by dehydration. This promotes the uptake of water from the collecting tubules thereby producing a reduced volume of hypertonic urine. Conversely, ADH secretion is inhibited by water overloading and an increased volume of hypotonic urine is thus produced.

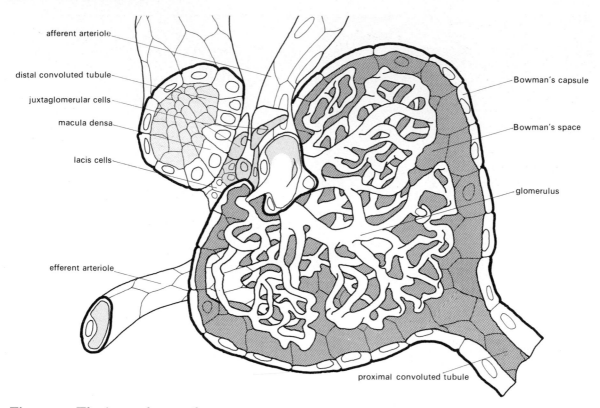

afferent arteriole

distal convoluted tubule

juxtaglomerular cells

macula densa

lacis cells

efferent arteriole

Bowman's capsule

Bowman's space

glomerulus

proximal convoluted tubule

Fig. 13.25 The juxtaglomerular apparatus

The juxtaglomerular apparatus (JGA) is involved in the regulation of systemic blood pressure.

The JGA is made up of the part of the afferent arteriole just before it enters Bowman's capsule, and a section of DCT of the same nephron which loops back to lie against the afferent arteriole at this point. The JGA has the following components:

(i) Juxtaglomerular cells: these cells are derived from the smooth muscle of the wall of the afferent arteriole and form a cuff of several layers around the afferent arteriole just before it enters the glomerulus. Juxtaglomerular cells have a prominent nucleus and the cytoplasm contains granules of the enzyme *renin*. It is thought that the juxtaglomerular cells are directly sensitive to the pressure of blood in the afferent arteriole. A decrease in systemic blood pressure stimulates the release of renin granules which activates the *renin-angiotensin-aldosterone mechanism*; this promotes an increase in systemic blood pressure (see Fig. 13.28).

(ii) Macula densa: this consists of modified DCT cells and is found where the juxtaglomerular cells and DCT are closely apposed. The cells of the macula densa are taller and have larger, more prominent nuclei than the other cells lining the DCT. The basement membrane between the macula and juxtaglomerular cells is extremely thin.

It is postulated that the cells of the macula densa are sensitive to the concentration of sodium ions in the fluid within the DCT. A decrease in systemic blood pressure results in decreased production of glomerular filtrate and hence decreased concentration of sodium ions in the fluid of the DCT; this stimulates the release of renin granules into the blood of the afferent arteriole via the juxtaglomerular cells. Consequently the JGA is thought to respond to systemic blood pressure changes via both mechano- and chemoreceptors.

(iii) Lacis cells (or **polkissen**): this small group of cells lies between the macula densa and Bowman's capsule at the point of entry of the afferent arteriole. These cells are thought to be extra-glomerular mesangial cells but their function is uncertain. Lacis cells may produce the hormone erythropoietin which promotes erythropoiesis in bone marrow (see Chapter 2). The stimulus for erythropoietin release is postulated to be a low concentration of oxygen in the blood of the afferent arteriole.

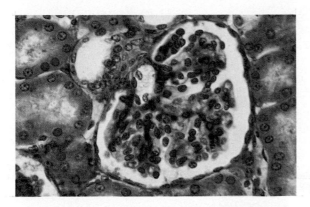

Fig. 13.26 Juxtaglomerular apparatus

(Azan × 320)

This section through the vascular pole of a renal corpuscle illustrates a juxtaglomerular apparatus. Note that the tall columnar cells of the macula densa have larger, more prominent, nuclei than the cells of the rest of the DCT. The juxtaglomerular cells, believed to be responsible for the secretion of renin, have a slightly granular cytoplasm.

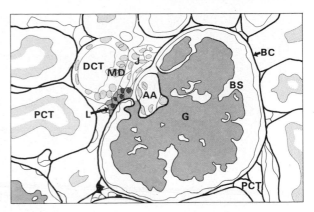

Fig. 13.27 Explanatory diagram for Fig. 13.26

G —glomerulus
BS —Bowman's space
BC —Bowman's capsule
MD —macula densa
J —juxtaglomerular cells
L —lacis cells
DCT —distal convoluted tubule
AA —afferent arteriole
PCT — proximal convoluted tubule

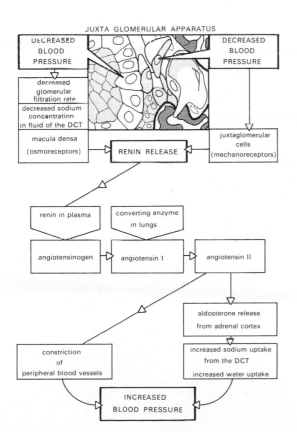

Fig. 13.28 Juxtaglomerular apparatus: control of blood pressure

This diagram summarises the mode of action of the juxtaglomerular apparatus. There are two circumstances in which renin is thought to be released into the bloodstream:

(i) A fall in systemic blood pressure; this may be sensed by pressure receptors (the juxtaglomerular cells) in the wall of the afferent arteriole.

(ii) A decrease in the concentration of sodium ions in the DCT which occurs when the glomerular filtration rate decreases due to a fall in blood pressure. This may be sensed by cells of the macula densa acting as chemoreceptors.

The enzyme renin, when liberated into the bloodstream, acts on the plasma globulin *angiotensinogen* to produce a polypeptide chain of ten amino-acids called *angiotensin I*. A further enzyme, called *converting enzyme*, cleaves two amino-acids from angiotensin I to form *angiotensin II* which is a potent vasoconstrictor.

Angiotensin II brings about an increased blood pressure in two ways: firstly, by constriction of peripheral blood vessels, and secondly by promoting the release of aldosterone from the adrenal cortex. Aldosterone increases blood pressure by promoting the reabsorption of sodium ions and therefore water from the DCT, thus expanding the plasma volume and hence increasing blood pressure.

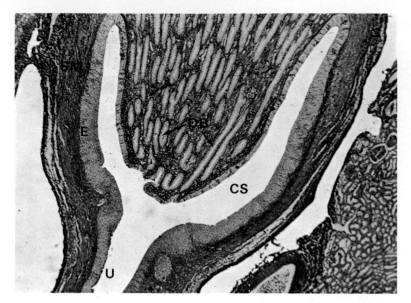

Fig. 13.29 Renal papilla
(*Monkey: LS: Azan × 30*)

The renal papilla forms the apex of the medullary pyramid where it projects into the calyceal space. The ducts of Bellini **DB**, the largest of the collecting ducts, converge in the renal papilla to discharge urine into the pelvicalyceal space **CS**. The renal pelvis is lined by urinary epithelium **E**, and the wall of the pelvis contains smooth muscle **SM** which contracts to force urine into the ureter **U**.

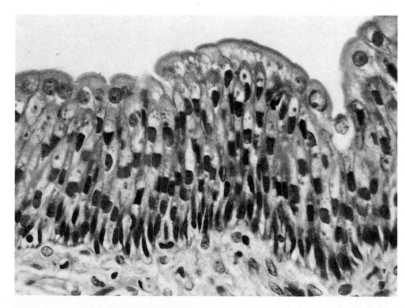

Fig. 13.30 Urinary epithelium
(*H & E × 480*)

Urinary epithelium, also called transitional epithelium or urothelium, is found only within the conducting passages of the urinary system for which it is especially adapted. The plasma membranes of the superficial cells are much thicker than most cell membranes and have a highly ordered substructure, thus rendering urinary epithelium impermeable to urine which is potentially toxic. This permeability barrier also prevents water from being drawn from the epithelium into hypertonic urine. The cells of urinary epithelium have highly interdigitating cell junctions which permit great distension of the epithelium without damage to the surface integrity (see also Fig. 4.16 and Fig. 4.17).

Urinary epithelium rests on a basement membrane which is often too thin to be resolved by light microscopy and was formerly thought to be absent. The basal layer is irregular and may be deeply indented by strands of underlying connective tissue containing capillaries. This unusual feature led early histologists to believe, mistakenly, that urinary epithelium contradicted the principle that epithelium never contains blood vessels.

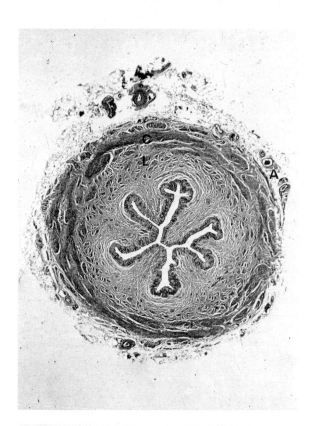

Fig. 13.31 Ureter
(TS: Masson's trichrome × 12)

The ureters are muscular tubes which conduct urine from the kidneys to the bladder. Urine is conducted from the pelvi-calyceal system as a bolus which is propelled by peristaltic action of the ureteric wall. Thus the wall of the ureter contains two layers of smooth muscle arranged into an inner longitudinal layer **L** and an outer circular layer **C**. Another outer longitudinal layer is present in the lower third of the ureter. The lumen of the ureter is lined by urinary epithelium which is thrown up into folds in the relaxed state. This allows the ureter to dilate during the passage of a bolus of urine. Surrounding the muscular wall is a loose connective tissue adventitia **A** containing blood vessels, lymphatics and nerves.

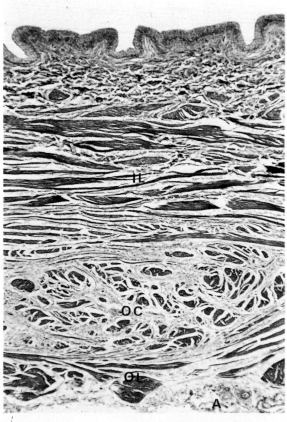

Fig. 13.32 Bladder
(TS: Masson's trichrome × 12)

The general structure of the bladder wall resembles that of the lower third of the ureters. The wall of the bladder consists of three loosely arranged layers of smooth muscle and elastic fibres which contract during micturition. Note the inner longitudinal **IL**, outer circular **OC** and outer longitudinal **OL** layers of smooth muscle. The urinary epithelium lining the bladder is thrown into many folds in the relaxed state. The outer adventitial coat **A** contains arteries, veins and lymphatics.

The urethra, the final conducting portion of the urinary tract, is discussed as part of the male reproductive tract in Chapter 15.

14. The endocrine glands

Introduction

Endocrine glands are the sites of synthesis and secretion of substances known as *hormones* which are disseminated throughout the body by the bloodstream where they act on specific *target organs*. In conjunction with the nervous system, hormones co-ordinate and integrate the functions of all the physiological systems.

Endocrine glands are in general composed of secretory cells of epithelial origin supported by connective tissue which is rich in blood and lymphatic capillaries. The secretory cells discharge hormones into the interstitial spaces from which they are rapidly absorbed into the circulatory system. Thus a characteristic feature of all endocrine glands is a very rich vascular supply. Unlike exocrine glands (see Chapter 4), endocrine glands have no duct system and are therefore called the *ductless glands*.

Reflecting their active synthetic function, endocrine secretory cells are generally characterised by prominent nuclei and prolific cytoplasmic organelles, especially mitochondria, endoplasmic reticulum, Golgi bodies and secretory vesicles.

Some endocrine glands exist in the form of discrete organs, e.g. pituitary, thyroid, parathyroid and adrenal glands. Other endocrine tissues are found in association with exocrine glands, e.g. pancreas, or within complex organs, e.g. kidney, testis, ovary, placenta, brain and the gastro-intestinal tract. This chapter deals with the pituitary, thyroid, parathyroid, adrenal, endocrine pancreas, pineal and the gastro-intestinal endocrine system; other endocrine tissues are discussed with the organs with which they are associated.

Pituitary gland

The *pituitary gland*, also known as the *hypophysis*, is a specialised appendage of the brain which secretes a variety of hormones. The hormones mediate non-nervous mechanisms by which the central nervous system integrates and controls many body functions. The pituitary hormones fall into two functional groups:

(a) hormones which act directly on non-endocrine tissues: growth hormone (GH), prolactin, antidiuretic hormone (ADH), oxytocin and melanocyte stimulating hormone (MSH);

(b) hormones which modulate the secretory activity of other endocrine glands, the so-called *trophic hormones:* thyroid stimulating hormone (TSH), adrenocorticotrophic hormone (ACTH) and the gonadotrophic hormones, follicle stimulating hormone (FSH) and luteinising hormone (LH). Thus the thyroid, adrenal cortex and gonads may be described as *pituitary-dependent endocrine glands*.

The secretion of all pituitary hormones is directly controlled by the hypothalmus; the activity of the hypothalmus, however, is under the influence of nervous stimuli from higher centres in the central nervous system, and is controlled by feedback from the levels of circulating hormones produced by the pituitary-dependent glands. Thus the pituitary gland plays a central role in integrating the nervous and endocrine systems.

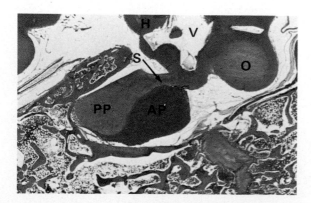

Fig. 14.1 Pituitary gland
(Monkey: H & E × 8)

This micrograph from a midline section through the brain and floor of the cranium illustrates the pituitary gland *in situ*. The pituitary is almost completely enclosed in a bony depression in the floor of the cranial cavity, called the *sella turcica*. The pituitary gland consists of two major components, the *anterior pituitary* **AP** and the *posterior pituitary* **PP**. The posterior pituitary is connected to the hypothalamus **H** via a short stalk, the *pituitary stalk* **S**. Note the close proximity of the third ventricle **V** above the hypothalamus and the close relationship of the optic chiasma **O** which lies anteriorly.

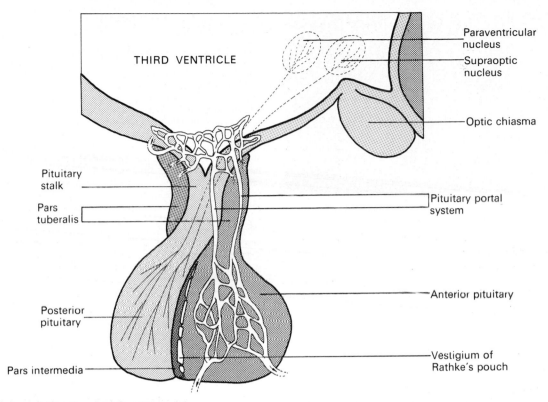

THIRD VENTRICLE

Paraventricular
nucleus

Supraoptic
nucleus

Optic chiasma

Pituitary
stalk

Pars
tuberalis

Pituitary portal
system

Anterior pituitary

Posterior
pituitary

Vestigium of
Rathke's pouch

Pars intermedia

Fig. 14.2 Pituitary gland

(sagittal section)

The anterior and posterior parts of the pituitary originate from different embryological sources and this is reflected in their structure and function.

(i) The posterior pituitary, also called the *neurohypophysis* or *pars nervosa*, is derived from a downgrowth of nervous tissue from the hypothalamus to which it remains joined by the pituitary stalk which is composed of nervous tissue.

(ii) The anterior pituitary arises as an epithelial upgrowth from the roof of the primitive oral cavity, known as *Rathke's pouch*. This specialised glandular epithelium is wrapped around the posterior pituitary and is often called the *adenohypophysis*. The adenohypophysis may contain a cleft or group of cyst-like spaces which represent the vestigial lumen of Rathke's pouch. This vestigial cleft divides the major part of the anterior pituitary from a thin zone of tissue lying against the posterior pituitary; this thin zone is known as the *pars intermedia*. An extension of the adenohypophysis surrounds the neural stalk and is known as the *pars tuberalis*.

The type and mode of secretion of the posterior pituitary differs greatly from that of the anterior pituitary. The posterior pituitary secretes two hormones: *antidiuretic hormone* (ADH), also called *vasopressin*, and the hormone *oxytocin*; both these hormones act directly on non-endocrine tissues. ADH is synthesised in the neurone cell bodies of the *supraoptic nucleus*, and oxytocin is synthesised in those of the *paraventricular nucleus* of the hypothalamus.

These hormones, bound to glycoproteins, pass down the axons of the hypothalamo-pituitary tract through the pituitary stalk to the posterior pituitary where they are stored in the distended terminal parts of the axons. Release of posterior pituitary hormones into the bloodstream is controlled directly by nervous impulses passing down the axons from the hypothalamus; this process is known as *neurosecretion*.

The anterior pituitary secretes both trophic and direct action hormones:

(a) trophic hormones: thyroid stimulating hormone (TSH), adrenocorticotrophic hormone (ACTH), and the gonadotrophic hormones, follicle stimulating hormone (FSH) and luteinising hormone (LH).

(b) direct action hormones: growth hormone (GH) and prolactin. (Recent evidence suggests that prolactin has a trophic action on the endocrine tissues of the ovary in some animals.)

Hypothalamic control of anterior pituitary secretion is mediated by specific hypothalamic releasing hormones such as *thyroid stimulating hormone releasing hormone* (TSHRH). These releasing hormones are conducted from the *median hypothalamic eminence* to the anterior pituitary by a unique system of portal veins.

The pars intermedia synthesises and secretes melanocyte stimulating hormone (MSH); in man, the physiological importance of this hormone and the control of its secretion is poorly understood.

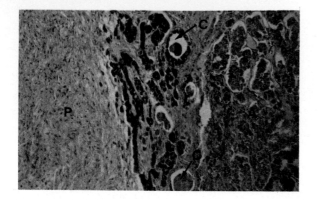

Fig. 14.3 Pituitary gland

(Isamine blue/eosin × 50)

This micrograph illustrates the three main zones of the pituitary gland: the anterior pituitary **A**, the pars intermedia **I** and the posterior pituitary **P**.

The anterior pituitary is composed of irregular branching cords of secretory cells supported by fine reticular connective tissue containing numerous capillary sinusoids. The various secretory cell types of the anterior pituitary have widely differing staining properties. The pars intermedia consists of cords of strongly basophilic cells, stained dark blue in this preparation. Within the pars intermedia are colloid-filled spaces **C**, which represent the remnants of the embryological cleft of Rathke's pouch. In man, the pars intermedia is poorly developed and cords of secretory cells may extend into the posterior pituitary. In contrast, the posterior pituitary does not exhibit the usual characteristics of endocrine tissues but contains the axons of neurosecretory cells, the cell bodies of which are located in the hypothalamus. These neurosecretory axons are supported by glial cells similar to those in the rest of the central nervous system (see Chapter 7).

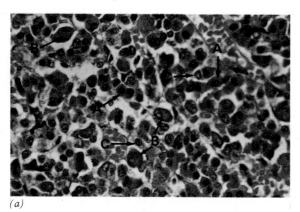

(a)

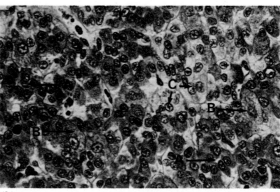

(b)

Fig. 14.4 Anterior pituitary

(a) H & E × 320 (b) Modified Azan × 320

The secretory cells of the anterior pituitary are classified into two groups according to their staining affinity: *chromophils* and *chromophobes*.

The chromophils are cells of variable size with strong affinity for histological dyes whereas the chromophobes are smaller cells which have little affinity for stains.

(i) Chromophils: traditionally, the chromophils have been subdivided into two groups, *acidophils* **A** and *basophils* **B**, because of their staining properties with a variety of histological methods such as that shown in (b). Note that in (b) acidophils are stained orange and basophils are stained blue. In H & E preparations, as in (a), the distinction between basophils and acidophils is much less obvious. Functionally, the acidophils are of two types: growth hormone-secreting cells and prolactin-secreting cells. Both these hormones are polypeptide in nature and are of the direct action type. There are three separate types of basophil each of which secretes one of the trophic glycoprotein hormones: TSH, FSH and LH.

(ii) Chromophobes: the chromophobes **C** are the smallest cell type in the anterior pituitary and contain few cytoplasmic granules; they have little affinity for either acidic or basic dyes. Some of the chromophobes secrete the polypeptide trophic hormone, ACTH. Most of the chromophobes, however, are thought to be degranulated or resting forms of chromophil cells.

All the cells of the anterior pituitary form cords of secretory cells which are surrounded by a rich network of sinusoidal capillaries. The basement membranes surrounding the clumps of epithelial cells are clearly demonstrated as blue-stained structures in preparation (b).

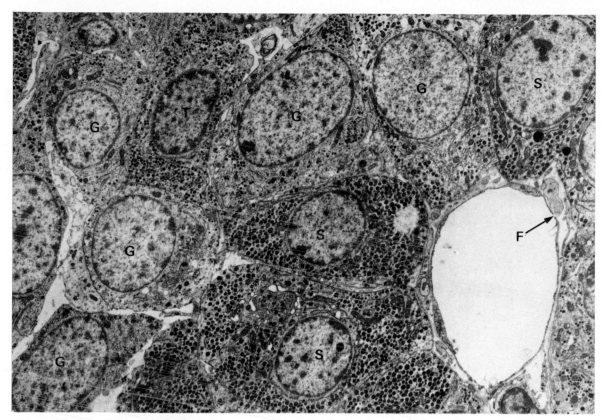

Fig. 14.5 Anterior pituitary
(EM × 4270)

The cells of the anterior pituitary may be differentiated in electron microscopy by the shape, size, electron density and texture of their secretory granules and by the characteristics of their cytoplasmic organelles. Gonadotroph cells **G**, a thyrotroph cell **T**, and several growth hormone secreting cells, often called somatotrophs **S**, are illustrated in this micrograph.

The endothelial lining of capillary sinusoids in endocrine tissues is characteristically fenestrated (see Fig. 6.12). Note the fenestrations **F** in the sinusoid seen in this micrograph. It is postulated that fenestrations facilitate passage of hormones into the sinusoids.

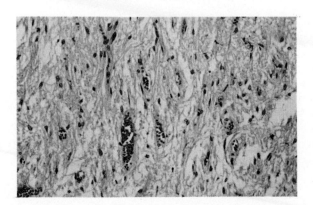

Fig. 14.6 Posterior pituitary
(H & E × 128)

The posterior pituitary contains the non-myelinated axons of neurosecretory cells, the cell bodies of which are located in the hypothalamus. The neurosecretory axons are supported by cells called *pituicytes* similar in structure and function to the neuroglial cells of the central nervous system (see Fig. 7.27). Most of the nuclei seen in this micrograph are those of pituicytes; the axons of the neurosecretory cells are indistinguishable from the cytoplasm of the pituicytes in H & E preparations. A rich network of fine, fenestrated capillaries pervades the posterior pituitary.

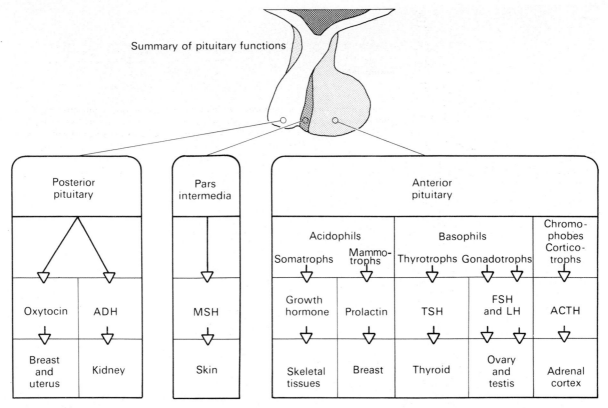

Fig. 14.7 Summary of pituitary functions

Thyroid gland

The thyroid gland is a lobulated endocrine gland lying in the neck in front of the upper part of the trachea. It is derived embryologically from an epithelial downgrowth of the primitive oral cavity.

The thyroid gland produces hormones of two types:

(i) Iodine-containing hormones *tri-iodothyronine* (T3) and *thyroxine* (T4); T4 is converted to T3 in the general circulation. T3 regulates the basal metabolic rate and has an important influence on growth and maturation particularly of nervous tissue. The secretion of these hormones is regulated by TSH secreted by the anterior pituitary.

(ii) The polypeptide hormone *calcitonin*; this hormone regulates blood calcium levels in conjunction with parathyroid hormone. Calcitonin lowers blood calcium levels by inhibiting the rate of decalcification of bone by osteoclastic resorption (see Fig. 9.14) and by stimulating osteoblastic activity. Control of calcitonin secretion is dependent only on blood calcium levels and is independent of pituitary and parathyroid hormone levels.

The thyroid gland is unique among the human endocrine glands in that it stores large amounts of hormones in an inactive form within extracellular compartments called follicles; in contrast, other endocrine glands store only small quantities of hormones in intracellular sites.

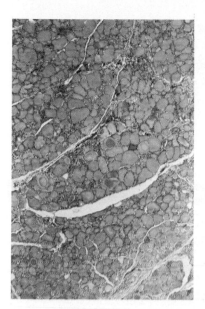

Fig. 14.8 Thyroid gland

(H & E × 8)

The functional units of the thyroid gland are the *thyroid follicles*, irregular, spheroidal structures composed of a single layer of cuboidal epithelial cells bounded by a basement membrane (see also Figs. 4.36 and 4.37). The follicles are variable in size and contain a homogeneous, colloid material which is stained pink in this preparation.

The thyroid gland is enveloped in an outer capsule of loose connective tissue and an inner capsule of fibro-elastic tissue. From the inner capsule, connective tissue septa extend into the gland dividing the gland into lobules, and conveying a rich blood supply, together with lymphatics and nerves.

This micrograph illustrates follicles of widely differing sizes, a characteristic of the normal active thyroid; the size of each follicle reflects its state of synthetic or secretory activity.

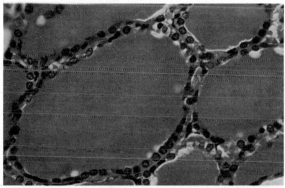

(a)

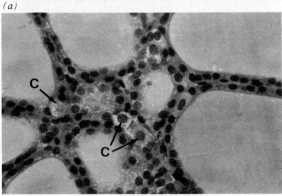

(b)

Fig. 14.9 Thyroid gland

(a) Human (b) Dog (H & E × 128)

Thyroid follicles are lined by a simple cuboidal epithelium which is responsible for the synthesis and secretion of the iodine-containing hormones T3 and T4. Thyroid follicles are filled with a glycoprotein complex called *thyroglobulin* or *thyroid colloid*, a substance which is a storage form of the thyroid hormones. In actively secreting thyroid glands, as in these micrographs, the follicles tend to be small and the amount of colloid diminished; the lining cells are tall and cuboidal reflecting active hormone synthesis and secretion. Conversely, the follicles of the less active thyroid are distended by stored colloid and the lining cells appear flattened against the follicular basement membrane.

A second secretory cell type is found in the thyroid gland either as single cells among the follicular cells or as small clumps in the interfollicular spaces. These so-called *parafollicular cells* were first described in the dog in which they have an extensive unstained cytoplasm and were therefore also called *'C' (clear) cells* **C**; this characteristic feature is seen in micrograph (b). In other mammals, including man, the cytological characteristics of parafollicular cells are similar to those of the dog but usually much less distinctive. Parafollicular cells synthesise and secrete the hormone calcitonin in direct response to raised blood calcium levels.

Parafollicular cells have a different embryological origin from the follicular cells and in some species constitute a discrete endocrine organ called the ultimo-branchial body.

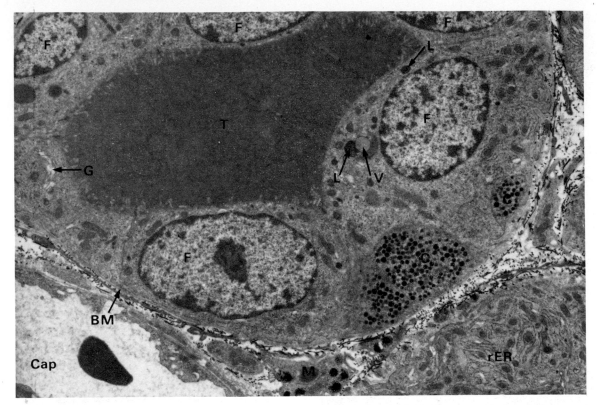

Fig. 14.10 Thyroid follicle

(Rat: EM ×6800)

This micrograph demonstrates a thyroid follicle composed of cuboidal follicular cells **F** surrounding a lumen containing the homogeneous colloid, thyroglobulin **T**. A basement membrane **BM** bounds the follicle. Two portions of the cytoplasm of a parafollicular or 'C' cell **C** are seen within the follicular epithelium; the cytoplasm contains numerous electron-dense secretory granules of the hormone, calcitonin. A fenestrated capillary **Cap** containing an erythrocyte is closely applied to the follicular basement membrane. Part of a mast cell **M** is seen in the interfollicular connective tissue.

Follicular cells concentrate iodide from the blood by means of an iodide pump in the basal plasma membrane. Within the cell, iodide is oxidised to iodine and transported to the follicular plasma membrane where it is released into the follicular lumen. The glycoprotein thyroglobulin is synthesised in the rough endoplasmic reticulum, packaged by the Golgi apparatus, then released into the follicular lumen by exocytosis. Within the follicular lumen (not within the follicular cells), iodine combines with tyrosine residues of the thyroglobulin to form the hormones tri-iodothyronine (T3) and thyroxine (T4) which remain bound to the glycoprotein in an inactive form.

Secretion of these hormones involves engulfment of the thyroglobulin-hormone complex to form cytoplasmic vacuoles; the vacuoles then fuse with lysosomes of the follicular cell cytoplasm and hydrolytic enzymes cleave the hormone from the thyroglobulin. The hormones are released in the basal cytoplasm from which they diffuse into the bloodstream. The synthetic and secretory activity of the thyroid gland is dependent on thyroid stimulating hormone (TSH) secreted by the anterior pituitary.

In this micrograph, rough endoplasmic reticulum **rER** is best demonstrated in the basal aspect of a secretory cell of an adjacent follicle. Mitochondria are closely associated with the endoplasmic reticulum and are also scattered throughout the cytoplasm. Golgi complexes **G** are a prominent feature. Small microvilli associated with the exocytosis of thyroglobulin and the endocytosis of thyroglobulin-hormone complex, protrude into the follicular lumen. In one cell a vacuole **V** of thyroglobulin-hormone complex is seen about to fuse with a large lysosome **L**. Electron-dense lysosomes are also seen scattered throughout the cytoplasm.

Parathyroid gland

The parathyroid glands are small, oval endocrine glands closely associated with the thyroid gland. In mammals, there are usually two pairs of glands, one pair situated on the posterior surface of the thyroid gland on each side.

The parathyroid glands regulate serum calcium and phosphate levels via *parathyroid hormone (parathormone)*. Parathyroid hormone raises serum calcium levels in three ways:

(i) Direct action on bone by increasing the rate of osteoclastic resorption and promoting breakdown of the bone matrix (see Chapter 9).

(ii) Direct action on the kidney by increasing the renal tubular reabsorption of calcium ions and inhibiting the reabsorption of phosphate ions from the glomerular filtrate.

(iii) Promotion of the absorption of calcium from the small intestine; this effect involves vitamin D.

Secretion of parathyroid hormone is stimulated by a decrease in blood calcium levels. In conjunction with calcitonin, secreted by the parafollicular cells of the thyroid gland, blood calcium levels are maintained within narrow limits. Parathyroid hormone is the most important regulator of blood calcium levels and is essential to life, whereas calcitonin may only provide a complementary mechanism for fine adjustment.

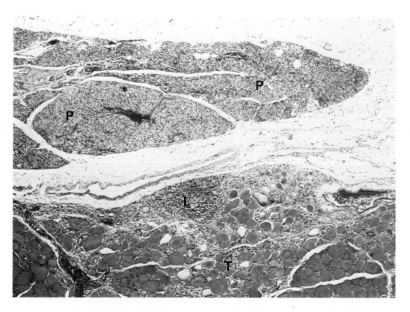

Fig. 14.11 Parathyroid gland

(H & E × 30)

This micrograph shows a parathyroid gland **P** characteristically embedded in the capsule of a thyroid gland **T**. The thin capsule of the parathyroid gland gives rise to delicate connective tissue septa which divide the parenchyma into dense, cord-like masses of secretory cells. The septa carry blood vessels, lymphatics and nerves.

Note that in this specimen, from a 55-year-old woman, there is some infiltration of the thyroid by lymphoid cells **L**; this is a normal feature of the ageing thyroid gland.

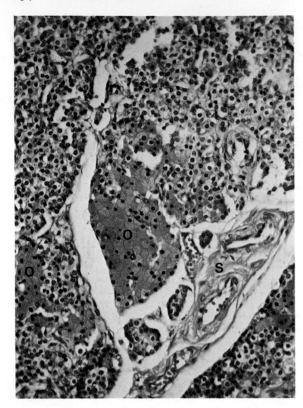

Fig. 14.12 Parathyroid gland
(H & E × 198)

The parathyroid gland contains secretory cells with two types of morphological characteristics:

(i) Chief or principal cells: these are the most abundant cells and are responsible for the secretion of parathyroid hormone. Chief cells have a prominent nucleus and relatively little cytoplasm which varies in staining intensity according to the degree of secretory activity of the cell. Actively secreting cells contain much rough endoplasmic reticulum and stain strongly; in contrast, inactive cells contain little rough endoplasmic reticulum and stain poorly.

(ii) Oxyphil cells: these are larger and much less numerous than chief cells and tend to occur in clumps. They have smaller, densely stained nuclei and strongly eosinophilic (oxyphilic) cytoplasm containing fine granules. Few oxyphil cells are found in the human parathyroid gland until puberty, after which they increase in number with age. Oxyphil cells do not secrete hormones except in certain pathological conditions and their function is poorly understood.

In this micrograph from a young adult, chief cells predominate; note the range of staining intensity from strong to very pale. Oxyphil cells **O** form clumps amongst the chief cells. Note the delicate septa **S** dividing the gland into small lobules and supporting a rich blood supply. With increasing age, adipocytes become characteristically scattered throughout the glandular tissue.

Adrenal gland

The adrenal or supra-renal glands are small, flattened endocrine glands which are closely applied to the upper pole of each kidney. In mammals, the adrenal gland contains two functionally different types of endocrine tissue which have distinctly different embryological origins; in some lower animals, these two components exist as separate endocrine glands. The two components of the adrenal gland are the *adrenal cortex* and *adrenal medulla*.

(i) The adrenal cortex: the adrenal cortex has a similar embryological origin to the gonads (see Chapters 15 and 16) and like the gonads, secretes a variety of *steroid hormones* all structurally related to their common precursor, *cholesterol*. The adrenal steroids may be divided into three functional classes; *mineralocorticoids*, *glucocorticoids* and *sex hormones*. The mineralocorticoids are concerned with electrolyte and fluid homeostasis. The glucocorticoids have a wide range of effects on carbohydrate, protein and lipid metabolism. Small quantities of sex hormones secreted by the adrenal cortex supplement gonadal sex hormone secretion.

(ii) The adrenal medulla: embryologically, the adrenal medulla has a similar origin to that of the sympathetic nervous system and may be considered as a highly specialised adjunct to the sympathetic nervous system. The adrenal medulla secretes the catecholamine hormones, *adrenaline (epinephrine)* and *noradrenaline (norepinephrine)*.

The control of hormone secretion differs markedly between the cortex and medulla. Adrenocortical activity is mainly regulated by the pituitary trophic hormone ACTH, and release of each of the adrenal corticosteroid hormones is controlled by various other circulating hormones and metabolites. In contrast, the secretion of adrenal medullary catecholamines is directly controlled by the sympathetic nervous system. The function of the adrenal medulla is to reinforce the action of the sympathetic nervous system under conditions of stress; the direct nervous control of adrenal medullary secretion permits a rapid response to stressful stimuli.

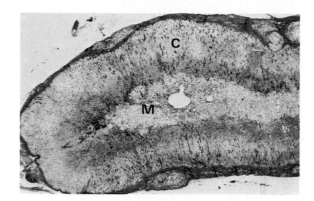

Fig. 14.13 Adrenal gland

(Azan × 8)

At low magnification, the adrenal gland is seen to be divided into an outer cortex **C** and a pale-stained inner medulla **M**. Dense fibrous tissue, stained blue in this preparation, invests the gland and often contains islands of cortical secretory tissue. A prominent vein is characteristically located in the centre of the medulla.

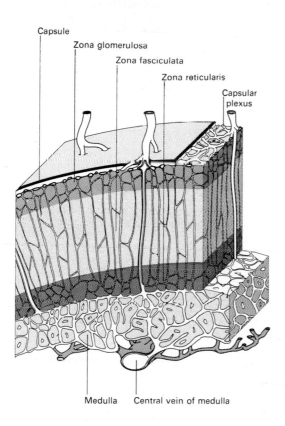

Capsule
Zona glomerulosa
Zona fasciculata
Zona reticularis
Capsular plexus

Medulla   Central vein of medulla

Fig. 14.14 Blood supply of the adrenal gland

The adrenal gland is supplied by three groups of arteries which form a plexus within the capsule of the gland.

The vascular system of the cortex consists of an anastomosing network of capillary sinusoids supplied by branches of the capsular plexus. The sinusoids descend between cords of secretory cells to drain, at the corticomedullary junction, into small veins which converge upon the central vein of the medulla.

The medulla is supplied by small arteries which descend from the capsular plexus through the cortex into the medulla where they ramify into a rich network of dilated capillaries surrounding the medullary secretory cells. The medullary capillaries also drain into the central vein of the medulla. Thus the secretory cells of the medulla are exposed to fresh arterial blood as well as blood rich in adrenocorticosteroids. The corticosteroids are believed to have an important influence on the synthesis of adrenaline by the medulla.

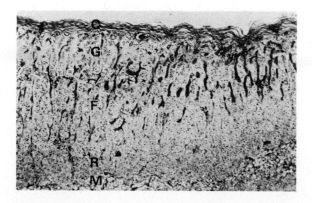

Fig. 14.15 Adrenal cortex

(Azan × 20)

At this magnification, the adrenal cortex can be seen to consist of three histological zones which are named according to the arrangement of the secretory cells: *zona glomerulosa, zona fasciculata, zona reticularis*.

The zona glomerulosa **G** lying beneath the capsule **C** contains secretory cells arranged in rounded clumps. The intermediate zona fasciculata **F** consists of parallel cords of secretory cells. The zona reticularis **R**, which lies adjacent to the medulla **M**, consists of closely packed, irregularly arranged, small cells.

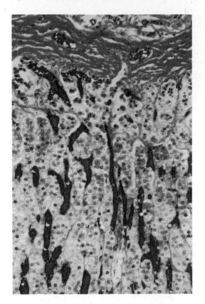

Fig. 14.16 Adrenal cortex: zona glomerulosa
(Azan × 128)

The secretory cells of the zona glomerulosa are arranged in irregular, ovoid clumps separated by delicate connective tissue trabeculae containing capillary sinusoids. The secretory cells have round, strongly stained nuclei and relatively little cytoplasm, thus giving rise to the moderately stained appearance of this zone when seen at lower magnification (see Fig. 14.13). The cytoplasm of the secretory cells contains much smooth endoplasmic reticulum, numerous mitochondria and triglyceride droplets which are the basic substrate for steroid synthesis. The abundance of smooth endoplasmic reticulum and small lipid droplets results in the relatively poor staining properties of the cytoplasm with routine staining methods.

The zona glomerulosa secretes the mineralocorticoid hormones, principally *aldosterone*. The major function of aldosterone is the regulation of body sodium and potassium ion levels by its stimulating action upon the sodium pump of cell membranes particularly in the renal tubules (see Chapter 13). Aldosterone also participates in blood pressure regulation via the renin-angiotensin hormone system controlled by the juxtaglomerular apparatus of the kidney (see Fig. 13.28). Aldosterone secretion is largely independent of ACTH but recent evidence suggests that it may be regulated by a hormone from the pineal gland.

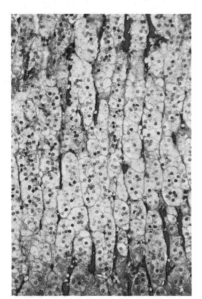

Fig. 14.17 Adrenal cortex: zona fasciculata
(Azan × 128)

The zona fasciculata is the intermediate and broadest of the three zones of the adrenal cortex. It consists of narrow cords of secretory cells, often only one cell thick, separated by connective tissue strands containing capillary sinusoids. The secretory cells are large with an abundant, poorly stained cytoplasm. The cytoplasm is even richer in smooth endoplasmic reticulum and lipid droplets than the zona glomerulosa and this may confer a foamy appearance to the cells.

The zona fasciculata secretes glucocorticoid hormones, principally *cortisol* which has numerous, wide-ranging metabolic effects. Reflecting the name glucocorticoid, an important metabolic effect is to increase blood glucose levels and the cellular synthesis of glycogen. These effects on carbohydrate metabolism are complemented by increased breakdown of proteins and liberation of lipid from tissue stores.

Control of cortisol secretion is maintained by the hypothalamus via the anterior pituitary hormone ACTH. By this means, many stimuli including stress, promote secretion of glucocorticoids which adjust body metabolism appropriately.

The zona fasciculata is probably also the site of secretion of small amounts of steroid sex hormones.

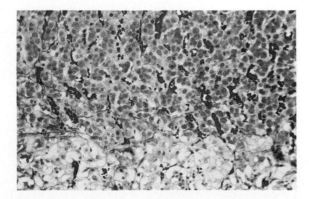

Fig. 14.18 Adrenal cortex: zona reticularis
(Azan × 128)

The zona reticularis is the thin, innermost zone of the adrenal cortex. It consists of an irregular network of branching cords and clumps of glandular cells separated by numerous wide capillary sinusoids. The glandular cells are much smaller than those of the adjacent zona fasciculata, and the cytoplasm, which contains few lipid droplets, stains more strongly.

The zona reticularis may be responsible for the secretion of small quantities of steroid sex hormones or alternatively, it may store, rather than synthesise, the hormones of the zona fasciculata. The two zones may thus constitute a single functional unit.

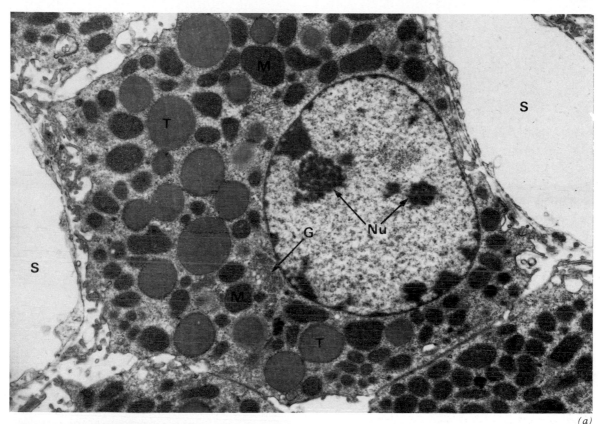

(a)

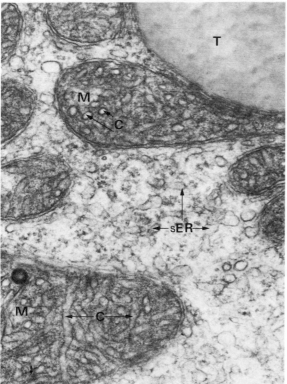

(b)

Fig. 14.19 Steroid-secreting cell (zona fasciculata)

(EM (a) ×8500 (b) ×110500)

These micrographs illustrate the typical ultrastructural features of steroid-secreting cells which are seen not only in the cells of the adrenal cortex but also in the steroid-secreting cells of the ovaries and testes (see Chapters 15 and 16). At low magnification, a secretory cell is seen intimately associated with fenestrated capillary sinusoids **S**. Note the numerous irregular projections of the secretory cell plasma membrane subjacent to the sinusoidal endothelium. The rounded secretory cell nucleus is characterised by more than one prominent nucleolus **Nu**.

The abundant cytoplasm contains many large triglyceride droplets **T**. Numerous irregularly shaped mitochondria **M** crowd the cytoplasm; these mitochondria have unusual tubular cristae **C**, clearly seen at high magnification. The cytoplasm contains a prolific system of smooth endoplasmic reticulum **sER** which forms a dense tubular network. A Golgi apparatus **G** is seen close to the nucleus.

Synthesis of steroids begins with the liberation of fatty acids from stored triglycerides. Mitochondrial oxidation of fatty acids provides acetate molecules for synthesis of cholesterol by the smooth endoplasmic reticulum. The basic steroid nucleus, cholesterol, is modified in the smooth endoplasmic reticulum or mitochondria depending on which steroid hormone is being synthesised.

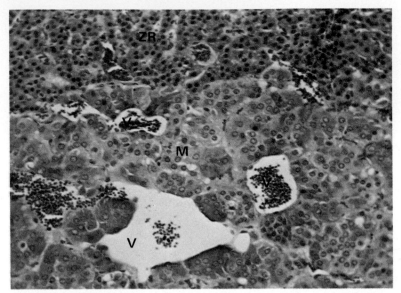

Fig. 14.20 Adrenal medulla
(H & E × 198)

The adrenal medulla **M** is composed of closely packed clumps of secretory cells supported by a fine reticular network containing numerous wide capillaries. Many venous channels **V** draining blood from the sinusoids of the cortex pass through the medulla towards the central medullary vein (see Fig. 14.14).

The secretory cells of the adrenal medulla have large, granular nuclei and extensive strongly basophilic cytoplasm. Note the contrasting eosinophilic cytoplasm of the adjacent zona reticularis **ZR** of the cortex.

The adrenal medulla secretes the catecholamine hormones noradrenaline and adrenaline under the direct control of the sympathetic nervous system. Unlike most of the endocrine glands, adrenal medullary hormones are not secreted continuously but are stored in cytoplasmic granules and released only in response to nervous stimulation in a manner similar to the release of neurotransmitter substances from nerve endings.

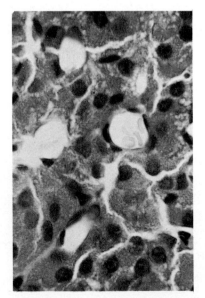

Fig. 14.21 Adrenal medulla
(H & E/Chrome salt fixation × 800)

When fixed in chrome salts, the stored catecholamine granules of adrenal medullary cells are oxidised to a brown colour; consequently the name *chromaffin cells* is often applied to the secretory cells of the adrenal medulla.

Like post-ganglionic sympathetic neurones, some adrenal medullary cells synthesise noradrenaline. Under the influence of cortisol secreted by the adrenal cortex, other medullary cells synthesise adrenaline by the addition of a further N-methyl group to noradrenaline.

Secretion of catecholamines by the adrenal medulla is controlled by preganglionic neurones of the sympathetic nervous system; thus the secretory cells of the adrenal medulla are functionally equivalent to the post-ganglionic neurones of the sympathetic nervous system. Acute physical and psychological stresses initiate release of adrenal medullary hormones; the released catecholamines act on adrenergic receptors throughout the body particularly in the heart and blood vessels, bronchioles, visceral muscle and skeletal muscle. Adrenaline has potent metabolic effects such as the promotion of glycogenolysis in liver and skeletal muscle, thus releasing a readily available energy source during stress situations.

The short-term response to acute stress of the adrenal medulla may be contrasted with the long-term response to chronic stress of the adrenal cortex.

The endocrine pancreas

The pancreas is not only a major exocrine gland (see Chapter 12) but it also has important endocrine functions.

The embryonic epithelium of the pancreatic ducts consists of both potential exocrine and endocrine cells. During development, the endocrine cells migrate from the duct system and aggregate around capillaries to form isolated clumps of cells scattered throughout the exocrine glandular tissue. The clumps of endocrine tissue are known as *islets of Langerhans*. The islets vary in size and are most numerous in the tail of the pancreas.

The endocrine pancreas mainly secretes two polypeptide hormones, *insulin* and *glucagon*, both of which play an important role in carbohydrate metabolism. Insulin promotes the uptake of glucose by most cells, particularly those of the liver, skeletal muscle and adipose tissue, thus lowering plasma glucose concentration. In general, glucagon has metabolic effects that oppose the actions of insulin. Apart from their role in carbohydrate metabolism these hormones have a wide variety of other effects on energy metabolism, growth and development.

Release of both insulin and glucagon is primarily controlled by the plasma concentration of glucose. The sympathetic and parasympathetic nervous systems innervate the islets of Langerhans but the significance of their influence is poorly understood.

A third polypeptide, somatostatin, is secreted by cells of the endocrine pancreas. Somatostatin has a wide variety of effects on gastro-intestinal function.

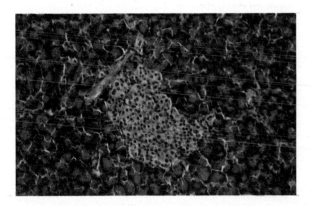

Fig. 14.22 Endocrine pancreas: Islet of Langerhans
(H & E × 128)

The islets of Langerhans are composed of clumps of secretory cells supported by a fine reticular network containing numerous fenestrated capillaries. A fine reticular capsule surrounds each islet. The endocrine cells are small with a poorly stained granular cytoplasm; in contrast, the large cells of the surrounding pancreatic acini stain strongly. This difference in staining intensity reflects the relatively greater amount of rough endoplasmic reticulum in the exocrine cells which secrete vast quantities of protein (see Figs. 12.56 to 12.59).

The endocrine pancreas contains secretory cells of three types, *alpha*, *beta* and *delta cells*, which secrete glucagon, insulin and somatostatin respectively. In H & E preparations, these cell types are indistinguishable from one another and special staining methods are required to differentiate between them.

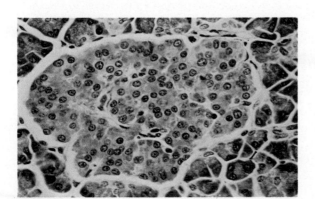

Fig. 14.23 Islet of Langerhans
(Gomori's chrome alum haematoxylin/phloxine method × 320)

This empirical staining method can be used to distinguish the alpha and beta cells of the endocrine pancreas. The alpha (glucagon-secreting) cells are stained pink and are much less numerous than the blue-stained beta cells (insulin-secreting). Generally the alpha cells tend to be distributed towards the periphery of the islets. Delta cells (somatostatin-secreting) cannot be differentiated from beta cells with this staining method.

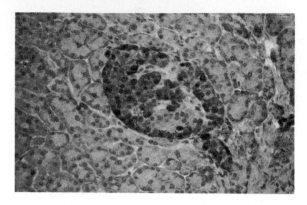

Fig. 14.24 Endocrine pancreas: glucagon cells

(Immunoperoxidase method × 128)

Immunohistochemical techniques may be used to demonstrate the presence of specific molecules within cells; in this preparation, such a method has been used to demonstrate glucagon within the alpha cells of a pancreatic islet. The sites of glucagon localisation within alpha cells appear as brownish deposits; note the characteristic peripheral distribution of alpha cells within the islet.

Pineal gland

The pineal gland is a small organ, 6 to 8mm long, which occurs as an evagination from the posterior part of the roof of the third ventricle in the midline. The pineal is connected to the brain via a short stalk containing nerve fibres many of which communicate with the hypothalamus. In reptiles and other lower vertebrates, the pineal lies at, or near, the skin surface where it functions as a photoreceptor organ; in such animals the pineal secretes a hormone, *melatonin*, which promotes lightening of skin colour. Melatonin acts on melanophores, pigmented cells analogous to melanocytes in mammals (see Chapter 8), to promote aggregation of dispersed pigment granules. In mammals, the function of the pineal is strongly disputed but at least three important functions may be attributable to the pineal:

 (i) The pineal may be involved in co-ordinating circadian and diurnal rhythms in many tissues, mediating its effects via the hypothalamus and pituitary gland.

 (ii) There is some evidence that the pineal secretes a hormone which inhibits growth and maturation of the gonads until puberty. After puberty the pineal undergoes partial involution.

 (iii) The pineal may secrete a trophic hormone which regulates the output of aldosterone from the adrenal cortex.

 Although the function of the pineal in mammals is poorly understood it has many histological features which suggest that it is an active endocrine gland.

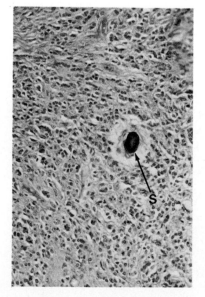

Fig. 14.25 Pineal gland

(H & E × 128)

The pineal consists of two main cell types: *pinealocytes* and *neuroglial cells*. Pinealocytes (pineal chief cells) are highly modified neurones which are arranged in clumps and cords surrounded by a rich network of fenestrated capillaries. In H & E preparations pinealocytes have round, granular nuclei with prominent nucleoli and poorly stained cytoplasm. With special silver impregnation methods, as used in neurohistology (see Chapter 7), pinealocytes appear to have many highly branched processes, some of which terminate near or upon blood vessels. The cytoplasmic granules of pinealocytes contain a variety of indole compounds, including melatonin which is not established as a hormone in mammals, and serotonin which acts as a neurotransmitter substance in parts of the central nervous system. The neuroglial cells, also called *interstitial cells*, are elongated cells which are dispersed between the clumps of pinealocytes and in association with capillaries.

 Myelinated sympathetic nerve fibres enter the pineal where they ramify as unmyelinated axons throughout the substance of the gland. A characteristic feature of the ageing pineal is the presence of basophilic extracellular bodies called *pineal sand* **S** consisting of concentric layers of calcium and magnesium phosphate within an organic matrix.

The gastro-intestinal endocrine system

Scattered in the mucosa of the gastro-intestinal tract, from the oesophagus to the anus, are a variety of endocrine cells which secrete peptide and amine hormones such as gastrin, secretin, CCK, serotonin and many others. These hormones constitute a balanced system of agonists and antagonists which collectively regulate and co-ordinate most aspects of gastro-intestinal activity (see Chapter 12).

The endocrine cells may be located at any level in the mucosa, from the base of glands to the tips of villi. The cells which are exposed to the tract lumen may be receptive to gastro-intestinal contents; these are termed the *open type*; other endocrine cells are deep to the surface, the *closed type*, and may be receptive to changes in the local tissue environment. The cells responsible for the secretion of a particular hormone tend to be located in a particular anatomical region in the tract but there is considerable overlap in distribution; for example, gastrin-producing cells are located mainly in the pyloric region of the stomach (see Fig. 12.27) although a few gastrin cells are found in the body of the stomach, the duodenum and the pancreas.

The presence of endocrine cells in the gastro-intestinal tract has long been demonstrable by staining with silver or chromium salts. Traditionally, the cells were divided into two types, *argentaffin cells* (silver reducing) and *argyrophil cells* (silver absorbing); since both these cell types could be stained specifically with chromium salts, the gastro-intestinal endocrine cells were collectively known as *enterochromaffin cells*. These classifications were subsequently found to be of little functional significance and currently the term enterochromaffin cell should only be applied to a specific cell type found throughout the tract in large numbers and which is responsible for the secretion of serotonin (5-hydroxytryptamine).

The various gastro-intestinal endocrine cells have many ultrastructural features in common but they may be divided into at least twelve different classes according to the shape, size and density of their secretory granules. On the basis of immunohistochemistry and other techniques, five or more gastro-intestinal hormones have been assigned to different ultrastructural cell types. Since gut hormones are a rapidly advancing field of research, there is considerable terminological confusion. It has been the practice for a cell type definitely known to produce a particular hormone to be known by the name of that hormone; for example gastrin-secreting cells are called *gastrin* or *G cells*. Difficulties have arisen where one cell type is found to produce more than one hormone. Another major problem has been the lack of agreement about which secretory products should be classified as hormones since some of the known secretory products have only local activity. An example is serotonin, a potent local smooth muscle constrictor, which is not generally recognised as a hormone since it does not normally have more distant effects; serotonin also acts as a neurotransmitter in the central nervous system. There are numerous candidates for the designation 'gastro-intestinal hormone' but only gastrin, secretin, cholecystokinin-pancreozymin (CCK) and enteroglucagon (an analogue of pancreatic glucagon) are universally accepted as such.

In summary, there is a spectrum of peptide and amine-secreting cells scattered throughout the gastro-intestinal tract which may be considered as a diffuse endocrine organ. The hormones produced by this organ have specific and overlapping activities which regulate and co-ordinate the function of the gastro-intestinal system.

The APUD cell concept

From comparative ultrastructural studies of endocrine tissues it became evident that the diverse group of peptide or amine hormone secreting cells have certain ultrastructural features in common. These cells have little rough endoplasmic reticulum, much smooth endoplasmic reticulum, numerous free ribosomes and small membrane-bound secretory granules. Subsequent histochemical investigation revealed that many of these cells share some common metabolic processes related to hormone synthesis. Amongst others, these processes include a high uptake of amine precursors and the ability to decarboxylate; on this basis, the descriptive term *APUD cell* (amine precursor uptake and decarboxylation) was applied and this group is now known to include at least the following diverse cells: adrenal medullary chromaffin cells, thyroid 'C' cells, all pancreatic endocrine cells, all gastro-intestinal hormone cells including enterochromaffin (serotonin) cells, ACTH and MSH cells of the pituitary, chemoreceptors of the carotid body and mast cells.

Further research has suggested that the APUD cells are part of an even more diverse group of cells which are all derived embryologically from neural crest tissue and therefore may be considered as highly modified neurones. Recently the term *paraneurone* has been proposed; in order to qualify for this description a cell should meet four requirements:

(i) the cell must produce substances identical with, or related to, known or suspected neurotransmitters and/or produce peptide substances with hormone-like activity;

(ii) the cell should possess synaptic vesicle-like structures or neurosecretory-like granules;

(iii) the cell should exhibit both receptor and secretory functions;

(iv) the cell should be of neuroectodermal origin.

At present, few cells have been shown to meet all these strict criteria; nevertheless, if further substantiated, the concept of a *paraneuronal system* may provide a more functional basis for understanding the often inter-related activities of a highly diverse group of cells.

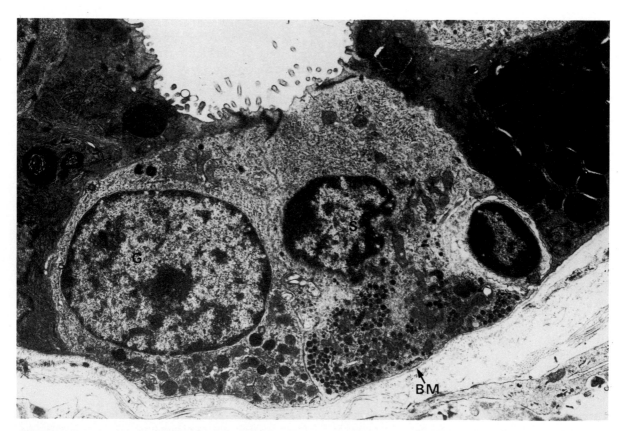

Fig. 14.26 Gastro-intestinal endocrine cells

(EM ×8300)

This micrograph shows two endocrine cells from the human pylorus, both of which exhibit the typical characteristics of open-type gastro-intestinal APUD cells. The endocrine cell **G** is a gastrin-secreting cell recognised on the basis of its large, moderately dense secretory granules. The adjacent endocrine cell **S** contains much smaller and more dense granules of the secretory product *somatostatin*; this substance has not yet been widely recognised as a hormone but appears to have a broad range of actions including the inhibition of insulin and glucagon secretion and inhibition of the secretion of many gastro-intestinal hormones. The open-type APUD cells are usually pyramidal in shape, the apex extending to the tract lumen and the base resting on the basement membrane **BM**. The apical surface forms a few microvilli which may receive stimuli from the tract lumen. Secretory granules are aggregated in the basal cytoplasm from which they are released into the capillaries of the lamina propria. Typically, the cytoplasm contains only a few short profiles of rough endoplasmic reticulum and numerous free ribosomes. The closed type of APUD cells are usually rounded and lack the polarity of the open-type but otherwise have similar ultrastructural features.

15. Male reproductive system

Introduction

The male reproductive system may be divided into four major functional components:

(i) The *testes* or male gonads, paired organs lying in the scrotal sac, are responsible for production of the male gametes, *spermatozoa*, and secretion of male sex hormones.

(ii) A paired system of ducts, each consisting of *ductuli efferentes, epididymis, ductus deferens* and *ejaculatory duct*, collect, store and conduct spermatozoa from each testis. The ejaculatory ducts converge on the *urethra* from which spermatozoa are expelled into the female reproductive tract during copulation.

(iii) Two exocrine glands, the paired *seminal vesicles* and the single *prostate gland*, secrete a nutritive and lubricating fluid medium called *seminal fluid* in which spermatozoa are conveyed to the female reproductive tract. Seminal fluid, spermatozoa and cells desquamated from the lining of the duct system comprise *semen*.

(iv) The *penis* is the organ of copulation. A pair of small accessory glands, the *bulbo-urethral glands of Cowper*, secrete a fluid which prepares the urethra for the passage of semen during ejaculation.

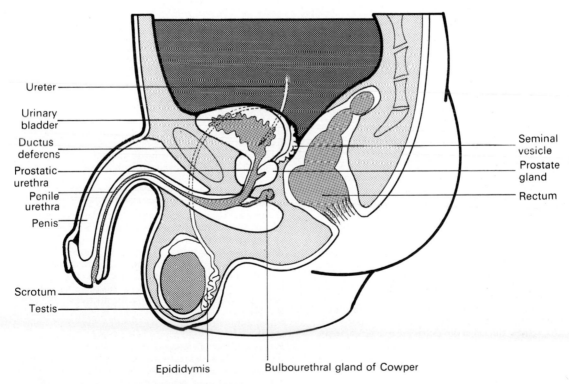

Fig. 15.1 Male reproductive system

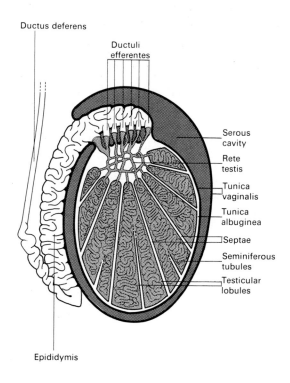

Ductus deferens

Ductuli efferentes

Serous cavity

Rete testis

Tunica vaginalis

Tunica albuginea

Septae

Seminiferous tubules

Testicular lobules

Epididymis

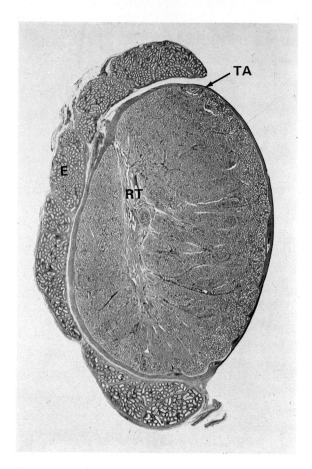

Fig. 15.2 Testis
(sagittal section)

During development, each testis with the first part of its duct system, blood vessels, lymphatics and nerves, descends along a tortuous path from the posterior wall of the peritoneal cavity to the scrotum. During migration, the testis carries with it an investing layer of peritoneum so that in the scrotum the testis is almost completely surrounded by a serous cavity which is an extension of the peritoneal cavity. This serous cavity protects the testis by allowing it to move freely in the scrotal sac; the lining of the cavity is known as the *tunica vaginalis*.

The testis is encapsulated by a dense, fibrous, connective tissue layer, the *tunica albuginea*, from which, at the posterior aspect, numerous ill-defined connective tissue septa divide the testis into about *250 testicular lobules*. Within each lobule are from one to four highly convoluted loops, the *seminiferous tubules*, in which spermatozoa are produced. The seminiferous tubules converge upon a plexus of spaces, the *rete testis*. From the rete testis, about twelve small ducts, called the *ductuli efferentes*, conduct spermatozoa to the extremely tortuous first part of the *ductus deferens* which is known as the *epididymis*.

Fig. 15.3 Testis
(Monkey: LS: H & E × 3)

This micrograph illustrates the gross morphological features of a testis cut in the sagittal plane so as to show the relationship of the epididymis **E** which lies on its posterior aspect. The testis is packed with numerous, coiled, seminiferous tubules which can just be seen in various planes of section at this magnification. Groups of about four seminiferous tubules are segregated into testicular lobules; the connective tissue septa are so delicate as to be barely seen at this magnification. The dense fibrous capsule which invests the testis, and which is continuous with many of the interlobular septa, is called the tunica albuginea **TA** since it appears white on gross examination. Spermatozoa pass from the seminiferous tubules into the rete testis **RT** which is connected to the epididymis via the ductuli efferentes at the upper posterior pole of the testis; the ductuli are not seen in this plane of section. The epididymis is a tightly coiled tube which forms a compact mass extending down the whole length of the posterior aspect of the testis. The epididymis is the major site of storage of newly formed spermatozoa. At the lower pole of the testis, the epididymal tube becomes continuous with the relatively straight ductus (vas) deferens which is not seen in this section.

Gametogenesis

In all somatic cells, cell division (mitosis) results in the formation of two daughter cells, each one genetically identical to the mother cell. Somatic cells contain a full complement of chromosomes (the diploid number) which function as homologous pairs (see Chapter 1). The process of sexual reproduction involves the fusion of specialised male and female cells called *gametes* to form a *zygote* which has the diploid number of chromosomes. Each gamete contains only half the diploid number of chromosomes; this half complement of chromosomes is known as the *haploid number*.

The production of haploid cells involves a unique form of cell division called *meiosis* which occurs only in the germ cells of the gonads during the formation of gametes; meiotic cell division is thus also called *gametogenesis*. Meiosis involves two cell division processes of which only the first is preceded by duplication of chromosomes.

(i) The first meiotic division results in the formation of two daughter cells; this process differs from mitosis in two important respects:

(a) Whereas in mitosis each chromosome divides at the kinetochore (centromere) liberating two chromatids which migrate to opposite ends of the mitotic spindle, in the first meiotic division there is no such separation of the chromatids but rather one chromosome of each homologous pair migrates to each end of the spindle. Thus at the end of the first meiotic division, each daughter cell contains a half complement of chromosomes, one chromosome being derived from each homologous pair of the mother cell.

(b) During the first meiotic division, and preceding the process described in (a) above, there is an exchange of alleles between the chromosomes of homologous pairs. This exchange, called *chiasma formation*, results in chromosomes with a different genetic constitution from those of the mother cell.

(ii) The second meiotic division merely involves splitting of each chromosome at the kinetochore to liberate chromatids which migrate to opposite poles of the spindle.

Thus, meiotic cell division of a single diploid germ cell gives rise to four haploid gametes. In the male, each of the four gametes undergoes morphological development into a mature spermatozoon whereas in the female, unequal distribution of the cytoplasm during meiosis results in one gamete gaining almost all the cytoplasm from the mother cell, whilst the other three acquire almost no cytoplasm; the large gamete matures to form an *ovum* and the other three, the so-called *polar bodies*, degenerate.

The primitive germ cells of the male, the *spermatogonia*, are present only in small numbers in the male gonads before sexual maturity. After sexual maturity, spermatogonia multiply continuously by mitosis to provide a supply of cells which then undergo meiosis to form male gametes. In contrast, the germ cells of the female, called *oogonia*, multiply by mitosis only during early fetal development thereby producing a fixed complement of cells with the potential to undergo gametogenesis. Gametogenesis in the female is discussed more fully in Chapter 16. The production of male gametes is called *spermatogenesis* and the subsequent development of the male gamete into a motile spermatozoon is called *spermiogenesis*; both these processes occur within the testes.

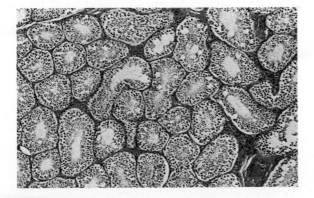

Fig. 15.4 Seminiferous tubules
(H & E × 50)

This micrograph illustrates seminiferous tubules cut in various planes of section. The seminiferous tubules are highly convoluted tubules lined by a stratified epithelium which consists of two distinct populations of cells:

(i) cells in various stages of spermatogenesis and spermiogenesis, collectively referred to as the *spermatogenic series*;

(ii) non-spermatogenic cells, called *Sertoli cells*, which support and nourish the developing spermatozoa.

In the interstitial spaces between the tubules, cells with an endocrine function, called *Leydig cells*, are found either singly or in clumps in the supporting connective tissue.

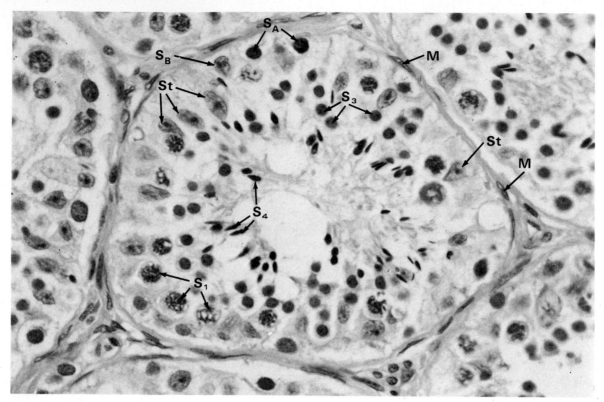

Fig. 15.5 Seminiferous tubule
(TS: H & E ×640)

This micrograph illustrates an active seminiferous tubule cut in transverse section. The processes of spermatogenesis and spermiogenesis occur in waves along the length of the tubule, taking about nine weeks to complete in man; thus in any one histological section all development phases are seldom represented.

Spermatogonia, the germ cells, are found in the basal layer of the seminiferous epithelium where they divide by mitosis giving rise to further spermatogonia (designated as Type A), and to spermatogonia which will proceed through meiosis to become spermatozoa (designated as Type B). Spermatogonia Type A S_A are characterised by a large, spheroidal or elliptical nucleus with fine, moderately condensed chromatin; nucleoli, which are associated with the nuclear envelope, and a nuclear vacuole may be prominent. Spermatogonia Type B S_B have a paler-stained nucleus, centrally located nucleoli, and no nuclear vacuole. Both types of spermatogonia have relatively little cytoplasm and this is poorly stained.

Spermatogonia Type B enter the first stages of meiotic division when they become known as *primary spermatocytes*. Primary spermatocytes S_1 are readily recognised by their extensive cytoplasm and large nuclei containing either coarse clumps or thin threads of chromatin; cells may be seen in chromosomal division. In man, the first meiotic cell division cycle takes approximately three weeks to complete, after which time the daughter cells become known as *secondary spermatocytes*. The smaller, secondary spermatocytes rapidly undergo the second meiotic division and are therefore much less commonly seen.

The gametes thus produced by meiosis, called *spermatids* S_3, then proceed through the long metamorphosis known as spermiogenesis to become recognisable as spermatozoa. As spermiogenesis proceeds, the nuclei of spermatids become smaller, more condensed and less granular until they assume the small pointed form of spermatozoa S_4 (see Fig. 15.7).

Throughout the entire developmental process from spermatogonia to spermatozoa, the daughter cells of each division remain connected to one another by narrow cytoplasmic bridges which only break down upon release of spermatozoa into the lumen of the tubule. This phenomenon has been used to explain the observation that synchronous development of spermatozoa occurs in waves throughout the seminiferous tubules.

During the developmental process, the cells of the spermatogenic series are supported by Sertoli cells **St**, the nuclei of which are usually found towards the basement membrane of the seminiferous tubule. The characteristic Sertoli cell nucleus is often triangular or ovoid in shape with a very prominent nucleolus and relatively homogeneous chromatin. Although not evident with light microscopy, Sertoli cells have an extensive cytoplasm which ramifies throughout the whole germinal epithelium enclosing all the cells of the spermatogenic series.

The basal layer of germinal cells is supported by a basement membrane beneath which are a variable number of layers of cells structurally similar to smooth muscle cells **M**. These cells have a contractile function in some mammalian species but their function in man is unknown.

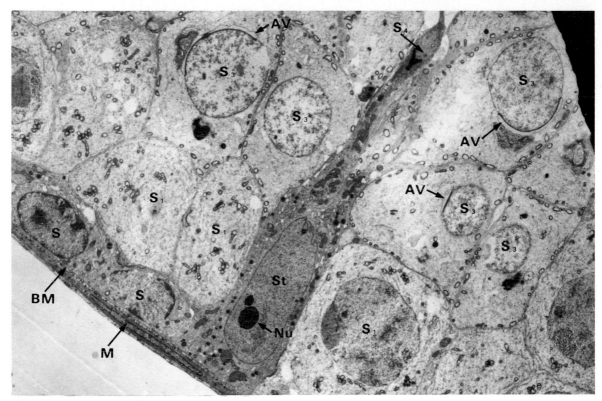

Fig. 15.6 Sertoli cell
(EM × 3400)

The intimate relationship of a Sertoli cell **St** to cells of the spermatogenic series is demonstrated in this electron micrograph.

The Sertoli cell rests on the basement membrane **BM** of the seminiferous tubule and its cytoplasm extends to the lumen of the tubule, thereby filling all the narrow spaces between the cells of the spermatogenic series. The cytoplasmic outline of the Sertoli cell is thus highly irregular and constantly changing to permit the progressive movement of developing spermatozoa towards the luminal surface. The ovoid nucleus of the Sertoli cell is characteristically orientated at right angles to the basement membrane and often exhibits a deep indentation; a large, dense nucleolus **Nu** is a constant feature and dense chromatin bodies are often associated with the nucleolus. The cytoplasm contains a moderate number of mitochondria, many lipid droplets, and relatively little rough endoplasmic reticulum. The presence of a highly ordered smooth endoplasmic reticulum suggests that Sertoli cells are, for some unknown reason, highly active in lipid biosynthesis.

Sertoli cells are postulated to act as 'nurse' cells, in some way providing structural and metabolic support for the developing spermatogenic cells. During spermiogenesis, Sertoli cells phagocytise excess cytoplasm cast off by spermatids.

Note in this micrograph the variety of cells of the spermatogenic series. Spermatogonia **S** rest upon the basement membrane beneath which is a slender smooth muscle-like (myoid) cell **M**. Above the germ cell layer, primary spermatocytes S_1 are seen; secondary spermatocytes are short-lived and therefore rarely seen. Spermatids S_3 in different phases of spermiogenesis are seen in the upper layers; these cells have developing acrosomal vesicles **AV** (see Fig. 15.7). At the luminal surface, the Sertoli cell envelops an almost fully formed spermatozoon S_4.

The control of spermatogenesis and spermiogenesis remains the subject of intense investigation; it is believed that Sertoli cells mediate some important regulatory mechanisms. It is well established that high concentrations of androgen hormones secreted by Leydig cells of the testicular interstitium (see Fig. 15.9) are essential for production and maturation of spermatogenic cells. Recent evidence suggests that Sertoli cells secrete an androgen-binding protein which concentrates androgens in seminiferous epithelium; production of this binding protein is believed to be dependent on the pituitary gonadotrophin, follicle-stimulating hormone (see Chapter 14).

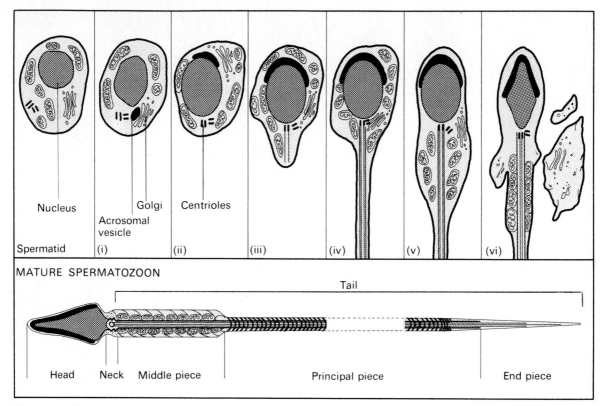

Fig. 15.7 Spermiogenesis

Spermiogenesis is the process by which spermatids, the gametes produced by meiotic division, are transformed into the potentially motile forms, the mature spermatozoa. This involves the following major stages:

(i) The Golgi apparatus elaborates a large vesicle, the *acrosomal vesicle*, which accumulates carbohydrates and hydrolytic enzymes.

(ii) The acrosomal vesicle becomes applied to one pole of the progressively elongating nucleus to form a structure known as the *acrosomal head cap*.

(iii) Both centrioles migrate to the end of the cell opposite to the acrosomal head cap and the centriole aligned parallel to the long axis of the nucleus elongates to form a flagellum which has a basic structure similar to that of a cilium (see Fig. 4.21).

(iv) As the flagellum elongates, nine coarse fibrils, which may contain contractile proteins, become arranged longitudinally around the core of the flagellum. Further rib-like fibrils then become disposed circumferentially around the whole flagellum.

(v) The cytoplasm migrates to surround the first part of the flagellum with the remainder of the flagellum appearing to project from the cell but in fact remaining surrounded by plasma membrane. This migration of cytoplasm thus concentrates mitochondria in the flagellar region.

(vi) As the flagellum elongates, excess cytoplasm is cast off and phagocytised by the enveloping Sertoli cell. The mitochondria become arranged in a condensed, helical manner around the fibrils which surround the first part of the flagellum.

The structure of fully formed spermatozoa varies in detail from species to species, but conforms to the basic structure seen in this diagram of a human spermatozoon.

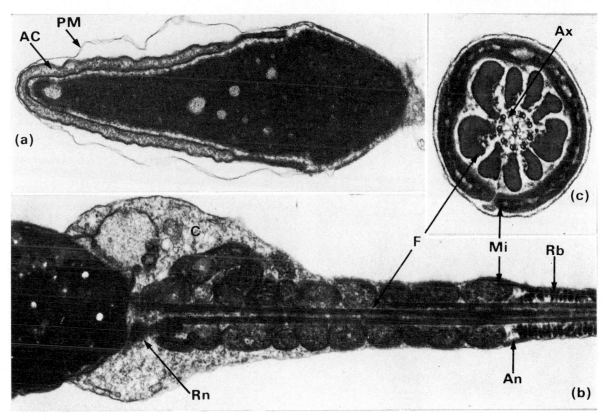

Fig. 15.8 Spermatozoon

(EM (a) Head LS ×14000 (b) Neck, middle piece and principal piece LS ×17000 (c) Middle piece TS ×48000)

The ultrastructural features of human spermatozoa are shown in these micrographs. The spermatozoon is an extremely elongated cell (about 65 μm long) consisting of three main components, the *head*, *neck* and *tail*. The tail is subdivided into three segments, the so-called *middle piece*, *principal piece* and *end piece* (see Fig. 15.7). The head is the most variable structure between different mammalian species. In man, the head is about 7 μm long and has a flattened pear-shape. The nucleus, which occupies most of the head, is composed of extremely condensed chromatin; in man, the nucleus is characterised by a variable number of clear spaces called *nuclear vacuoles* which are areas of dispersed chromatin. Surrounding the anterior two-thirds of the nucleus is the acrosomal cap **AC**, a flattened, membrane-bound vesicle containing a range of glycoproteins and a variety of hydrolytic enzymes, principally *hyaluronidase*; these enzymes disaggregate the cells of the corona radiata and dissolve the zona pellucida during penetration of the ovum at fertilisation (see Chapter 16). Note the plasma membrane **PM** which has become partially separated during preparation.

The neck is a very short segment which connects the head with the tail. It contains vestiges of the centrioles, one of which gives rise to the axoneme **Ax** of the flagellum. The axoneme has the standard 'nine plus two' arrangement of microtubule doublets seen in cilia (see Fig. 4.21). The axoneme of the neck is surrounded by several condensed fibrous rings **Rn**. In human spermatozoa, a significant amount of cytoplasm **C** often remains in the neck region.

The middle piece, the first part of the tail, is about the same length as the head and consists of the flagellar axoneme surrounded by nine coarse outer fibrils **F** arranged longitudinally. External to this core, elongated mitochondria **Mi** are arranged in a tightly packed helix; the mitochondria are thought to generate the energy required for flagellar movement. A fibrous thickening beneath the plasma membrane, called the anulus **An**, prevents mitochondria from slipping into the principal piece.

The principal piece, which constitutes most of the tail length, consists of a central core, comprising the axoneme and the nine longitudinal fibrils continuing from the middle piece. Surrounding this core are numerous fibrous ribs **Rb** arranged in a circular manner. Two of the longitudinal fibrils of the core are fused with the surrounding ribs so as to form anterior and posterior columns extending throughout the length of the principal piece. This arrangement divides the principal piece longitudinally into two functional compartments, one containing three coarse fibrils and the other containing four. Although little is known of the mechanism of flagellar motion, it has been suggested that this asymmetry accounts for the more powerful stroke of the tail in one direction, the so-called 'power stroke'; this can easily be observed in fresh, live preparations of spermatozoa viewed with the light microscope. The end piece, not shown in these micrographs, is merely a short tapering portion of the tail containing the axoneme only.

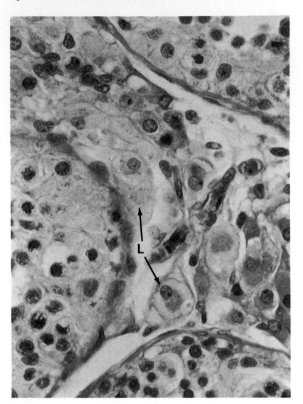

Fig. 15.9 Interstitial cells of the testis (Leydig cells)

(H & E × 480)

Leydig cells, responsible for secretion of the male sex hormones, are the principal cell type found in the connective tissue between seminiferous tubules. Leydig cells **L** occur singly or in clumps and are intimately associated with rich plexuses of blood and lymph capillaries which surround the seminiferous tubules. These large cells have an extensive, eosinophilic cytoplasm containing variable numbers of lipid vacuoles; the ultrastructural features closely resemble those of the steroid-secreting cells of the adrenal cortex (see Fig. 14.19). In man, but no other species, Leydig cells also contain elongated cytoplasmic crystals, called *crystals of Reinke*, which are large enough to be seen with light microscopy when suitably stained; these crystals become more numerous with age but their function is completely unknown.

Testosterone is the principal hormone secreted by Leydig cells. Testosterone is not only responsible for the development of male secondary sexual characteristics at puberty but is also essential for the continued function of the seminiferous epithelium (see Fig. 15.6). The secretory activity of Leydig cells is controlled by the pituitary gonadotrophic hormone, luteinising hormone, often referred to as *interstitial cell stimulating hormone (ICSH)* in the male.

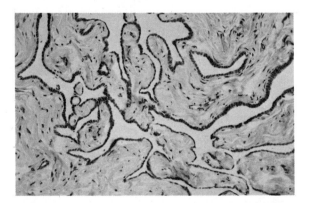

Fig. 15.10 Rete testis

(H & E × 128)

The seminiferous tubules converge upon the so-called *mediastinum testis* which consists of a plexiform arrangement of spaces, the *rete testis*, supported by highly vascular, collagenous connective tissue. The rete testis is lined by a single layer of cuboidal epithelial cells some of which may possess a flagellum. Flagellar activity is presumed to aid the progress of spermatozoa which do not become motile until after maturation is completed in the epididymis.

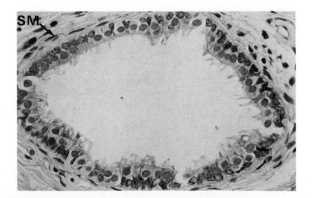

Fig. 15.11 Ductulus efferens

(H & E × 320)

The rete testis drains into the head of the epididymis via approximately twelve convoluted ducts, the *ductuli efferentes*. The ductuli are lined by a single layer of epithelial cells some of which are tall, columnar and ciliated and others which are short and non-ciliated; both cell types often contain a brown pigment of unknown composition. Ciliary action in the ductuli propels spermatozoa towards the epididymis. A thin band of circularly arranged smooth muscle **SM** surrounds each ductulus.

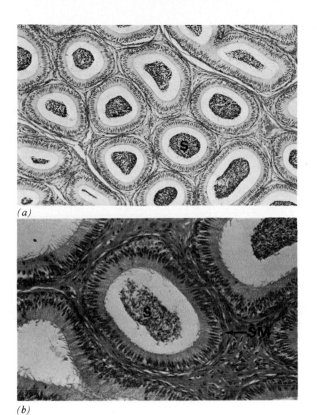

(a)

(b)

Fig. 15.12 Epididymis

(H & E (a) × 50 (b) × 128)

The epididymis is a long, extremely convoluted duct extending down the posterior aspect of the testis to the lower pole where it becomes the ductus deferens. The major function of the epididymis is thought to be the accummulation and storage of spermatozoa **S** during which time the spermatozoa develop motility. The epididymis is a tube of smooth muscle **SM** lined by a pseudostratified epithelium. From the proximal to the distal end of the epididymis, the muscular wall increases from a single, circular layer to three layers organised in the same manner as in the ductus deferens (see Fig. 15.13). The smooth muscle at the proximal end exhibits slow, rhythmic contractility; this activity gently moves spermatozoa towards the ductus deferens. Distally, the smooth muscle is richly innervated by the sympathetic nervous system which produces intense contractions of the lower part of the epididymis during ejaculation.

The epithelial lining of the epididymis shows a gradual transition from a tall, pseudostratified columnar form proximally, to a shorter pseudostratified form distally. The principal cells of the epididymal epithelium bear tufts of very long microvilli, inappropriately called stereocilia (see Fig. 4.23); stereocilia are thought to be involved in absorption of a vast excess of fluid accompanying the spermatozoa from the testis. The ultrastructure of the cells strongly suggests an additional secretory function but the nature of epididymal secretory products, if any, remains unknown. Occasional lymphocytes may be seen within the epithelium.

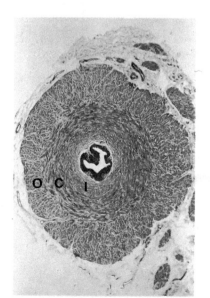

Fig. 15.13 Ductus deferens

(H & E × 20)

The ductus (or vas) deferens, which conducts spermatozoa from the epididymis to the urethra, is a thick-walled muscular tube consisting of inner **I** and outer **O** longitudinal layers and a thick intermediate circular layer **C**. Like the distal part of the epididymis, the ductus deferens is innervated by the sympathetic nervous system and contracts strongly to expel its contents into the urethra during ejaculation. The ductus deferens is lined by a pseudostratified epithelium similar to that of the epididymis (see Fig. 15.12); the epithelial lining and its supporting lamina propria are thrown into longitudinal folds which permit expansion of the duct during ejaculation. The dilated distal portion of each ductus deferens, known as the *ampulla*, receives a short duct draining the seminal vesicle, thus forming the short ejaculatory duct; the ejaculatory ducts from each side converge to join the urethra as it passes through the prostate gland.

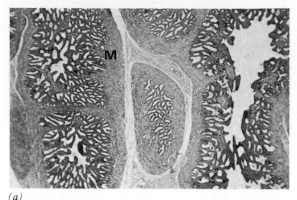

(a)

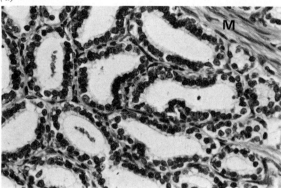

(b)

Fig. 15.14 Seminal vesicle

(H & E (a) × 20 (b) × 320)

Each seminal vesicle is a highly convoluted, glandular outpocketing of the associated ductus deferens. The central lumen of each seminal vesicle is highly irregular and recessed giving a honeycomb appearance at low magnification. The prominent muscular wall **M** is arranged into inner circular and outer longitudinal layers. The epithelial lining is simple, usually pseudostratified in man, and consists of secretory cells which produce a yellowish, viscid, alkaline fluid containing fructose, fibrinogen and vitamin C; this secretion contributes to the nutritive and supporting fluid of semen. Although not thought to store spermatozoa, seminal vesicles are often seen to contain spermatozoa which have probably entered by reflux from the ampulla. The smooth muscle of the seminal vesicles is supplied by the sympathetic nervous system; during ejaculation, muscle contraction forces secretions from the seminal vesicles into the urethra via the ampullae.

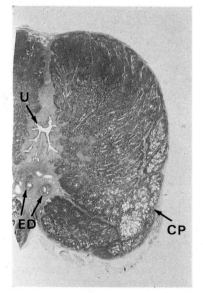

Fig. 15.15 Prostate gland

(Dog: H & E × 3)

The prostate is a large gland which surrounds the bladder neck and the first part of the urethra in the midline; the wall of the prostatic urethra is formed by the substance of the prostate gland. As seen in this micrograph, the prostate gland consists of glandular lobules, up to fifty in all, which converge to open via about twenty separate ducts into irregular outpockets of the prostatic urethra **U** throughout its length. In addition to prostatic glandular tissue proper, numerous, small *paraurethral glands* (not seen in this micrograph) open into the prostatic urethra throughout its length, and it is these glands and their supporting connective tissue which increase greatly in size as a normal part of the ageing process of human males; this process, known as *benign prostatic hypertrophy*, may cause obstruction of urinary outflow by occluding the prostatic urethra. Note in this micrograph, the ejaculatory ducts **ED** which join the prostatic urethra just before its exit from the prostate gland.

The secretory product of the prostate, which makes up about seventy-five per cent of the seminal fluid, is thin and milky; it is rich in citric acid and hydrolytic enzymes, notably fibrinolysin, which liquefies coagulated semen after it has been deposited within the female genital tract.

The supporting stroma and capsule **CP** of the prostate gland consists of dense fibro-elastic connective tissue which contains numerous smooth muscle fibres. The smooth muscle of the prostate, like that of the seminal vesicles and the rest of the tract, is innervated by the sympathetic nervous system which stimulates powerful contractions during ejaculation.

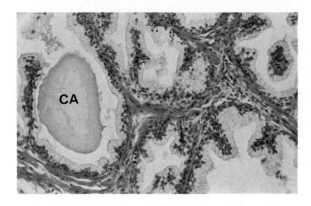

Fig. 15.16 Prostate gland
(H & E ×128)

The prostatic glandular epithelium varies from inactive, low cuboidal to active, pseudostratified columnar depending on the degree of stimulation by androgens from the testis. The histological appearance seen in this micrograph is that of highly active secretory cells. The secretory product is stored temporarily within the gland and often forms amorphous masses called *corpora amylacea* **CA**, one of which is seen in this section from a young man. With increasing age, these bodies become progressively calcified to form lamellated deposits called *prostatic concretions* or *prostatic salt*.

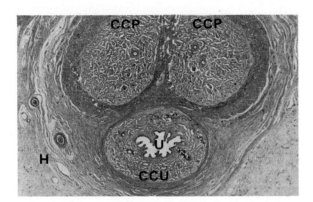

Fig. 15.17 Penis
(TS: H & E ×8)

This transverse section through the penis of an adult human male demonstrates the general arrangement of the penile tissues. The penis consists of three cylindrical masses of erectile tissue: the paired *corpora cavernosa penis* **CCP** in the upper aspect, and the midline *corpus cavernosum urethrae* **CCU** (formerly called the *corpus spongiosum*) which surrounds and supports the penile urethra **U**. Condensed fibro-elastic tissue invests the cavernous bodies, being thickest around the corpora cavernosa penis which are incompletely separated by a midline septum. This dense connective tissue is continuous with the very loose hypodermis **H** which allows the thin penile skin to move freely over the underlying structures. Note the prominent blood vessels of the hypodermis.

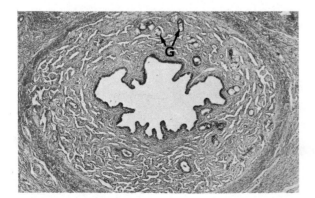

Fig. 15.18 Corpus cavernosum urethrae
(TS: H & E ×20)

At higher magnification, more detail of the urethra **U** and surrounding erectile tissue can be seen. The erectile tissue of the penis consists of broad vascular lacunae or cavernous sinuses supported by trabeculae of fibro-elastic connective tissue containing smooth muscle fibres. The lacunae are lined by the usual vascular endothelium. The penile urethra has an irregular outline due to the presence of deep outpocketings which are continuous with the ducts of simple acinar glands, the *paraurethral glands* **G**.

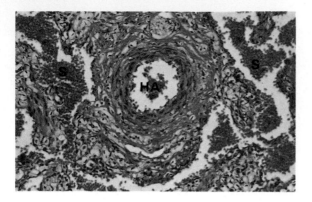

Fig. 15.19 Penile erectile tissue
(H & E × 128)

The vascular sinuses **S** of the cavernous bodies of the penis are directly supplied by numerous anastomosing thick-walled arteries and arterioles; these vessels are called *helicine arteries* **HA** since they follow a spiral course in the flaccid state. Blood drains from the sinuses via veins which lie immediately beneath the dense fibro-elastic tissue investing the cavernous bodies. During erection, dilatation of the helicine arteries, which is mediated by the parasympathetic nervous system, results in engorgement of the vascular sinuses which enlarge, thus compressing and restricting venous outflow. Engorgement of the corpus cavernosum urethrae tends to collapse the penile urethra, but this is overcome by the extremely forceful contractions of the seminal tract during ejaculation.

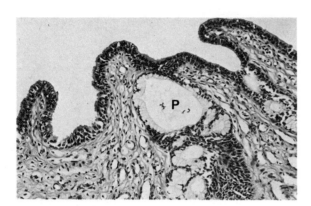

Fig. 15.20 Penile urethra
(H & E × 128)

Apart from the prostatic urethra which is lined by urinary epithelium, the male urethra is lined by stratified or pseudostratified columnar epithelium; small areas of stratified squamous epithelium may be found along the length of the penile urethra in human adult males. The external opening *(urethral meatus)* is always lined by stratified squamous epithelium.

The urethra is lubricated by mucous secretions from the paraurethral glands **P** and the bulbo-urethral glands of Cowper which have a similar, but more discrete, organisation.

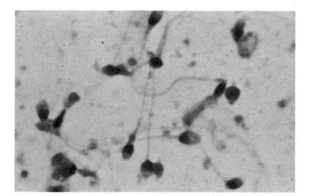

Fig. 15.21 Semen
(H & E × 800)

Semen, the product of ejaculation, consists of spermatozoa and seminal fluid which is derived principally from the seminal vesicles and prostate gland. The volume of each human ejaculate is about 3·5 ml, containing from 50 to 150 million spermatozoa per ml. In normal fertile human males, up to twenty-five per cent of the ejaculated spermatozoa are abnormal or degenerate forms. By the time of ejaculation, spermatozoa have matured and acquired the property of motility; they remain incapable of fertilising an ovum until after undergoing an incompletely understood process called *capacitation*, within the female genital tract. Metabolites for motility are provided in the form of fructose and citrate in the seminal fluid. Note that desquamated cells, prostatic concretions and other tract debris are normal constituents of semen.

16. Female reproductive system

Introduction

The female reproductive system has the following major functions:

(i) the production of female gametes, the *ova*, by a process called *oogenesis*;

(ii) the reception of male gametes, the spermatozoa;

(iii) the provision of a suitable environment for the fertilisation of ova by spermatozoa;

(iv) the provision of an environment for the development of the fetus;

(v) a means for the expulsion of the developed fetus to the external environment;

(vi) nutrition of the newborn.

These functions are all integrated by hormonal and nervous mechanisms.

The female reproductive system may be divided into three structural units on the basis of function: the ovaries, the genital tract and the breasts.

The *ovaries*, paired organs lying in the pelvic cavity, are the sites of oogenesis. In sexually mature mammals, ova are released by the process of *ovulation* in a cyclical manner either seasonally or at regular intervals throughout the year. The cyclical ovulations are suspended during pregnancy. The process of ovulation is controlled by the cyclical release of gonadotrophic hormones from the anterior pituitary (see Chapter 14). The ovaries themselves have an endocrine function; they secrete the hormones *oestrogen* and *progesterone* which co-ordinate the activities of the genital tract and breasts with the ovulatory cycle.

The *genital tract* extends from near the ovaries to open at the external surface and provides an environment for reception of male gametes, fertilisation of ova, development of the fetus, and expulsion of the fetus at birth. The genital tract begins with a pair of *uterine tubes*, also called *oviducts* or *Fallopian tubes*, which conduct ova from the ovaries to the *uterus* where fetal development occurs.

Fertilisation of ova by spermatozoa occurs within the uterine tubes. The uterus is a muscular organ, the mucosal lining of which undergoes cyclical proliferation under the influence of ovarian hormones. This provides a suitable environment for implantation of the fertilised ovum. At birth, or *parturition*, strong contractions of the muscular uterine wall expel the fetus through the *cervix* into the birth canal or *vagina*. The vagina is an expansile muscular tube specialised for the passage of the fetus to the external environment and the reception of the penis during coitus. At the external opening of the vagina are thick folds of skin which constitute the *vulva*.

The breasts are highly modified apocrine sweat glands which, in the female, develop at puberty and regress at menopause. During pregnancy the breasts undergo structural changes in preparation for milk production or *lactation*.

In the non-pregnant state, the female reproductive system undergoes continuous cyclical changes from puberty to menopause. When ovulation is not followed by the implantation of a fertilised ovum, the proliferated mucosal lining regresses and a new ovulation cycle commences. In humans, the proliferated uterine mucosa is shed in a period of bleeding known as *menstruation*; the first day of bleeding marks the beginning of a new cycle of proliferation of the uterine mucosa which is known as the *menstrual cycle*. In humans, the menstrual cycle is usually of twenty-eight days duration and ovulation usually occurs at the midpoint of the cycle. The ovulatory and menstrual cycles are integrated by hormones secreted by the ovaries; ovarian hormones also promote cyclical changes in all other parts of the female reproductive system.

In other animals, the proliferated uterine mucosa is absorbed rather than shed and the female is receptive to the male only during the period of ovulation known as *oestrus* (or heat). The remaining part of the cycle is called the *dioestrus* and the whole cycle is known as the *oestrus cycle*.

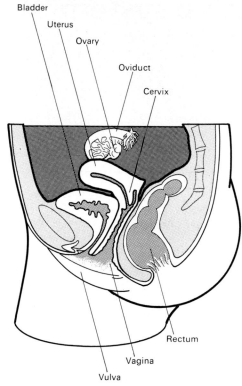

Fig. 16.1 Human female reproductive system

(sagittal section)

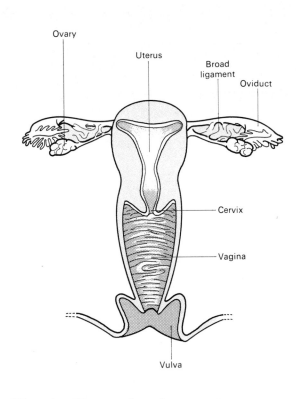

Fig. 16.2 Human female reproductive system

(coronal view)

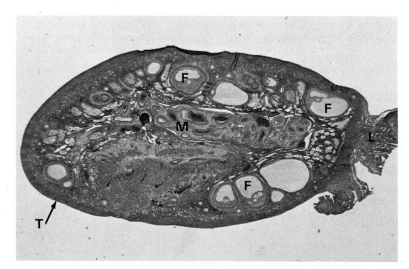

Fig. 16.3 Ovary

(Monkey: Azan × 12)

The ovaries are flattened, oval organs encapsulated in a fibrous connective tissue layer called the *tunica albuginea* **T**. The body of the ovary consists of spindle-shaped cells, reticular fibres and ground substance which together constitute the *ovarian stroma*. In the peripheral zone of the stroma, known as the *cortex*, are numerous follicles **F** which contain female gametes in various stages of development. The central zone of the ovarian stroma, the *medulla* **M**, is highly vascular and contains few follicles. The blood vessels of the ovary, together with autonomic nerves and lymphatics, pass in the *broad ligament* **L** to enter the ovary at the *hilum*.

Follicular development

During early fetal development, primordial germ cells called *oogonia* migrate into the ovarian cortex where they multiply by mitosis. By the fourth and fifth months of fetal development in the human, some oogonia enlarge and assume the potential for development into mature gametes. At this stage they become known as *primary oocytes* and commence the first stage of meiotic division (see Chapter 15). By the seventh month of fetal development, primary oocytes become encapsulated by a single layer of flattened *follicular cells*, of epithelial origin, to form *primordial follicles*. This encapsulation arrests the first meiotic division and no further development of the primordial follicle then occurs until after the female reaches sexual maturity. The remaining phases of meiotic division occur during follicular development leading to ovulation and fertilisation. Thus all the female germ cells are present at birth and the process of meiotic division is completed between 15 and 50 years later. In contrast, in males, meiotic division of germ cells commences only after sexual maturity and sperm formation is accomplished within about two months (see Chapter 15). Female germ cells may undergo degeneration (*atresia*) at any stage of follicular maturation.

During each ovarian cycle, up to twenty primordial follicles are in some way activated to undergo the maturation process; nevertheless, usually only one follicle reaches full maturity and is ovulated whilst the remainder undergo atresia before the point of ovulation. The reason for this apparent wastage is unclear; during maturation, however, the follicles have an endocrine function which may be far beyond the capacity of a single follicle.

Follicular maturation involves changes in the oocyte, the follicular cells and the surrounding stromal tissue. Follicular maturation is stimulated by the gonadotrophic hormone FSH secreted by the anterior pituitary (see Chapter 14).

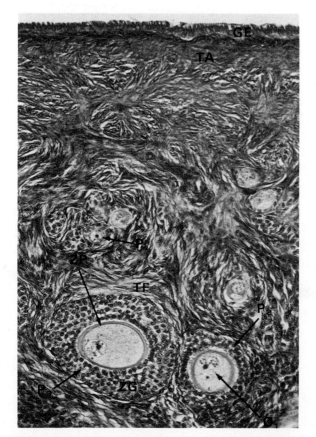

Fig. 16.4 Ovarian cortex

(Azan ×120)

In the mature ovary, undeveloped follicles exist as *primordial follicles* P_1 which are composed of a *primary oocyte* surrounded by a single layer of flattened follicular cells. The primary oocyte has a large nucleus, a prominent nucleolus and little cytoplasm. When stimulated to develop, the primordial follicle enlarges to form a *primary follicle* P_2 in which the oocyte O_1 has greatly enlarged and the follicular cells have become cuboidal. A homogeneous glycoprotein layer, the *zona pellucida* ZP, develops between the oocyte and the surrounding follicular cells. During this stage of follicular maturation the surrounding connective tissue stroma begins to form an organised layer around the follicle called the *theca folliculi* TF. With further development, the primary follicle P_3 continues to enlarge and the follicular cells proliferate to form a layer several cells thick called the *zona granulosa* ZG. The external connective tissue layer, the theca, begins to differentiate into two layers, the *theca interna* and *theca externa*.

Note also in this micrograph, the fibrous tunica albuginea TA and the single layer of cuboidal epithelial cells on the surface of the ovary. This epithelial layer is continuous with the mesothelial lining of the peritoneal cavity and is called the *germinal epithelium* GE from the mistaken belief that these cells were the origin of the female germ cells.

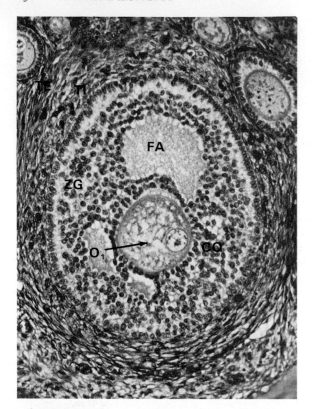

Fig. 16.5 Secondary follicle

(Azan × 120)

Primary follicles continue to develop until the stage at
which they become known as *secondary follicles*. Secondary
follicles are usually situated deeper in the ovarian cortex
and are recognised by the following features: the zona
granulosa **ZG** has proliferated greatly and a space, called
the *follicular antrum* **FA**, appears in which follicular fluid
accumulates. At this stage the oocyte O_1 has almost reached
its mature size and becomes situated eccentrically in a
thickened area of the granulosa called the *cumulus oophorus*
CO. The theca interna **TI** and the theca externa **TE** are
now well defined.

By this stage, the cells of the theca interna have
differentiated into typical steroid secreting cells (see Fig.
14.19) and have commenced the secretion of oestrogen
hormones. Oestrogens promote proliferation of the uterine
mucosa in readiness for the implantation of a fertilised
ovum. The theca externa is merely composed of connective
tissue and has no endocrine function.

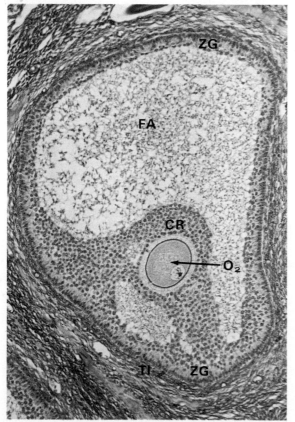

Fig. 16.6 Graafian follicle

(Azan × 75)

Approaching maturity, further growth of the oocyte ceases
and the first meiotic division is completed just before
ovulation. At this stage the oocyte becomes known as the
secondary oocyte and commences the second meiotic
division. The first polar body, containing very little
cytoplasm, remains inconspicuously within the zona
pellucida (see Chapter 15). The follicular antrum **FA**
enlarges markedly and the zona granulosa **ZG** forms a layer
of even thickness around the periphery of the follicle. The
cumulus oophorus diminishes leaving the oocyte O_2
surrounded by a layer several cells thick, the *corona radiata*
CR, which remains attached to the zona granulosa by thin
bridges of cells. Before ovulation these bridges break down
and the oocyte, surrounded by the corona radiata, floats free
inside the follicle.

At ovulation, the mature follicle ruptures and the ovum,
comprising the secondary oocyte, zona pellucida and corona
radiata, is expelled into the peritoneal cavity near the
entrance to the uterine tube. The second meiotic division of
the oocyte is not completed until after penetration of the
ovum by a spermatozoon.

During the process of follicular maturation the amount of
oestrogen secreting tissue, the theca interna **TI**, increases
progressively and there is a corresponding rise in the level
of circulating oestrogens. Atresia of all but the follicle
destined to ovulate probably accounts for the fall in
circulating oestrogens which occurs just prior to ovulation
(see Fig. 16.19).

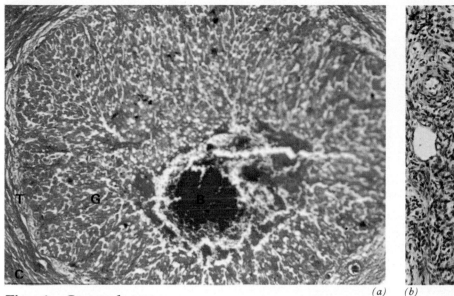 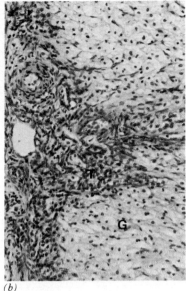

(a)   (b)

Fig. 16.7 Corpus luteum

(H & E (a) ×75 (b) ×128)

Following ovulation the ruptured follicle collapses and fills with a blood clot and the three layers of the follicular wall become re-organised to form a temporary endocrine gland, the *corpus luteum*. Under the influence of luteinising hormone (LH) secreted by the anterior pituitary (see Chapter 14), the cells of the former zona granulosa increase greatly in size and begin secretion of the steroid hormone progesterone. The cytoplasm of these cells contains a bright yellow pigment which gives rise to the name *granulosa luteal cells* and the name corpus luteum to the whole structure. Progesterone promotes exocrine secretion by glands in the mucosal lining of the uterus, which are now greatly proliferated under the influence of the oestrogens secreted by the theca interna cells of the follicle before ovulation. This provides a suitable environment for the implantation of a fertilised ovum.

The cells of the former theca interna also increase in size but to a lesser extent. Although interrupted by ovulation, these cells continue to secrete oestrogens, which are necessary to maintain the proliferated uterine mucosa. These cells become known as *theca luteal cells* or *paraluteal cells*.

The blood clot, granulosa luteal and theca luteal layers are invaded by capillaries from the former theca externa to form a rich vascular network characteristic of endocrine glands (see Chapter 14).

The corpus luteum is dependent on the secretion of LH from the anterior pituitary; however, rising levels of progesterone inhibit LH secretion. Without the continuing stimulus of LH, the corpus luteum cannot be maintained and 12 to 14 days after ovulation it regresses to form the functionless *corpus albicans* (see Fig. 16.9). Once the corpus luteum regresses, secretion of both oestrogens and progesterone ceases. Without these hormones the mucosal lining of the uterus collapses with the onset of menstruation.

Implantation of a fertilised ovum in the uterine wall interrupts the integrated ovarian and menstrual cycles. After implantation, a hormone called *human chorionic gonadotrophin* (HCG) is secreted into the maternal circulation by the developing placenta. HCG, which has an analogous function to that of LH, maintains the function of the corpus luteum in secreting oestrogens and progesterone until about the twelfth week of pregnancy. After this time, the corpus luteum of pregnancy slowly regresses to form the functionless corpus albicans and the placenta takes over the major role of oestrogen and progesterone secretion until parturition.

At low magnification, the remnant of the blood clot **B** is seen in the centre of the corpus luteum, surrounded by a broad zone of granulosa luteal cells **G**. Peripherally, a thin zone of theca luteal (paraluteal) cells **T** can be seen. The corpus luteum is bounded by a connective tissue zone **C** representing the theca externa of the antecedent Graafian follicle.

At higher magnification, granulosa luteal cells **G** may be compared with theca luteal (paraluteal) cells **T**. Granulosa luteal cells have a relatively large amount of pale-stained cytoplasm containing numerous lipid droplets which give rise to the vacuolated appearance seen in this preparation; lipid is utilised in the synthesis of the steroid hormone, progesterone.

Theca luteal (paraluteal) cells form a thin zone around the periphery of the granulosa luteal layer with finger-like extensions of the theca luteal layer extending into the granulosa luteal layer. Theca luteal cells are smaller, with a more densely staining, less vacuolated cytoplasm: these cells are responsible for the secretion of oestrogens.

The ultrastructure of the endocrine cells of the corpus luteum is characteristic of all steroid secretory cells (see Fig. 14.19).

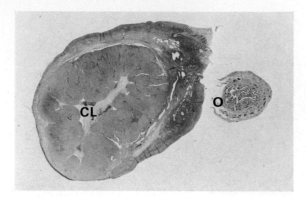

Fig. 16.8 Corpus luteum of pregnancy

(H & E × 3)

The corpus luteum of pregnancy is a much larger structure than the corpus luteum of the ovarian cycle but has a similar basic organisation; the corpus luteum of pregnancy produces oestrogens and progesterone for approximately the first trimester of pregnancy and then slowly regresses. In this micrograph the corpus luteum **CL** occupies most of the ovarian stroma. Note the adjacent oviduct **O**.

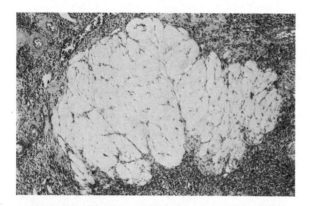

Fig. 16.9 Corpus albicans

(H & E × 20)

The corpus albicans is the inactive fibrous tissue mass which forms following the involution of a corpus luteum. The secretory cells of the degenerate corpus luteum autolyse and are phagocytised by macrophages. The vascular supporting tissue regresses to form a relatively acellular scar which eventually merges with the surrounding ovarian stroma.

In the human ovary, corpora albicantes are a dominant feature, increasing in number with age and often appearing to occupy almost the whole ovarian stroma.

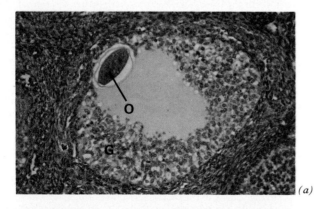

(a)

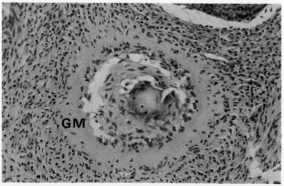

(b)

Fig. 16.10 Atretic follicles

(a) Azan × 128 (b) H & E × 128

The process of follicular atresia (degeneration) may occur at any stage in the development of the ovum. By the sixth month of development the fetal ovary contains approximately six million primordial follicles, four million of which undergo atresia by the time of birth. Atresia continues until puberty when less than half a million follicles remain and thereafter follicular atresia continues at a slow rate amongst primordial follicles.

In addition, with each ovarian cycle approximately twenty follicles begin to mature, usually all but one become atretic at some stage before complete maturity. The biological significance of this remarkable wastage is poorly understood.

The histological appearance of atretic follicles varies enormously, depending on the stage of development reached and the progress of atresia. The atretic follicle seen in (a) is a secondary follicle in early atresia; the oocyte **O** has degenerated and the granulosa cells **G** have begun to disorganise. Advanced atresia, as seen in (b) is characterised by gross thickening of the basement membrane between the granulosa cells and the theca interna forming the so-called 'glassy membrane' **GM**. Atretic follicles are ultimately replaced completely by fibrous connective tissue.

DEVELOPMENT OF HUMAN OVA

DEVELOPMENTAL EVENTS	DEVELOPMENTAL STAGE

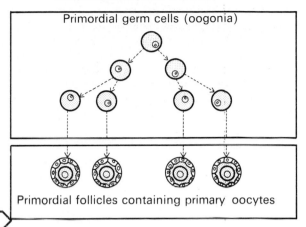

Primordial germ cells (oogonia)

Migration to ovarian cortex
6th week of fetal development

Multiplication by mitosis

Some oogonia develop the potential
to become mature female gametes.
Encapsulation by follicular cells
First stage of meiotic division
arrested

Primordial follicles containing primary oocytes

> BIRTH

No further follicular development until
sexual maturity

> SEXUAL MATURITY

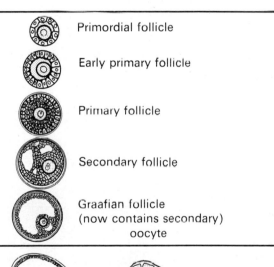

Secretion of pituitary gonadotrophins
FSH & LH
Some primordial follicles develop
towards maturity with each ovarian
cycle

Primordial follicle

Early primary follicle

Increasing secretion of oestrogen
progressively inhibits release
of FSH and promotes LH release

Primary follicle

Secondary follicle

First meiotic division completed
Second meiotic division commences
High levels of oestrogen inhibit
FSH release and promotes large
release of LH

Graafian follicle
(now contains secondary)
oocyte

> OVULATION

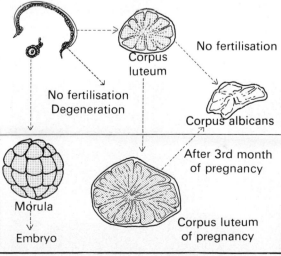

Progesterone secretion by
corpus luteum maintained by LH

Corpus
luteum

No fertilisation

No fertilisation
Degeneration

Inhibition of LH secretion by progesterone

Corpus albicans

> FERTILISATION

After 3rd month
of pregnancy

Morula

> IMPLANTATION

Corpus luteum of pregnancy maintained
by HCG secreted by developing embryo

Embryo

Corpus luteum
of pregnancy

Fig. 16.11 Summary of follicular development

The genital tract

The genital tract comprises the oviducts, uterus and the vagina, all of which have the same basic structure; a wall of smooth muscle, an inner mucosal lining and an outer layer of loose connective tissue. The mucosal and muscular components vary greatly according to their location and functional requirements; the whole tract undergoes cyclical changes under the influence of ovarian hormones released during the ovarian cycle.

The cyclical changes in the genital tract facilitate the entry of ova into the oviduct, the passage of spermatozoa into the oviduct, the passage of the fertilised ovum into the uterus and the implantation and development of the fertilised ovum in the mucosal lining of the uterine wall. Implantation of a fertilised ovum results in the secretion of hormones which inhibit the ovarian cycle and produce the gross changes in the genital tract necessary for fetal development and parturition.

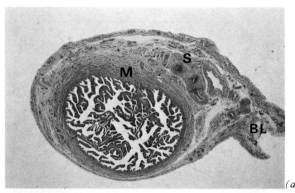

(a)

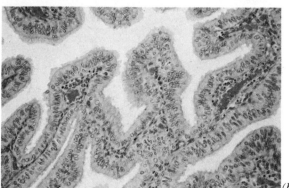

(b)

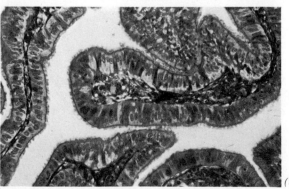

(c)

Fig. 16.12 Oviduct

(a) H & E × 10 (b) H & E × 128 (c) Azan × 128

The oviducts (also called uterine tubes or Fallopian tubes) conduct ova from the surface of the ovaries to the uterine cavity and are also the site of fertilisation by spermatozoa.

The ovarian end of the tube moves so as to overlie the site of rupture of the Graafian follicle at ovulation; finger-like projections called *fimbriae*, extending from the end of the tube, envelop the ovulation site and direct the ovum into the tube.

Movement of the ovum down the tube is mediated by gentle peristaltic action of the longitudinal and circular smooth muscle layers **M** of the oviduct wall and is aided by a current of fluid propelled by the action of the ciliated epithelium lining the tube.

The mucosal lining of the oviduct is thrown into a labyrinth of branching folds which occupy the entire lumen of the main part of the tube called the *ampulla*. The epithelial-lined folds provide a suitable environment for fertilisation to take place. The highly vascular connective tissue serosa **S** is continuous with the broad ligament **BL**.

The oviduct epithelium consists of a single layer of columnar cells which are of two types: ciliated and non-ciliated. The non-ciliated cells, which are stained blue in (c), produce a secretion which is propelled towards the uterus by the ciliated cells. This secretion may have a role in the nutrition and protection of the ovum. The ratio of ciliated to non-ciliated cells and the height of the cells undergoes cyclical variations under the influence of ovarian hormones. The epithelial folds are supported by a highly vascular connective tissue core, the collagen of which is stained blue in (c).

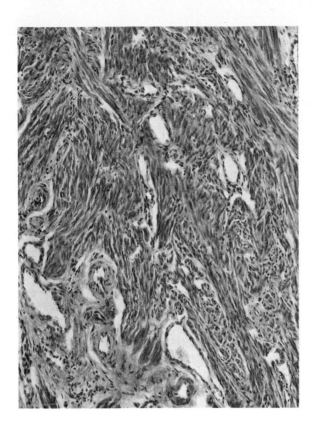

Fig. 16.13 Uterus: myometrium
(H & E × 198)

The uterus is that part of the genital tract in which the fertilised ovum develops. Its mucosal lining, called the *endometrium*, provides the environment for fetal development; the smooth muscle wall, the *myometrium*, plays the dominant role in expulsion of the fetus during parturition.

In the non-pregnant uterus, the myometrium is composed of interlacing bundles of long, smooth muscle fibres arranged in ill-defined layers; within the muscle is a rich network of arteries and veins supported by dense connective tissue. During pregnancy, under the influence of oestrogen, the myometrium increases greatly in size by both cell division and cell growth.

At parturition, strong contractions of the myometrium are reinforced by the action of the hormone oxytocin secreted by the posterior pituitary (see Chapter 14). These contractions expel the fetus from the uterus into the vagina and also constrict the blood supply to the placenta, thus precipitating its detachment from the uterine wall.

The human menstrual cycle

The endometrium, the mucosal lining of the uterine cavity, consists of a simple columnar ciliated epithelium supported by a broad, highly cellular, connective tissue stroma containing many simple tubular glands. Under the influence of the hormones oestrogen and progesterone, secreted by the ovary during the ovarian cycle, the endometrium undergoes regular cyclical changes so as to offer a suitable environment for implantation of a fertilised ovum. For successful implantation, the fertilised ovum requires an easily penetrable, highly vascular tissue and an abundant supply of glycogen for nutrition until vascular connections are established with the maternal environment.

The cycle of changes in the endometrium proceeds through two distinct phases, proliferation and secretion, which involve both the epithelium and supporting connective tissue stroma.

(i) The proliferative phase: the endometrial stroma proliferates to form a deep, richly vascularised stroma resembling primitive mesenchyme (see Fig. 3.1). The simple tubular glands proliferate to form numerous glands which begin secretion coincident with ovulation. The proliferative phase is initiated and sustained until ovulation by the increasing production of oestrogens from developing ovarian follicles.

(ii) The secretory phase: release of progesterone from the corpus luteum after ovulation promotes production of copious, thick, glycogen-rich secretion by the proliferated endometrial glands.

Unless implantation of a fertilised ovum occurs, the continuing production of progesterone is inhibited by negative feedback via the anterior pituitary, thus suppressing LH release leading to involution of the corpus luteum. In the absence of progesterone, the endometrium is unable to be maintained and most of it is shed during the period of bleeding known as menstruation. Activation of FSH secretion initiates a new cycle of follicular development and oestrogen secretion; this, in turn, initiates a new cycle of proliferation of the uterine mucosa from the remnants of the endometrium of the previous cycle. Although the process of menstruation represents the end point of the cycle of endometrial changes, the first day of menstruation is the most easily recognisable point and is usually taken to mark the first day of the 28-day menstrual cycle. Menstruation is usually completed by the fifth day, after which the proliferative phase continues until about the fourteenth day. Ovulation, which usually occurs at the fifteenth day, marks the beginning of the secretory phase which culminates in menstruation about the twenty-eighth day.

The endometrium is divided into three histologically and functionally distinct layers; the deepest or basal layer, the *stratum basalis*, adjacent to the myometrium, undergoes the least dramatic changes during the menstrual cycle and is not shed during menstruation. The broad, intermediate layer is characterised by a stroma with a spongy appearance and is called the *stratum spongiosum*. The thinner, superficial layer which has a compact stromal appearance is known as the *stratum compactum*. The compact and spongy layers exhibit dramatic changes throughout the cycle and are both shed during menstruation; hence they are jointly referred to as the *stratum functionalis*.

The arrangement of the arterial supply of the endometrium has important influences on the menstrual cycle. Branches of the uterine arteries pass through the myometrium and immediately divide into two different types of arteries: *straight arteries* and *spiral arteries*. Straight arteries are short and pass a small distance into the endometrium then bifurcate to form a rich plexus supplying the stratum basalis. Spiral arteries are long, coiled, and thick walled and pass to the surface of the endometrium giving off numerous branches which give rise to a rich capillary plexus around the glands and in the stratum compactum. Unlike the straight arteries, the spiral arteries are highly responsive to the hormonal changes of the menstrual cycle. The withdrawal of progesterone secretion at the end of the cycle causes the spiral arteries to constrict and this precipitates an *ischaemic phase* which immediately precedes menstruation.

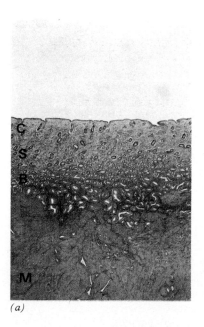

(a)

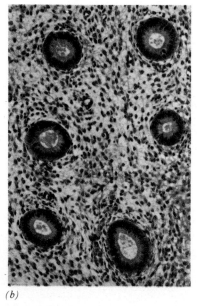

(b)

Fig. 16.14 Endometrium: early proliferative phase

(H & E (a) ×8 (b) ×128)

The low-magnification micrograph illustrates the myometrium **M** and the relatively thin endometrium consisting of the stratum basalis **B**, stratum spongiosum **S** and stratum compactum **C**. At this early proliferative stage, the stroma of the stratum functionalis (spongiosum plus compactum) has proliferated but the simple tubular glands have as yet barely proliferated into the stratum compactum.

At high magnification the proliferating glandular epithelium is seen to consist of low columnar cells. Occasional mitotic figures can be seen. Note the highly cellular connective tissue stroma, almost devoid of collagen fibres, which resembles primitive mesenchyme.

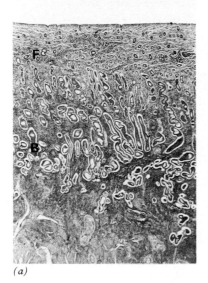

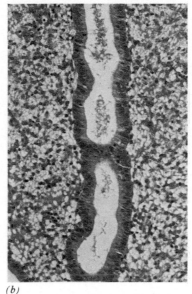

(a)   (b)

Fig. 16.15 Endometrium: late proliferative phase

(H & E (a) ×8 (b) ×128)

By the late proliferative stage the glands have extended to open on to the endometrial surface and the endometrium has doubled in thickness. Note that in contrast to the stratum functionalis **F**, the appearance of the stratum basalis **B** is little changed when compared with the early proliferative phase.

At high magnification many mitotic figures are usually evident in both the glandular epithelium and the connective tissue stroma. At this stage the glandular epithelium may have a pseudostratified appearance.

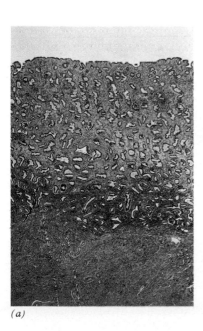

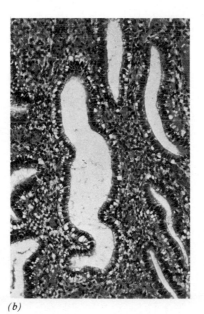

(a)   (b)

Fig. 16.16 Endometrium: early secretory phase

(H & E (a) ×8 (b) ×128)

Ovulation marks the onset of the secretory phase; endometrial proliferation continues for several days, however. At low magnification the gland configuration may appear similar to the late proliferative phase; at high magnification the characteristic feature of early secretory endometrium becomes evident, that is, *basal vacuolation*.

Under the influence of progesterone, the glandular epithelium is stimulated to synthesise glycogen. Initially the glycogen accumulates to form vacuoles in the basal aspect of the cells, thus displacing the nuclei towards the centre of the now tall columnar cells.

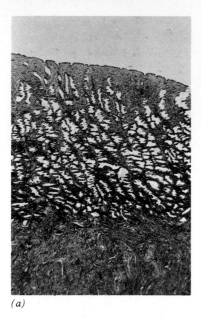

(a)

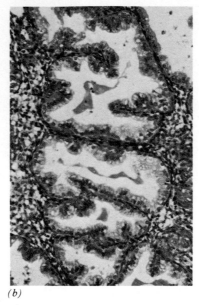

(b)

Fig. 16.17 Endometrium: late secretory phase

(H & E (a) ×8 (b) ×128)

At low magnification, the late secretory phase is characterised by a saw-tooth appearance of the glands which contain copious, thick, glycogen-rich secretions.

At high magnification, basal vacuolation is not evident in the glandular epithelium since active secretion is taking place. Mitotic figures are rarely seen. Note the highly vascular connective tissue stroma which has become infiltrated with leucocytes.

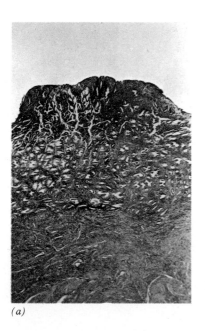

(a)

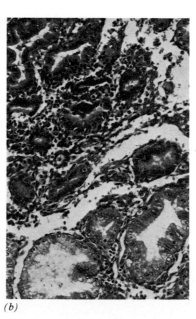

(b)

Fig. 16.18 Endometrium: onset of menstruation

(H & E (a) ×8 (b) ×128)

In the absence of implantation of a fertilised ovum, degeneration of the corpus luteum results in cessation of oestrogen and progesterone secretion. This event initiates phases of spasmodic constriction in the spiral arterioles. The resulting ischaemia is initially manifest by degeneration of the superficial layers of the endometrium and leakage of blood into the stroma. This is clearly seen at low magnification.

Further ischaemia leads to degeneration of the whole stratum functionalis which is progressively shed as *menses*. Menses is thus composed of blood, glandular epithelium and stromal elements. Normally menses is unable to clot due to the local release of inhibitory (anticoagulant) factors. At high magnification the degenerating endometrium is seen to be heavily infiltrated by leucocytes.

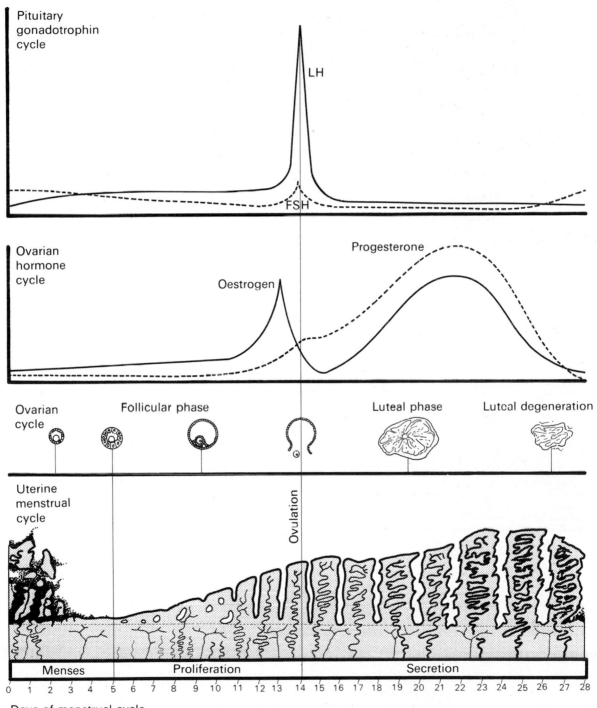

Fig. 16.19 The hormonal integration of the ovarian and menstrual cycles

Fig. 16.20 Uterine cervix

(H & E × 128)

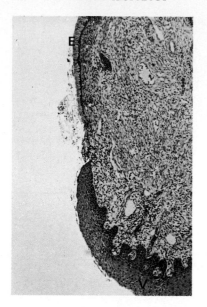

The neck of the uterus protrudes into the upper part of the vagina. The vaginal portion of the cervix **V** is lined by a stratified squamous epithelium which is identical with vaginal epithelium. The entrance to the uterine cavity, the *endocervical canal*, is lined by a simple, tall columnar, mucus-secreting epithelium **E** containing numerous highly branched tubular glands which also secrete mucus. The endocervical mucus glands are not seen in this micrograph; they are more prolific higher up the canal. The junction between the simple columnar and stratified squamous epithelia of the cervix is extremely abrupt.

During the menstrual cycle the numerous glands of the endocervix undergo cyclic changes in secretory activity. During the proliferative phase of the menstrual cycle, rising levels of oestrogen promote increasing secretion of thin cervical mucus which facilitates the entry of spermatozoa into the uterus around the period of ovulation. Following ovulation, under the influence of progesterone, the cervical mucus becomes highly viscid. This viscid mucus forms a plug which inhibits the entry of micro-organisms from the vagina and is a particularly important protective barrier should pregnancy occur.

The connective tissue underlying the cervical epithelium differs from that of the rest of the uterus in that it has a high content of collagen fibres which interlace with smooth muscle fibres of the myometrium. The subepithelial stroma of the cervix is frequently infiltrated with leucocytes.

Fig. 16.21 Vagina

(LS: Masson's trichrome × 50)

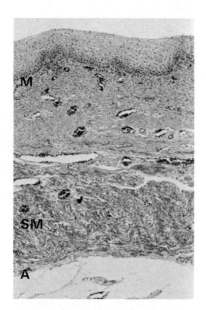

The wall of the vagina, or birth canal, conforms to the general structure of the whole genital tract; that is, it has a mucosal lining **M**, smooth muscle **SM** and outer adventitial **A** layers. In the relaxed state, the vaginal wall collapses to obliterate the lumen and the vaginal epithelium is thrown up into folds. The dense lamina propria contains many elastic fibres, has a rich plexus of small veins and is devoid of glands. The vagina is lubricated by cervical mucus and a fluid transudate from the rich vascular network of the lamina propria. The smooth muscle bundles of the muscular layer are arranged in ill-defined circular and longitudinal layers; the longitudinal layers predominate especially in the outer region.

The combination of a muscular layer and a highly elastic lamina propria permits the gross distension which occurs during parturition. Conversely after coitus, involuntary contraction of the smooth muscle layer ensures that a pool of semen remains in the cervical region. Thick elastic fibres in the outer adventitial layer also facilitate these functions.

Fig. 16.22 Vagina

(Masson's trichrome × 128)

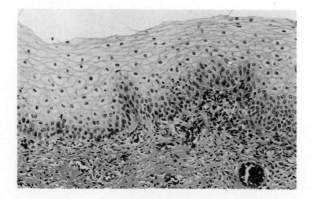

This micrograph illustrates the stratified squamous epithelium which lines the vagina. During the menstrual cycle, this epithelium undergoes cyclical changes which includes slight keratinisation of the superficial cells; histological examination of cells scraped from the surface provides a useful means for estimation of the time of the last ovulation. Throughout the cycle, the superficial cells produce glycogen which is anaerobically metabolised by commensal bacteria in the vagina to form lactic acid; this inhibits the growth of pathogenic micro-organisms.

The mammary glands

The breasts, or mammary glands, are highly modified apocrine sweat glands (see Fig. 8.16) which develop embryologically along two lines, the *milk lines*, extending from the axillae to the groin. In humans, usually only one gland develops on each side of the thorax although accessory breast tissue may be found anywhere along the milk lines.

The breasts of both sexes follow an identical course of development until puberty, after which the female breasts develop under the influence of pituitary, ovarian and other hormones. Until the menopause, the breasts undergo cyclical changes in activity which are controlled by the hormones of the ovarian cycle. After menopause, the breasts, like the other female reproductive tissues, undergo progressive atrophy and involution.

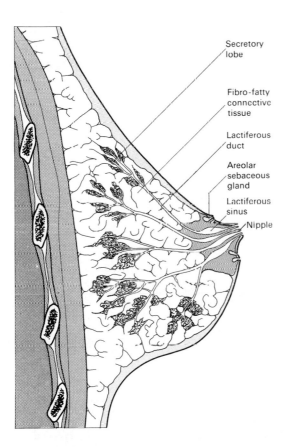

Secretory lobe

Fibro-fatty connective tissue

Lactiferous duct

Areolar sebaceous gland

Lactiferous sinus

Nipple

Fig. 16.23 Structure of the breast

This highly schematic diagram illustrates the general organisation of the breast. Each breast consists of from fifteen to twenty five independent glandular units called *breast lobes,* each consisting of a compound tubulo-acinar gland (see Fig. 4.25). The lobes are arranged radially at different depths around the *nipple* or *mammary papilla*. A single large duct, the *lactiferous duct,* drains each lobe via a separate opening on the surface of the nipple. Just before each duct opens on to the surface the duct forms a dilatation called the *lactiferous sinus.* The nipple contains bands of smooth muscle orientated parallel to the lactiferous ducts and circularly near the base; contraction of this muscle causes erection of the nipple.

Each breast lobe is divided into a variable number of lobules; the lobules consist of a system of ducts, *the alveolar ducts,* from which large numbers of secretory alveoli develop during pregnancy. The lobules are separated from each other by loose connective tissue whereas each lobe is separated by dense connective tissue often containing a large amount of adipose tissue.

The skin surrounding the nipple, the *areola,* is pigmented and contains sebaceous glands which are not associated with hair follicles. The secretions of these glands probably help to protect the nipple and areola during suckling.

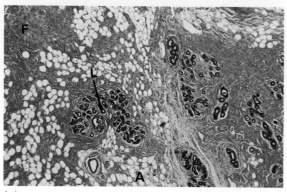

(a)

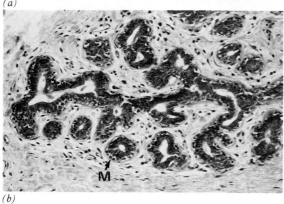

(b)

Fig. 16.24 Resting breast

(H & E (a) × 20 (b) × 128)

These micrographs show breast tissue from a non-pregnant woman of reproductive age. At low magnification, the lobules **L** of the breast are seen to form islands of glandular tissue within an extensive mass of dense fibrous **F** and adipose **A** connective tissue. At higher magnification, the lobules are seen to consist of alveolar ducts lined by a cuboidal epithelium supported by a prominent basement membrane. Like sweat glands, a discontinuous layer of myoepithelial cells **M** lies between the duct-lining cells and the basement membrane. In the resting breast, the duct epithelium undergoes cyclical changes under the influence of ovarian hormones. Early in the cycle, the duct lumina are not clearly evident but later in the cycle the lumina become more prominent and may contain an eosinophilic secretion.

The interlobular connective tissue is usually dense and fibrous whereas the connective tissue within the lobule is loose, highly cellular, rarely contains fat, and has a rich capillary network. This loose intralobular connective tissue may facilitate proliferation and expansion of breast alveoli during pregnancy.

Resting – fat
rare see lumen

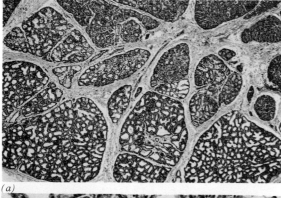

(a)

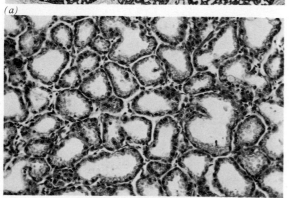

(b)

Fig. 16.25 Proliferating breast

(H & E (a) × 20 (b) × 128)

These micrographs demonstrate the histological changes which occur in the breast during pregnancy. Under the influence of oestrogens and progesterone produced by the corpus luteum, and later by the placenta, the alveolar duct epithelium proliferates to form numerous secretory alveoli. Breast proliferation also depends on prolactin, a prolactin-like hormone produced by the placenta called human placental lactogen (HPL), thyroid hormone and corticosteroids. At low magnification, the breast lobules are seen to have expanded greatly at the expense of the interlobular connective tissue.

As pregnancy progresses the alveoli begin to secrete a protein-rich fluid called *colostrum*, the accumulation of which dilates the alveolar and duct lumina. Colostrum is the form of breast secretion available during the first few days of suckling; it contains a laxative substance and maternal antibodies which are thought to confer passive immunity to some diseases on the newborn. Unlike milk, colostrum contains little lipid. Breast secretion is controlled by the hormone prolactin secreted by the anterior pituitary. During pregnancy, prolactin secretion progressively increases but its activity is suppressed by high levels of circulating oestrogens and progesterone.

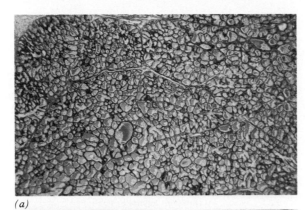

(a)

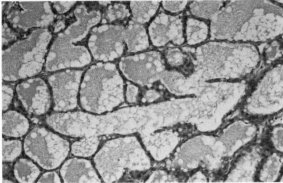

(b)

Fig. 16.26 Lactating breast

(H & E (a) ×20 (b) ×128)

After parturition the levels of circulating progesterone and oestrogens fall, thus promoting prolactin activity. Prolactin stimulates milk production (lactation) in conjunction with several other hormones. During lactation the breast consists almost entirely of glandular tissue; the alveoli are widely dilated by milk and most of the interlobular connective tissue disappears, as can be seen in (a).

Milk contains large quantities of protein, lipid, vitamins and sugars such as lactose. The protein constituents are synthesised and secreted by the usual process of merocrine secretion (see Chapter 4) whereas lipid is secreted as large, membrane-bound droplets which also contain a small quantity of cytoplasm. Lipid accumulates as droplets within the apical cytoplasm before release into the duct system. This form of secretion represents true apocrine secretion (see Chapter 4).

Milk production proceeds for as long as suckling continues and may even occur for some years after childbirth. This process is mediated by a neuro-hormonal reflex involving nipple stimulation by suckling and release of prolactin from the anterior pituitary. A different neuro-hormonal reflex promotes milk expulsion from the breasts; this reflex, also initiated by suckling, causes the release of the hormone oxytocin from the posterior pituitary. Oxytocin causes contraction of the myoepithelial cells which embrace the secretory alveoli and ducts, thus propelling milk into the lactiferous sinuses. Withdrawal of the suckling stimulus, and hence the release of pituitary hormones at weaning, results in regression of the lactating breast and resumption of the ovarian cycle.

Index